The Iris

THE IRIS
Understanding the Essentials

New Insight on Structural Details
Applications for New Diagnostic Modalities
Potentials and Possibilities to Change the Color of The Eye

BY K.T. MOAZED, MD

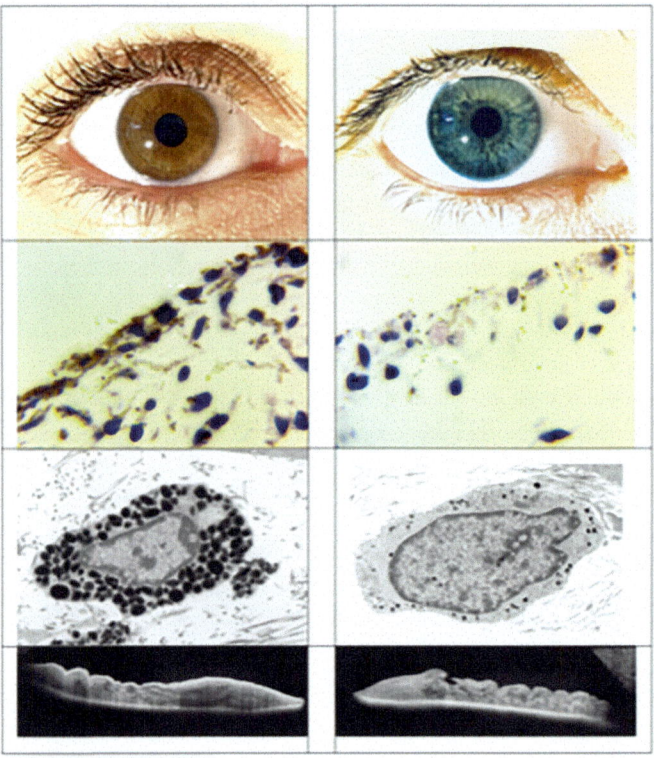

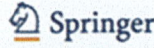 Springer

Kambiz Thomas Moazed

The Iris

Understanding the Essentials

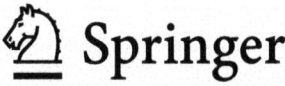 Springer

Kambiz Thomas Moazed, MD
Former Associate Clinical Professor
Columbia University
New York, NY
USA

ISBN 978-3-030-45755-6   ISBN 978-3-030-45756-3   (eBook)
https://doi.org/10.1007/978-3-030-45756-3

This Springer imprint is published by the registered company Springer Nature Switzerland AG
The registered company address is: Gewerbestrasse 11, 6330 Cham, Switzerland

Preface

This book is a result of my observations and studying of human Iris for 35 years. This includes a year of fellowship at the eye pathology department and Stanford University in California, a year of fellowship at the eye pathology department of Harvard University at Massachusetts Eye & Ear Infirmary and my ophthalmology residency training at Harvard University, and 25 years of eye pathology teaching at Colombia University in New York.

This book, for the first time, provides a comprehensive insight into the iris which has been a neglected part of the eye and has not been focused on as compared to the other parts of the eye such as cornea lens, retina and the optic nerve.

The goal of this book is to combine the different aspect of scientific information from different fields of science such as histology, molecular biology, electron microscopy and diagnostic modalities, etc. This effort is to construct a new concept as a whole for diagnosis and treatment of the large variety of diseases that affects the iris of the eye.

There is a special focus and emphasize on the iris pigmentation and its associated structural differences related to variation in eye color and the future strategies to make changes in the color of the eye.

In this book the current information and new concepts has been summarized that would be useful for ophthalmologists, clinicians, researchers, medical students, pharmaceutical companies and ophthalmic equipment manufacturing industries. It would help the reader to have a better understanding of the iris in order to open the door for future research projects and discoveries regarding this organ.

The contents of this book have been chosen to summarize and to focus on important issues and pearls in hope that one can look at the iris with a better understanding of its complexity and diverse structure. The references are provided for more comprehensive look at the specific issues if needed.

New York, NY, USA   Kambiz Thomas Moazed, MD

Contents

Chapter 1
Embryology of Iris

Abstract The formation of the iris is an interaction between neural ectoderm, neural crest and mesoderm. It starts from formation of the optic cup from neural ectoderm which invaginates into itself to form the posterior double layer of iris pigment epithelium. The neural crest origin melanoblasts, will migrate into the stromal tissue that is formed by the periocular mesenchyme. The stroma of the iris is formed from mesoderm as part of anterior chamber formation and regression and disappearance of the endothelium on the front surface of the iris by birth.

The focus here is to explain the Iris structural development and not intended to teach embryology of the eye, as it can be reviewed in many embryology textbooks and articles including Iris development as part of anterior segment formation.

The purpose of this chapter is to focus on embryological evolution of the eye relevant to the unusual structure of the iris. This is to explain for example, why there is no epithelium on the surface of the iris and why there is a double layers of pigment epithelium on the back part of the iris.

To understand the process of Iris development we have to briefly discuss the development of the embryonic eye as a whole [4, 10].

The first sign of the eye formation is the single walled Primary optic vesicles which in humans starts at fourth weeks of gestation on either side of the forebrain. It moves outwards to finally meet the surface ectoderm [6].

The distal portion of the optic vesicles invaginates inward to form a double layered optic cup. The gap that forms in the wall during this process will carry essential blood vessels (hyloid vasculature) and is called choroidal fissure. Failure to complete this process will end up with colobomas in the infero-nasal quadrant of the eye.

At the same time the surface ectoderm gets thicker at the top to form lens placode, which invaginates inside to form the lens vesicle.

The neural crest component of the secondary mesenchyme goes between the cornea and the newly formed primitive lens to form the corneal stroma, corneal endothelium, anterior chamber angle and iris stroma [9].

K. T. Moazed, *The Iris*, https://doi.org/10.1007/978-3-030-45756-3_1

Anterior chamber cavity is then formed by the beginning of the 20th week of gestation the anterior chamber of the eye is formed which is a closed cavity with an endothelial lining [5].

The primitive iris that is formed by folding of the tip of the optic cup with iris pigment epithelium (IPE) in the back and secondary mesenchyme as stroma in front. The anterior part of the primitive iris is located more anteriorly at this stage which will become the location for the future trabecular meshwork.

In the final weeks of gestation, the primordial endothelial lining the pupillary space, anterior surface of the iris and the angle structures undergoes fenestration and gradually disappears. The iris insertion moves posteriorly to uncover the trabecular meshwork. At birth, the iris insertion is normally has reached the scleral spur. The iris continues to migrate posteriorly until the first postnatal year.

Any arrest in this process will cause multiple anomalies called Anterior Segment Dysgenesis (ASD) that is summarized below:

• Developmental disorders following inactivation of TGFb signaling [17]
• Mechanisms of anterior segment dysgenesis [26]
• Deletion of Tcs1 disrputs ciliary body and iris development [12]
• Aniridia [13]
• Posterior embryotoxon [28]
• Axenfeld Rieger syndrome [27]
• Iridogoniodysplasia [1]
• Iris dysplasia [16]
• Congenital Glaucoma [21]
• Iridocorneal endothelial (ICE) syndrome [29]
• Congenital hereditary endothelial dystrophy [20]
• Posterior polymorphous syndrome [11]
• Peter's anomaly [2]

There is a spectrum of developmental anomalies that overlapping one another and makes the classification challenging.

Anterior segment dysgenesis (ASD) conditions are the result of dominantly inherited genetic mutations. In recent years many of these genes has been identified, the process that is continued today:

• Mutation (Phe112Ser) in the FOXC1 gene [14]
• Rieger Syndrome Associated With PITX2 Mutations [22]
• Transcription Factor Gene FOXC1 Causes Iris Hypoplasia [18]

Overview of iris development for better understanding of this complex process we focus on the process again from a different angle.

As was discussed before, the development of the iris involves in a series of interactions between neural ectoderm, neural crest origin cells and mesoderm. The neural ectoderm after formation of the optic cup will invaginate and form the double layer of iris pigment epithelium (IPE) which is located on the posterior surface of the iris. The neural crest origin melanoblasts will migrate into the stromal tissue that is formed by the periocular mesenchyme [9].

The origin of muscular structures of the iris, the dilator and the sphincter muscles are also from neural ectoderm [14].

There are very unique structural characteristics of iris that makes it a valuable study tool.

Important highlights of reviewing the embryology of the iris are as follows:

- Anterior Border layer of iris is formed from large gaps between Mesenchymal cells.

There is no epithelium or endothelium (the endothelium on the front surface of the iris completely regress and disappear during the formation of the anterior chamber on the front surface of the iris) [10].

- Remnants of the blood vessels at the pupil forming the anterior tunica vasculosa lentis which disappear by birth, but its remnants can be seen in some adults [24].
- There is no anterior limiting membrane on the front surface of the iris and the fibroblasts and melanocytes are immersed and float in the Aqueous Humor of the anterior chamber.
- Iris stroma forms from accumulation of connective tissue, collagen fibers, vascular tissue, nerve fibers, melanocytes and macrophages.
- The Iris pigment epithelium (IPE) is located on the posterior surface of the iris facing the lens of the eye and is formed by double layer of pigment epithelium folded on itself that lays on top of each other head to head (tête á tête). Figure 1.9
- As the result of folding of the optic cup the location of the basement membrane is on the most posterior part of the Iris facing the lens and on the anterior it separates RPE from the stroma.
- These folded 2 layers of the original optic cup continue to differentiate to different cellular structures with different functions accordingly.

The inner invaginated layer of the optic cup will form:

1. The retina.
2. The nonpigmented layer of the epithelium of the ciliary processes.
3. The anterior layer of the Iris pigment epithelium (IPE).

The outer layer of the optic cup will form:

1. The Retinal pigment epithelium (RPE).
2. The pigmented layer of the epithelium of the ciliary processes.
3. The posterior layer of the iris pigment epithelium (IPE).

There is always a possibility that these two folded layers get separated in the posterior pole by different factors which would lead to the condition called retinal detachment. This separation between the sensory retina and retinal pigment epithelium can happen with the tear in the retina and leaking the intraocular fluid in the subretinal space which is called Rhegmatogenous retinal detachment which is the most common type. Other conditions are due to injury inflammation or malignancy causes the accumulation of fluid or blood in the subretinal space which is called nonrhegmatogenous retinal detachment.

It is important to emphasize that the basement membrane of the IPE is located on the either sides of the double pigmented layer as the consequence of the folding optic cup on itself due to invagination. As the result the IPE cells are in a head to head position (tête á tête). In order to understand it better, it is necessary to review the formation of the neural tube, the origin of the optic cup. As embryonic ectoderm folds to form the neural tube its basement membrane will locate on the outside so when the optic cup forms from it, the basement membrane already located on the outside. And as it invaginates into itself the basement membrane stays on either side of Iris Pigment epithelium (IPE) (Fig. 1.10).

The reason to emphasize the location of the basement membrane (BM) in the iris is the recent new concepts that revealed many interactions between iris melanocytes and BM. As will be discussed in the chapters on electron microscopy and molecular biology of this book, BM not only have a anchoring function but also control migration and proliferation and melanin production of the melanocytes.

To simplify:

- Neural ectoderm provides the Iris pigment epithelium (IPE) and the iris muscles (the sphincter and the dilator)
- The mesoderm provides the stromal fibroblasts, stromal connective tissue, collagen fibers and the blood vessels.
- Neural crest provides stromal melanocytes.

Pigment Cell Development and Migration

MITF gene provides instructions for making a specific protein that is called microphthalmia-associated transcription factor or melanocyte inducing transcription factor (MITF). This protein in combination with other proteins plays an essential role in development, survival, migration and differentiation of melanocytes [3].

MITF-M an isoform of MITF is regulated by multiple transcription factors including PAX3, SOX10, LEF, CREB.

Wnt signaling is critical for melanocyte development by promoting the interaction between ß-catenin with LEF1/TCF, which induces the MITF-M promotor.

A very thorough review of molecular biology of the eye development is well described and highly recommended to access [8].

The iris development starts with surface ectoderm suppresion of WNTs which will activate WNT/beta-catenin signaling in which cooperate with Pax6 [7].

Multiple genes are involved in this process.

Developmental biology of the melanocytes can be reviewed in the article "Biology of Waardenburg syndrome" [25].

The Pigmented cells and melanocytes of the iris also have different embryonic origins, as we mentioned earlier [15].

- The stromal melanocytes (ISM) are originated from neural Crest that migrate via mesoderm to their final destination on the surface of the iris and some in deeper layers of stroma.
- The Iris pigment epithelium (IPE) is originated from neural ectoderm by formation of optic vesicle and later on the optic cup.
- Macrophages containing pigment are originating from hematopoietic stem cells (HSCs) emerge from the aorta-gonad-mesonephros. Later they migrate to the

fetal liver, which then serves as the major hematopoietic organ during the remainder of embryonic development.
- Schwann cells from ventral migration of Neural crest origin. They are the supportive system (Glial cells) of the neurons [23].

The Developmental Timetable of the Iris in Brief

- By 3rd week of gestation the surface ectoderm is formed (Fig. 1.1).
- Between 3rd and 4th week the neural groove is developing (Fig. 1.2).
- By 4th week of gestation the Neural tube formation is completed (Fig. 1.3).
- By 5th week of gestation the optic vesicles are formed (Figs. 1.4 and 1.5).
- Between the 5th and 12th week of gestation the optic cup is formed by invagination of the optic vesicle and penetration of the surface ectoderm inside the optic cup to form the lens vesicle and the location of the basement membrane (BM) (Fig. 1.6).
- Pigmentation begins to appear at 10th week post-natal and is complete by age 7 months.
- By 12th week of gestation The Optic cup begins to enlarge and elongate and grows between the lens and cornea (Fig. 1.6).
- The Iris starts to form by elongation of the optic cup between the lens and the cornea by the end of the 12th weeks of gestation. This is due to invasion of the primary mesenchyme that surrounds the optic cup by Neural Crest cells to form secondary Mesenchyme (Fig. 1.6).
- By 20th week of gestation, the Iris and anterior chamber are formed (Fig. 1.7).
- The tip of the invaginated optic cup forms the pupil and the 2 layers of the invaginated optic cup forms the posterior pigment epithelium of the iris with the location of the basement membrane (BM) on either side (Figs. 1.8 and 1.9)
- The sphincter muscle pulls away from pupillary zone of epithelium and differentiates into smooth muscle.
- By 24th week of gestation, Iris dilator muscle fibers develop within pigment epithelium.
- By birth the Sphincter and the Dilator muscles are completed (Fig. 1.10).

The sphincter muscle separates and differentiates from epithelium into the smooth muscle by the end of the fifth month. Neural crest cells migrate between the surface ectoderm and the lens vesicle [3].

- The dilator muscle develops from anterior layer of iris pigment epithelium by the end of the 6th month [14].
- The Sphincter and the Dilator muscles originate from neural ectoderm are completed by birth.
- The distinctive formed structures of the iris are completed by the end of the 8th month, with formation of anterior chamber and there is a complete endothelial lining over the primitive anterior chamber and the surface of the iris.
- The primordial endothelial lining undergoes fenestration and progressively disappears form pupillary space, surface of the iris and the angle structures by the final weeks of gestation to the first week after birth.

Fig. 1.1 Formation of surface ectoderm and the location of the basement membrane around 3rd week of gestation

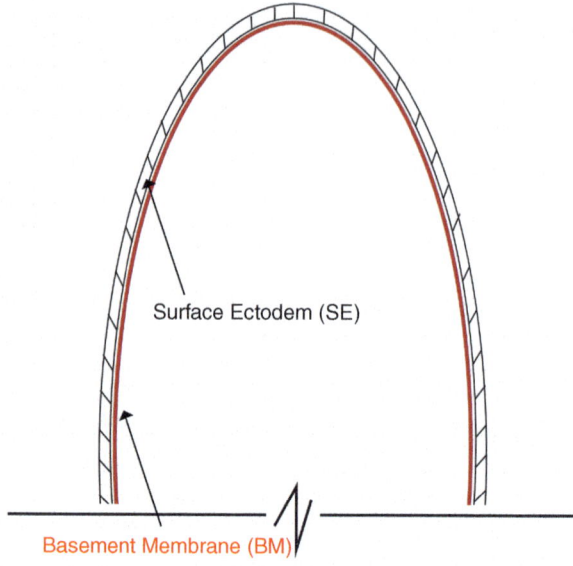

Fig. 1.2 Formation of the neural groove between 3rd and 4th week of gestation and location of basement membrane (BM)

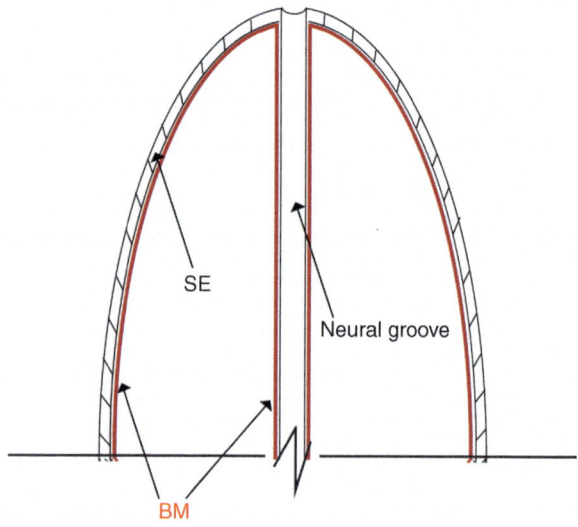

- Iris pigmentation begins to appear at 10 weeks and continues to be completed by the first year after birth. There are different pigment cells from different embryonic origins. Iris pigment epithelium originates from neural ectoderm. Iris stromal melanocytes originate from neural crest. Pigmented macrophages originate from mesenchyme.
- The Iris insertion reposition itself to the scleral spur by the end of gestation and continues its posterior migration till the end of the first year after birth.
- Iris stroma forms from accumulation of collagen fibers form mesenchyme.
- The blood vessels and nerves form from mesoderm and neural crest [23].

Fig. 1.3 Closure of the neural groove and formation of the neural tube at fourth week of gestation and related position of the basement membrane (BM)

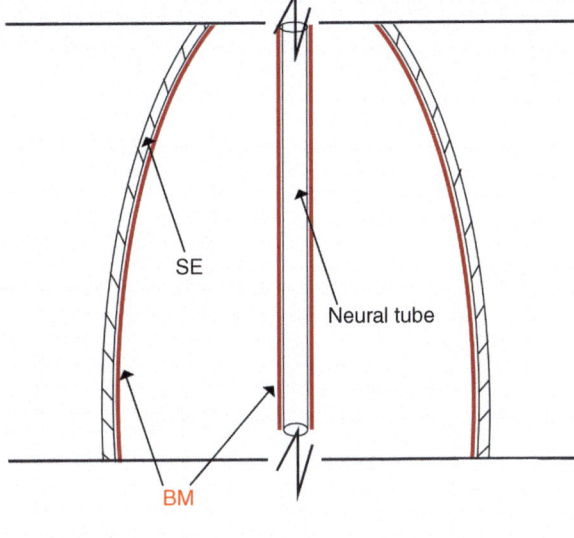

SE

Neural tube

BM

Fig. 1.4 Formation of the optic vesicle from neural tube by the 5th week of gestation and the location of the basement membrane (BM)

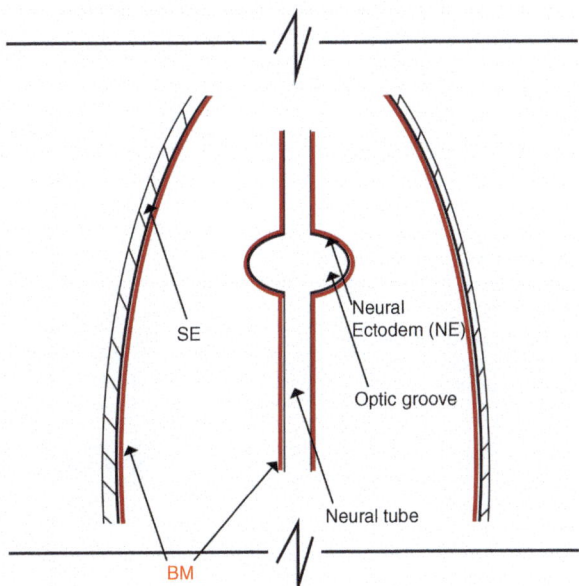

SE

Neural Ectodem (NE)

Optic groove

Neural tube

BM

The Embryonic Vascular System

At About 4 weeks of gestation, hyaloid artery enters the eye at the optic disc. In the iris it branches to form a network of capillaries called Tunica Vasculosa Lentis. Its branches interconnect with the capillaries from anterior pupillary membrane. These vascular membranes disappear by an orderly programmed cell death shortly before birth. The remnants of the pupillary membrane can often be seen as Pupillary strands.

Fig. 1.5 Enlargement of the optic vesicle and its movement towards the surface ectoderm and the location of the basement membrane (BM)

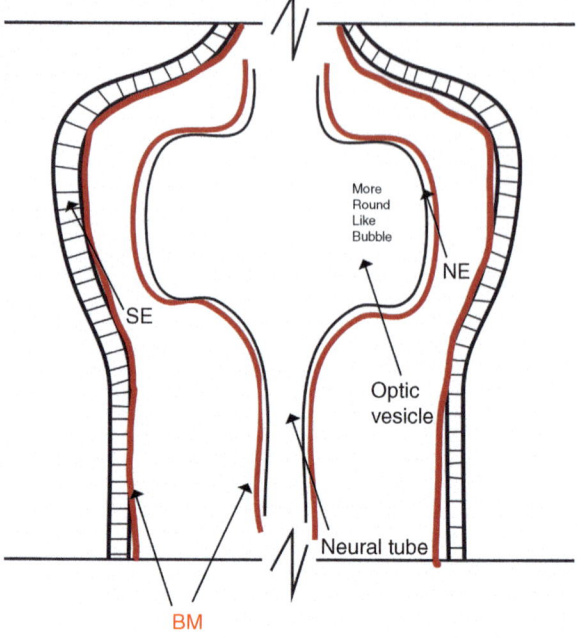

Fig. 1.6 Formation of the optic cup by invagination of the optic vesicle and penetration of the surface ectoderm inside the optic cup to form the lens vesicle by the 12th week of gestation and the location of the basement membrane (BM)

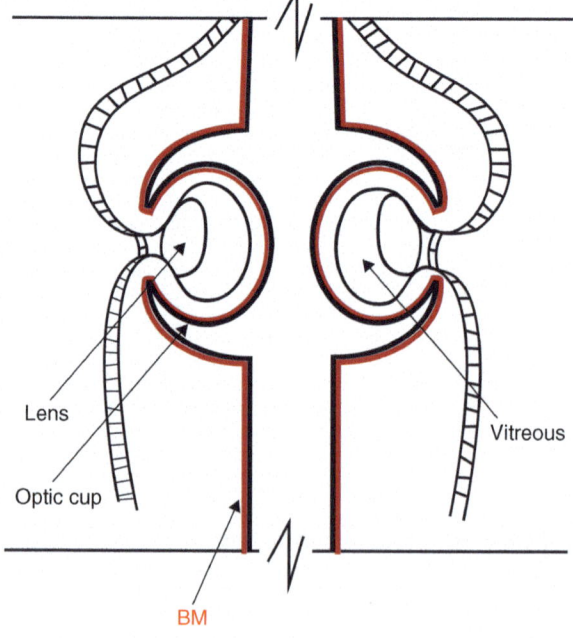

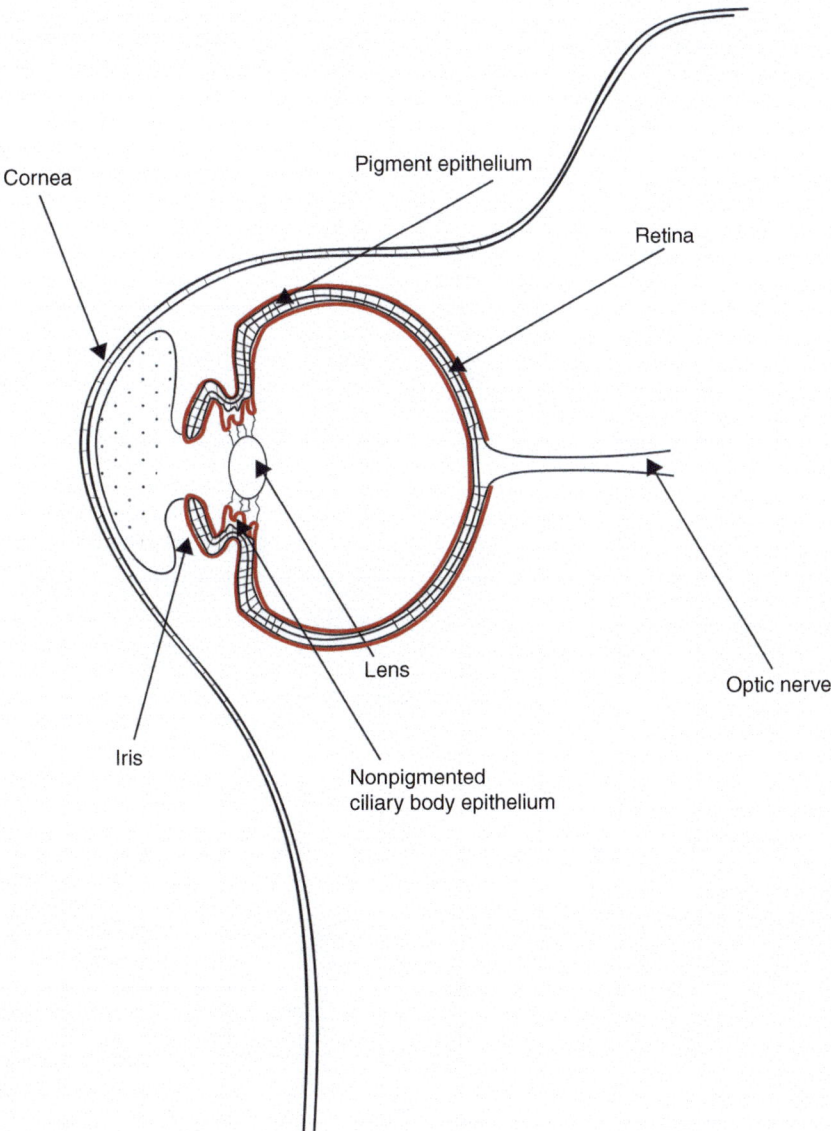

Fig. 1.7 By 20th week of gestation, the Iris and anterior chamber are formed. The tip of the invaginated optic cup forms the pupil and the 2 layers of the invaginated optic cup forms the posterior pigment epithelium of the iris with the location of the basement membrane (BM) on either side

Fig. 1.8 Closeup schematic view of the iris. With double layers of the optic cup lay on top of each other on the back of the iris and the stroma generated by mesoderm covers the front of the iris with attention to the position of the basement membrane (BM)

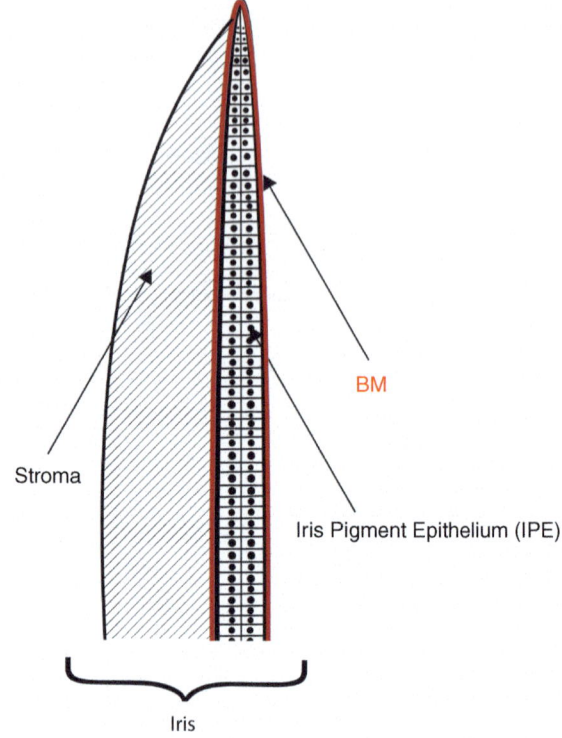

Stroma

BM

Iris Pigment Epithelium (IPE)

Iris

Fig. 1.9 Further closeup view of the double layers of the iris pigment epithelium on the posterior surface of the iris and the location of the basement membrane (BM)

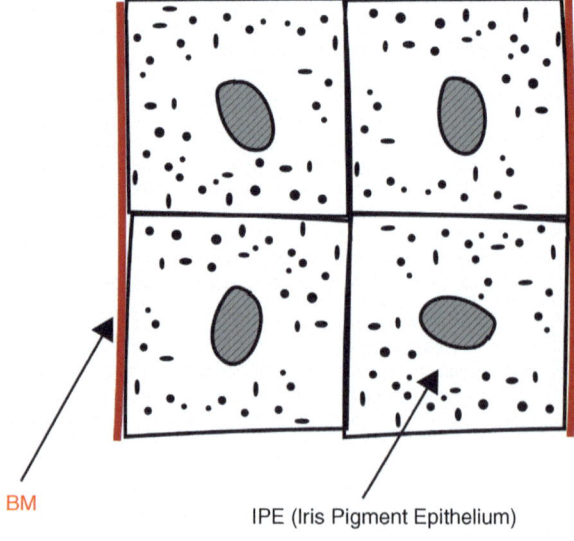

BM

IPE (Iris Pigment Epithelium)

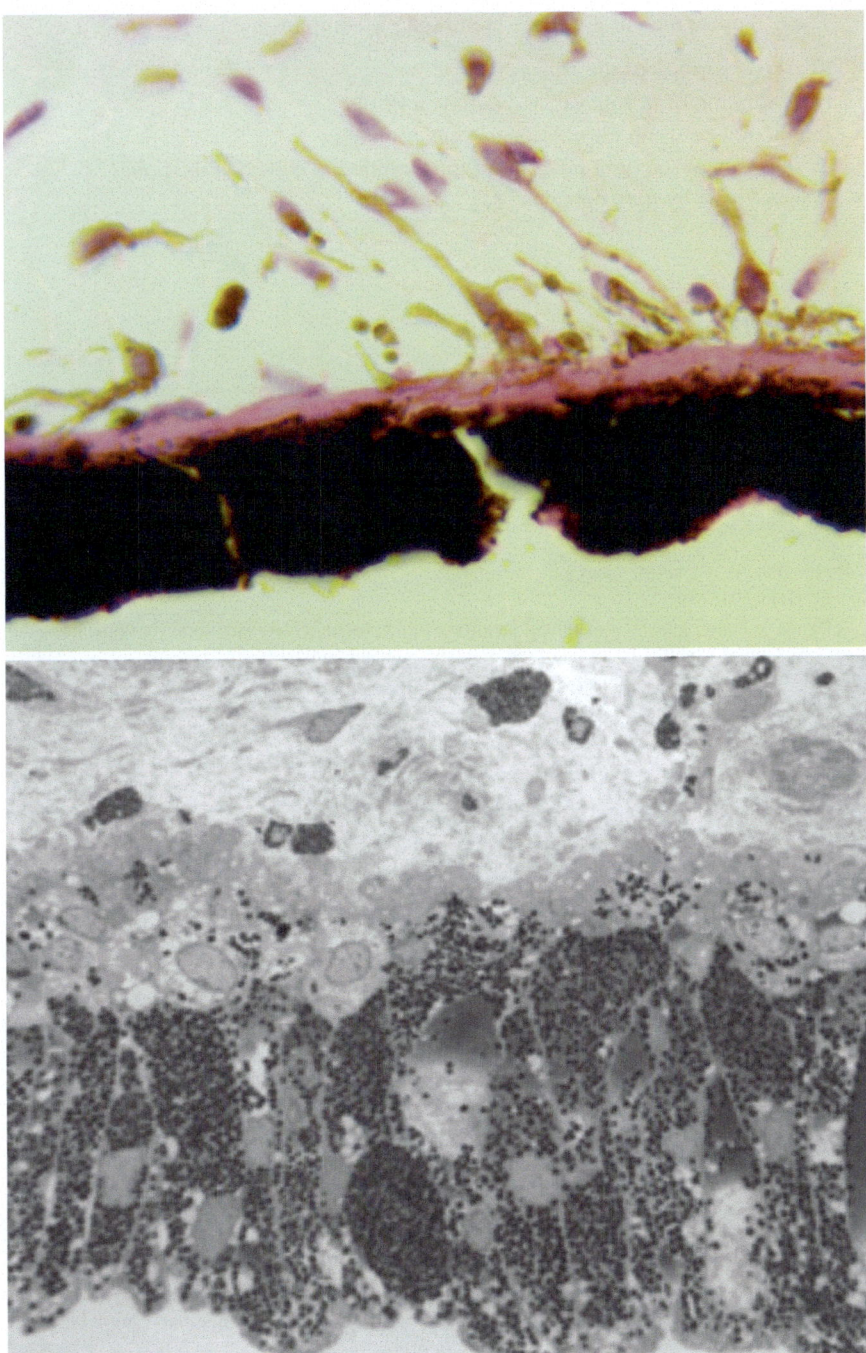

Fig. 1.10 Light and electron microscopy of the posterior surface of the iris. The double layers highly pigmented of iris pigment epithelium below. The dilator muscle in the middle and the loose connective tissue of the iris stroma on top of each picture

The disappearance of pupillary membrane is complex and is orchestrated by:

- Synthetic activity of fibroblasts
- Degeneration of fibroblasts and collagen fibrils
- Interaction between fibroblasts and macrophages
- Destruction of the tight junction of the endothelial cells by macrophages
- Phagocytosis by macrophages [22]

Bibliography

1. Alward W. Axenfeld-Rieger syndrome in the age of molecular genetics. Am J Ophthalmol. 2000;130(1):107–15.
2. Bhandari R, Ferri S, Whittaker B, Liu M, Lazzaro DR. Peters anomaly: review of the literature. Cornea. 2011;30(8):939–44.
3. Bonaventure J, Domingues MJ, Larue L. Cellular and molecular mechanisms controlling the migration of melanocytes and melanoma cells. Pigment Cell & Melanoma Research. 2013;26(3):316–25.
4. Douglas B. Anterior segment development relevant to glaucoma. Int J Dev Biol. 2004;48:1015–29.
5. Evans A. Expression of the homeobox gene Pitx2 in neural crest is required for optic stalk and ocular anterior segment development. Hum Mol Genet. 2005;14(22):3347–59.
6. Fuhrman S. Eye morphogenesis and patterning of the optic vesicle. Curr Top Dev Biol. 2010;93:61–84.
7. Fuhrmann S. Wnt signaling in eye organogenesis. Organogenesis. 2014;4(2):60–7.
8. Fujimura N. WNT/β-Catenin signaling in vertebrate eye development. frontiers in cell and developmental biology. 2016;4.
9. Gage P. Fate maps of neural crest and mesoderm in the mammalian eye. Invest Ophthalmol Vis Sci. 2005;46:4200–8.
10. Gage PJ. Signaling "cross-talk" is integrated by transcription factors in the development of the anterior segment in the eye. Dev Dyn. 2009;238(9):2149–62.
11. de Godoy FRM , Qahtani EA, Lyons CJ. Posterior polymorphous corneal dystrophy in X linked Alport syndrome. Revista Brasileira de Oftalmologia. 2016;75(5):396–7.
12. Hägglund, A. 2017. "A novel mouse model of anterior segment dysgenesis (ASD): conditional deletion of Tsc1 disrupts ciliary body and iris development." Dis Model Mech 2017 10: 245–257.
13. Hingorani M, Hanson I, van Heyningen V. Aniridia. European Journal of Human Genetics. 2012;20(10):1011–7.
14. Honkanen RA, Nishimura DY, Swiderski RE, Bennett SR, Hong S, Kwon YH, Stone EM, Sheffield VC, Alward WLM. A family with Axenfeld–Rieger syndrome and Peters Anomaly caused by a point mutation (Phe112Ser) in the FOXC1 gene. American Journal of Ophthalmology. 2003;135(3):368–75.
15. Hu D-N, Simon JD, Sarna T. Role of ocular melanin in ophthalmic physiology and pathology. Photochemistry and Photobiology. 2008;84(3):639–44.
16. Idrees F. A review of anterior segment dysgeneses. Surv Ohthalmol. 2006;51(3):213–31.
17. Ittner LM, Wurdak H, Schwerdtfeger K, Kunz T, Ille F, Leveen P, Hjalt TA, Suter U, Karlsson S, Hafezi F, Born W. Compound developmental eye disorders following inactivation of TGFβ signaling in neural-crest stem cells. J Biol. 2005;4(3):11.
18. Lehmann OJ, Ebenezer ND, Jordan T, Fox M, Ocaka L, Payne A, Leroy BP, Clark BJ, Hitchings RA, Povey S, Khaw PT, Bhattacharya SS. Chromosomal duplication involving the

forkhead transcription factor gene FOXC1 causes iris hypoplasia and glaucoma. The American Journal of Human Genetics. 2000;67(5):1129–35.

19. Matsuo N, Smelser GK. Electron microscopic studies on the pupillary membrane: the fine structure of the white strands of the disappearing stage of this membrane. Investigative Ophthalmology & Visual Science. 1971;10:108–19.

20. Mullaney P. Congenital hereditary endothelial dystrophy associated with glaucoma. Ophthalmology. 1995;102(2):186–92.

21. Nishimura D. The forkhead transcription factor gene FKHL7 is responsible for glaucoma phenotypes which map to 6p25. Nat Genet. 1998;19:140–7.

22. Perveen R, Lloyd IC, Clayton-Smith J, et al. Phenotypic variability and asymmetry of Rieger syndrome associated with PITX2 mutations. Invest Ophthalmol Vis Sci. 2000;41(9):2456–60.

23. Pilar G, Nunez R, McLennan IS, Meriney SD. Muscarinic and nicotinic synaptic activation of the developing chicken iris. The Journal of Neuroscience. 1987;7(12):3813–26.

24. Roberts DK, Newman TL, Roberts MF, Wilensky JT, Remnants of the anterior tunica vasculosa lentis and long anterior lens zonules. Journal of Glaucoma. 23(7):441–5.

25. Saleem MD. Biology of human melanocyte development, Piebaldism, and Waardenburg syndrome. Pediatric Dermatology. 2019;36(1):72–84.

26. Sewden J. Molecular and developmental mechanisms of anterior segment dysgenesis. Camb Ophthalmol Symp Eye. 2007;21:1310–8.

27. Shields B. Axenfeld-Rieger syndrome. A spectrum of developmental disorders. Surv Ohthalmol. 1985;29(6):387–409.

28. Sim K. Posterior embryotoxon may not be a forme fruste of Axenfeld-Rieger's Syndrome. J Am Assoc Pediatr Opthalmol S. 2004;8(5):504–6.

29. Sliva L. The iridocorneal endothelial syndrome. Surv Ohthalmol. 2018;63(5):665–76.

Chapter 2
Iris Anatomy

Abstract The anatomy of iris is reviewed with focus on its relevance to medical and surgical interventions.

The Iris is composed of, from front to the back, anterior surface, Stroma, sphincter and dilator muscle and posterior double layers of iris pigment epithelium.

Anterior surface which is part of the stroma and stroma structure are extremely variable in different individuals, but the iris muscles and posterior double layered iris pigment epithelium is relatively constant. These anterior anatomical variations are like fingerprints, and are very unique in each individual. The use of new technologies such as optical coherence tomography (OCT) and Implementation of the collected anatomical information will facilitate treatment modalities, for example the use of laser for the treatment of eye diseases such as glaucoma.

The purpose here is also to improve the technologies of displaying exact anatomical variations of the iris. By doing so we hope to fabricate generation of a more specific equipment to evaluate the iris structure to improve the diagnostic modalities and surgical results.

In this chapter we focus on the specifications of iris structure relevant to medical and surgical interventions including use of laser, nanoparticles, electromagnetic, and small molecules. There is an emphasize on facilitating the performance of laser surgery on the iris to prevent narrow angle glaucoma.

The anatomy of iris at a glance may appear very simple. It consists of, from front to the back of the eye:

- Anterior surface
- Stroma
- Sphincter and dilator muscles
- Double layered Pigment epithelium

Anterior surface which is part of the stroma is extremely variable in different individuals, but the iris muscles and posterior double layered pigment epithelium is relatively constant.

K. T. Moazed, *The Iris*, https://doi.org/10.1007/978-3-030-45756-3_2

Fig. 2.1 Wolfflin nodules prominent from 3 o'clock to 5 o'clock of a very blue iris

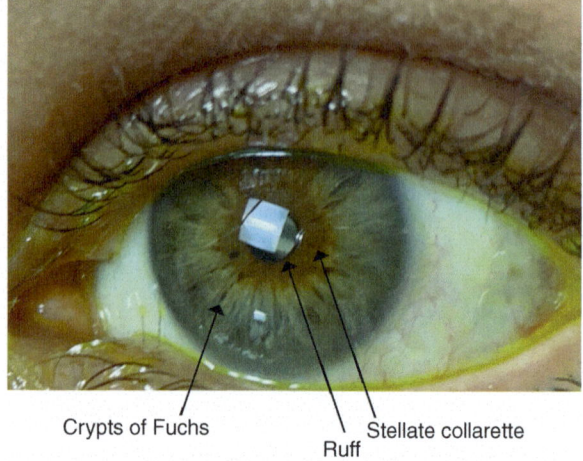

Crypts of Fuchs   Stellate collarette
                              Ruff

Fig. 2.2 The ruffs and pigmented stellate collarette are prominent in this iris. The Crypts of Fuchs can be seen at 360°

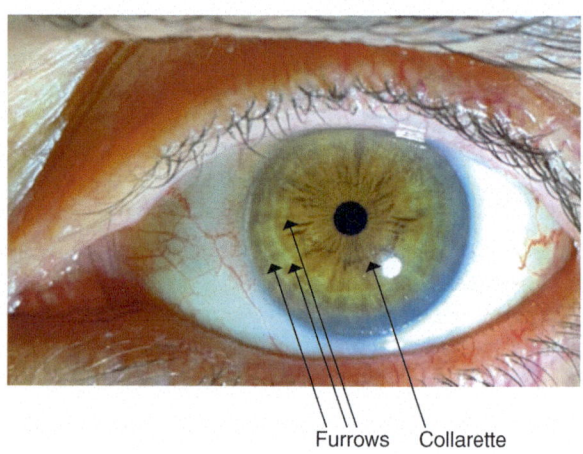

Furrows   Collarette

The anatomical variations in the anterior surface of the iris are very unique in each individual.

These variations can appear as:

- Stellate collarette (Figs. 2.1 and 2.2).
- Pupillary zone with outlines by stellate collarette as its outer border. Collarette which is the thickest part of the iris and holds the minor vascular circle.
- The ciliary zone which has smooth inner portion surrounded by middle furrowed section which contains the crypts of Fuchs which oriented radially and contraction furrows circular lines.
- Crypts of Fuchs are areas of defect in the stroma due to embryonic regression of the mesoderm and formation of the anterior chamber (Figs. 2.1 and 2.3).
- Wolfflin nodules that are white or orange nodules at the very superficial layer which is prominent in light iris color people (Fig. 2.4).
- Brushfield spots are seen in children with trisomy 21 (Down syndrome) very similar to Wolfflin nodules but in the brown iris is very noticeable.

Fig. 2.3 The circular furrows are seen as three concentric rings on this iris

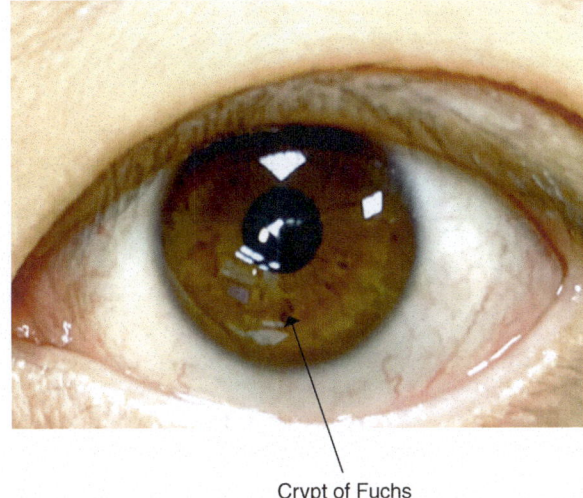

Crypt of Fuchs

Fig. 2.4 Brown iris with prominent Crypts of Fuchs. There is a poor view due to absorbed reflected light by pigment melanin

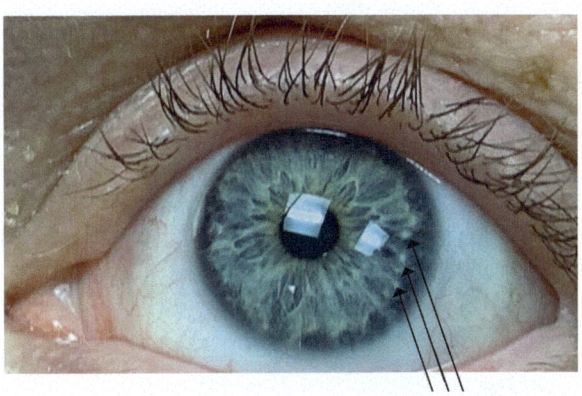

Wolfflin nodules

- Iris Freckles superficial pigmented spots that can change in size due to sun exposure and aging [17] (Fig. 2.12).

The Iris is located in front of the crystalline lens and divides the eye into anterior and posterior chambers (Fig. 2.11). Its central hole "pupil" constantly changes in diameter by sophisticated neural network in order to control the amount of light to reach the retina.

The iris has many anatomical functions which are as follows:

- Formation of diaphragm to permit the light entrance only through the pupil.
- Adjusting the depth of focus and depth perception.
- Reduce light aberration in the eye refracting system
- Formation of the dark room in its anterior section.
- Absorb and reflect incoming light spectrum by its melanin content.
- Sexual selection influence by its color diversity.

Fig. 2.5 Very dark iris. Most of the reflected light is absorbed by melanin, making it hard to see the details

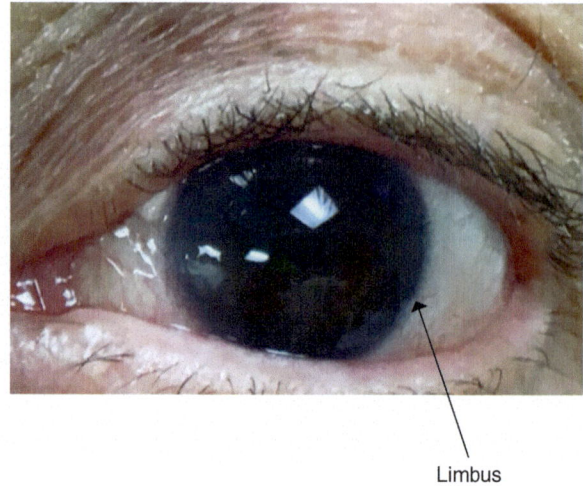

Limbus

Iris shape, Color, thickness and diameter varies tremendously in people (Fig. 2.5) even in the same ethnical background groups to the point that it is used for identification and security systems in many institutions and industries. Iris recognition system camera and software unites are getting more and more sophisticated and complex and being used in more places in recent times.

In a thorough publication by Edwards et al. [6] on analysis of iris surface features in populations of diverse ancestry, they have elegantly described the shape and color of the iris by its anthropological aspect and correlating the anatomical diversity and color variations in different ethnical backgrounds.

Functional Aspects of Iris Anatomy

Initially the discussion of iris anatomy in this chapter is based on its relevance to Ophthalmic surgery and imaging systems, specifically the optical coherence tomography (OCT) (Fig. 2.6).

The use of OCT in recent years have revolutionized the field of medicine specially in the field of ophthalmology.

OCT of the anterior chamber, even though is not specific for the iris but can distinguish the anatomical differences between different color eyes, for example, a blue iris has no pigment on the anterior surface but has the same posterior demarcation of iris pigment epithelium as in the brown iris (Fig. 2.7). (Comparison OCT images can be seen on the first page image at the beginning of the book)

OCT topographic demarcations:

Anatomical demarcation of the iris relevant to its tissue specifications in order to facilitate the desired interventions.

1. Functional anatomy is based on the relevance to surgical procedures, laser interventions and imaging techniques such as Optical Coherence Tomography (OCT).
2. Histological separation lines relevant to OCT.

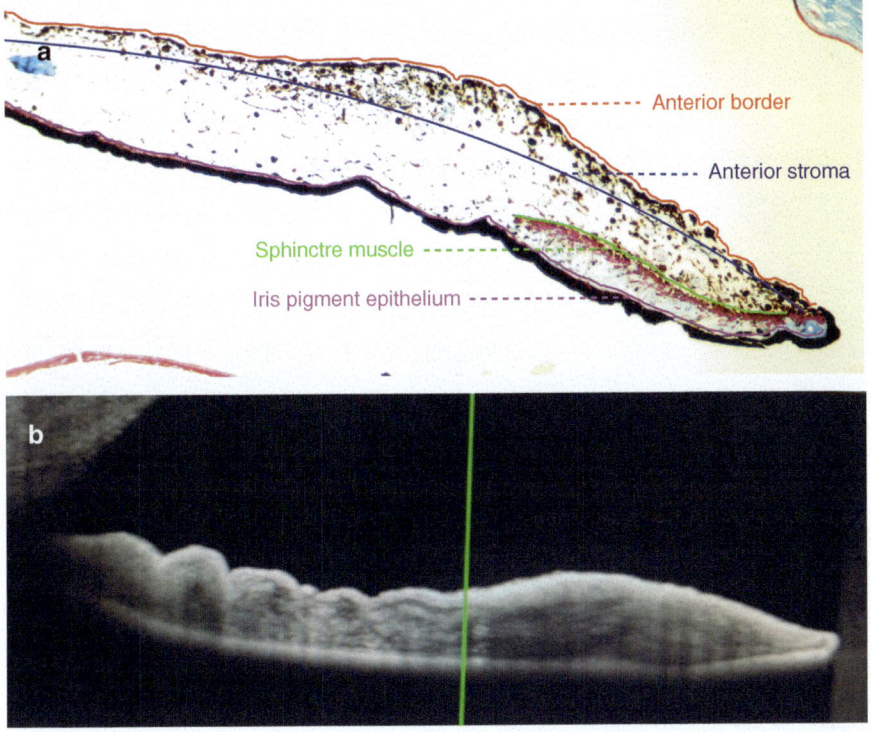

Fig. 2.6 (a) Light microscopy of the iris with recommended demarcation lines with pigment on the anterior surface and on the posterior iris pigment epithelium. (b) OCT of the iris with demarcation of pigment on the anterior stroma and posterior iris pigment epithelium

Fig. 2.7 OCT of a blue eye with no pigment on the anterior surface but the same posterior demarcation of iris pigment epithelium as in the brown iris (the iris and OCT images belong to the same patient)

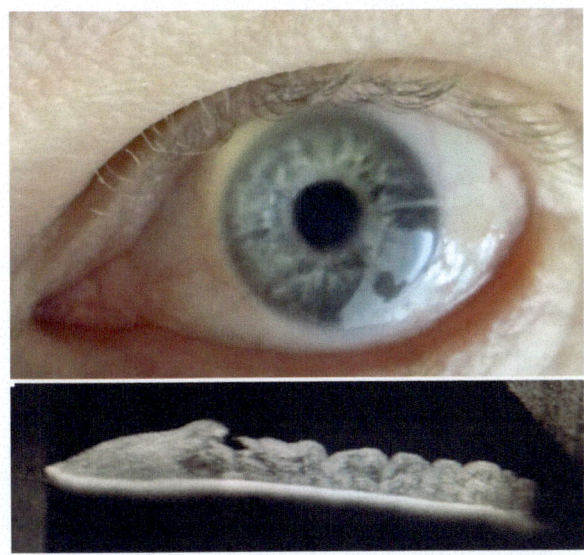

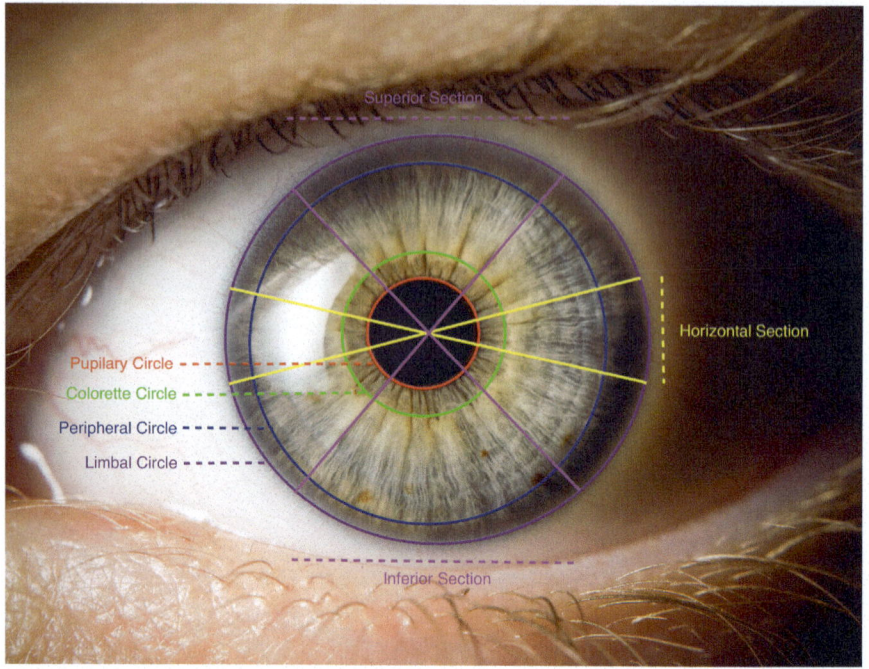

Fig. 2.8 Our recommended iris demarcations. These are compartments to be used for laser surgery on the iris

3. The computer-generated anterior border red demarcation.
4. The anterior stroma with high density of melanocytes with blue demarcation.
5. Anterior border of sphincter muscle green line demarcation.
6. Anterior border of iris pigment epithelium purple line (Fig. 2.8).

The presentation of segmenting the different areas of iris is illustrated in the Fig. 2.8 in this chapter.

1. The horizontal section (Yellow) line is the locations to avoid laser applications to prevent pain and hemorrhage during surgery since the innervation of the iris is highest in these areas. Long ciliary arteries enter the iris at 3:00 and 9:00 O'clock positions.
2. The thinnest part of the iris that is very suitable for laser iridotomy is marked as blue circle.
3. The Location of pigment cells in the stroma is necessary for pigment ablation and is marked by (green circle).
4. Surgical limbus for anatomical iris periphery (purple circle).
5. Quadrant section lines for topography in pink

The Iris superficial structures and measurements from center to the periphery:

• Pigmented ruff at the pupil margin which is the anterior border and the termination of folded iris pigment epithelium from the posterior surface of the iris.

It has close association with the sphincter muscle. It also has been referred to as physiological Ectropion Uveii or mamelons of Gallemaerts and Kleefeld. The ruff is essentially the anterior lip of neuroectodermal optic cup and in normal individuals measures between 0.03 and 0.06 mm with a regular pattern (Fig. 2.1).

Changes in pigmentary ruff and pathologic Ectropion Uveii can be seen in many conditions such as Pseudoglioma, Rubeosis Irides, essential iris atrophy, Uveitis and malignant tumors of the iris.

- The peripheral or marginal cribriform area that can be seen only by gonioscopy or anterior segment OCT (AS-OCT). The very preferred area for laser iridotomy due to its very thin thickness.
- At the very periphery, iris continues with the trabecular meshwork which drains the aqueous humor out of the eye and back to the circulation.

Iris diameter varies between 12 and 13 mm and the circumferential diameter is around 37–38 mm.

Iris thickness at the very periphery is very thin in about 0.2 mm (Fig. 2.9).

Thinnest part of the Iris is at its attachment to the ciliary processes and the angle structures (Fig. 2.10).

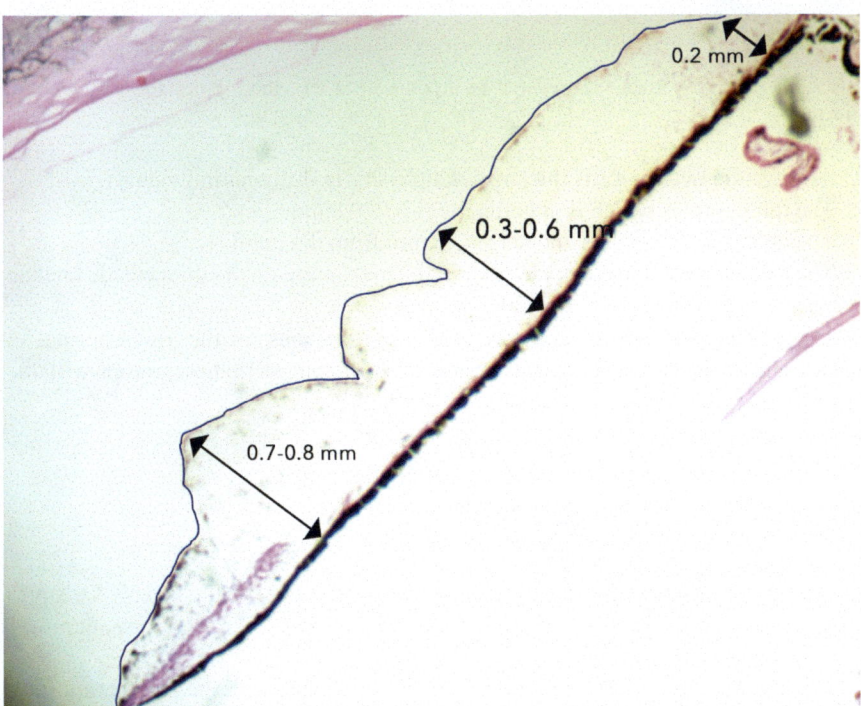

Fig. 2.9 The average diameters of iris thickness vary in different individuals according to the eye color

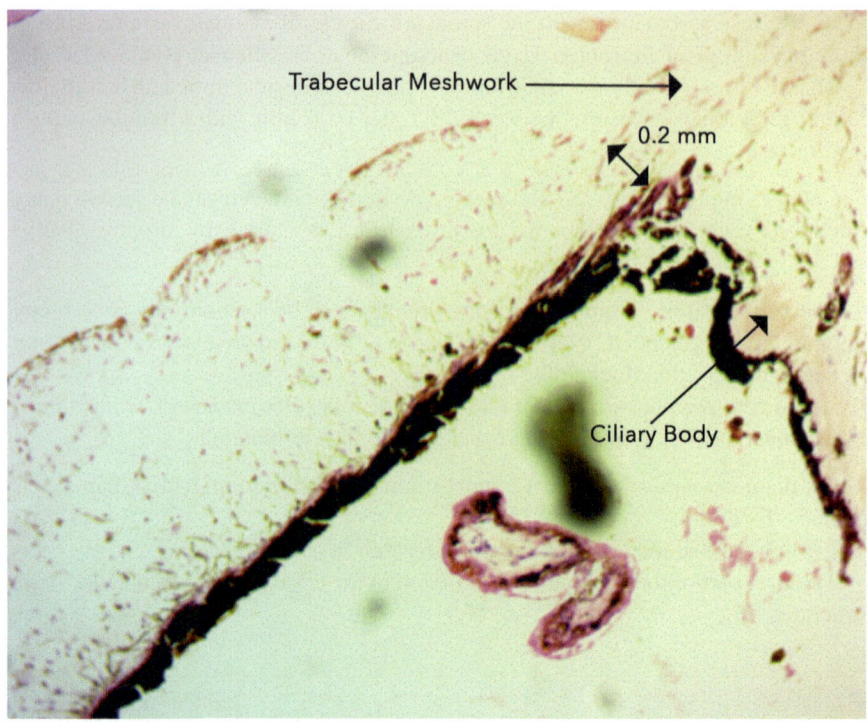

Fig. 2.10 Thinnest part of the iris is at its attachment to the ciliary processes and the angle structures

Average diameters of iris thickness which vary in different individuals.
The thickest part which is at collarette is 0.7–0.8 mm.
The collarette average is about 1.2–1.5 mm from the pupil.
The Ciliary zone thickness varies from 0.3 to 0.6 mm, on the thinner side on blue eyes and on the thicker side on dark color eyes.
In one study the authors compared the mean thickness of the iris in normal vs albino persons and revealed the difference of the thickness in these groups with the latter being thinner [14].

Posterior Surface of the Iris

The posterior surface of the iris is carpeted with the dense double layers of iris pigment epithelium (IPE). It has multiple folds that is necessary for its constant movement and changing diameter.
The smaller radial folds at pupillary margin continues with the pigmentary ruff.
The smaller circumferential folds are non-continuous and branching.

The large radial folds which extends to the iris base (The structural folds of Schwalbe).

Blood Supply

The iris blood supply originates from the major arterial circle located in the corona ciliaris located near the iris root which sends branches to the iris. The arteries enter the iris in an acute angle then branch and travel in the anterior part of stroma to reach the collarette which then form an incomplete minor circle of Iris.

The sphincter muscle and the pupillary zone are supplied by many smaller branches from the minor circle. From the minor circle the branches will supply the pupillary margin and extend posterior to supply sphincter muscle and the posterior surface of the iris.

Venus channels follows the almost similar pattern except the lack of major circle and drains into the vortex veins and the ciliary plexus.

Nerve Supply and Neural Network

- Sensory nerve supply originates from the long ciliary nerve which is the first branch of trigeminal nerve. The nerve fibers infiltrating the stroma and end with unmyelinated terminals. This explains the almost instant anesthesia after application of the anesthetic eye drops.
- Sympathetic nerve fibers are the postganglionic fibers from superior cervical ganglion which also travels along the long ciliary nerves and will innervate the dilator muscle. Some of these fibers make synapses with the melanocytes of the stroma, and act as vasomotor function on the iris blood vessels.
- Parasympathetic post ganglionic fibers originate from short ciliary nerves that arise from ciliary ganglion that innervates the sphincter muscle.

Iris Muscles

- The dilator muscle that is a very thin layer and is the extension of the iris pigment epithelium and is located between the stroma and iris pigment epithelium (IPE).
- They contain alpha exciting and beta 2 relaxing receptors. The dilator muscle lacks the cholinergic, serotoninergic, dopaminergic and histamine receptors.
- The sphincter muscle is a millimeter band located at the pupillary margin and has muscarinic cholinergic receptors but lack the adrenergic receptors [15].

Anterior and post. Chambers are separated by iris (Fig. 2.11).

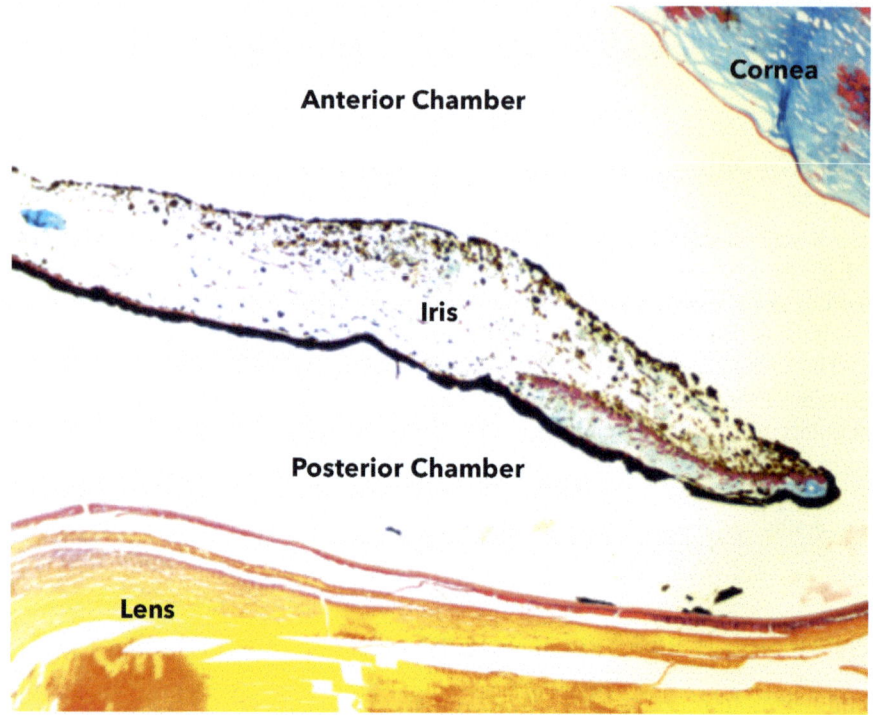

Fig. 2.11 Anterior and posterior chambers are separated by the iris

Our recommended iris demarcations. These are compartments to be used for laser surgery on the iris (Fig. 2.8).

Iris Anatomical Significance in Iris Intervention

Recognition of iris anatomy is an important factor in variety of anatomical malformations and pathological conditions.

Glaucoma is one of the leading causes of blindness in the world. It is estimated that there is over 60 million people are affected worldwide and the numbers are increasing [5].

There are many different types of glaucoma and the treatment is different with each category (Fig. 2.12).

The two main types of glaucoma are:

- Open angle glaucoma
- Angle closure glaucoma.

Fig. 2.12 Iris freckles. Superficial pigmented spots that can change in size due to sun exposure and aging

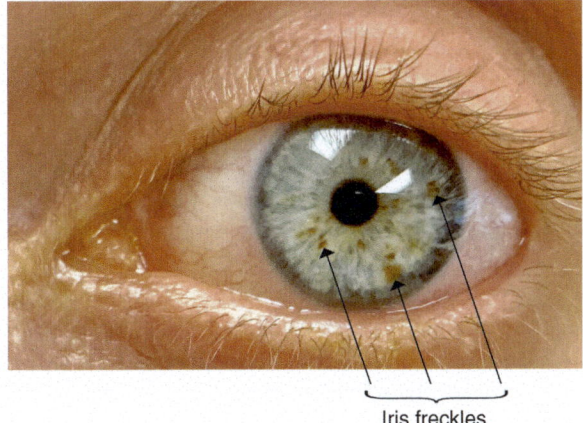

Iris freckles

There are many other types of glaucoma that are not as common, including:

- Normal tension glaucoma
- Congenital glaucoma
- Irido-Corneal Endothelial Syndrome (ICE)
- Secondary glaucoma

  - Pigmentary glaucoma
  - Uveitic glaucoma
  - Traumatic glaucoma
  - Neovascular glaucoma
  - Pseudoexfoliative glaucoma

Standard treatment for open angle glaucoma is different in many parts of the world but basic mode of treatment in US is to start with topical eye drops, followed by laser treatment and as the glaucoma progresses the surgical interventions from filtering procedures to tube implants are considered.

The anatomical target identifications for laser surgery and filtering procedures are crucial for desired outcome.

The 2 common modes of laser surgery for open angle glaucoma are:

- Argon Laser Trabeculoplasty (ALT) which laser beam is aimed to the trabecular meshwork based on thermal and coagulation property of laser to facilitate the drainage system.
- Selective Laser Trabeculoplasty (SLT) which is done by use of cool low energy nanosecond laser pulses which selectively targeting the pigmented cells only.
- Laser Cyclophotocoagulation that different forms of laser used to coagulate ciliary body and decrease the production of the aqueous humor.
- Laser Peripheral iridotomy (LPI) using argon or YAG laser to open a full thickness hole in the iris and It has been used for treatment of narrow angle glaucoma also, in pigmentary glaucoma, but recent studies are questioning its effect on the latter [13].

The standard treatment for narrow angle glaucoma and acute angle Closure Glaucoma is to perform laser peripheral iridotomy or surgical iridectomy to facilitate to flow of the aqueous humor from posterior chamber to the anterior chamber of the eye.

This is basically making a puncture hole in the iris to prevent capture of the aqueous humor in the posterior chamber and prevent acute raise in intraocular pressure that if not treated can cause blindness.

The laser iridotomy is performed by using Argon laser or YAG laser to which would make a safety valve on the iris.

The laser iridotomy is also indicated for the patients with narrow iridocorneal angle as a preventative procedure to protect them against the glaucoma attack.

The standard evaluation of the angle of the eye is a part of standard examination by the eye specialists and is called Gonioscopy. This is done by placing a contact mirrors with an angle to provide view of the angular structures (Gonioscopy) [7].

Recently there has been a major role for the OCT to evaluate and measure the angular degree and structure [16]. However, their images are crude and primitive with current OCT programs. There is a need for an OCT to give a 3-dimensional topography of the iris with thickness assessment in order to locate the best possible spot for laser and surgical interventions.

There is very essential for an integrated iris scanner or Iris topography to map the surface of the iris and evaluate the thickness of different areas of the iris to show the best possible place for the laser procedures.

As was mentioned earlier the two major sub-types of glaucoma are being discussed here:

The most common type is the chronic Open Angle Glaucoma (COAG) which is usually due to decrease drainage of the aqueous humor even though the iridocorneal angle is open.

Treatment usually begins with topical medications followed by laser treatment of the angle and/or the ciliary body to increase the drainage or decrease the aqueous formation respectively.

Primary Angle Closure Glaucoma (PACG) is the second most common glaucoma.

The main mechanism of (PACG) is the blockage of aqueous flow from the posterior chamber to the anterior chamber of the eye which is called pupillary block. This would cause the iris to move forward and close the iridocorneal angle which is responsible for the drainage of the aqueous humor outside the globe. As the result the pressure inside the eye increases to the point that would cause permanent damage to the optic nerve that can cause blindness if not immediately treated.

The treatment before the laser era was surgery, by performing a surgical incision at the limbus of the eye to enter the anterior chamber. The peripheral iris is then pinched with forceps and is pulled out of the eye and is cut with a small scissors. The surgical wound is then to be closed with a suture. This is called peripheral iridectomy and still is used during the glaucoma filtering surgery of the eye.

By introduction of the laser, the procedure can be done much faster and easier without the need to surgically opening the eye due to the good penetration of the laser energy through the clear cornea.

Like in any other surgical procedures there are possibilities of complications with laser iridotomy. These problems can be minimized by creating a special type of interactive process to identify and localize the feasible area for laser treatment.

There are many factors involved in laser iridotomy procedure:

- Corneal transparency: This can be affected by corneal scar, edema or other opacities such as (Arcus Senilis or band keratopathy).
- Iris thickness: The location of the crypts of Fuchs, folds, furrows, ridges, corona, freckles, and the collarette.
- Iris color: Iris pigment absorbs the laser energy and can affect the outcome. The darker the color of the eye the more laser energy is needed [10].
- Ethnic background: There is a large variation in structure, the thickness and as a result the color of the iris. These variations can also affect the pathology and diseases of the eye for example, there is an increase incidence of the Primary Angle-Closure Glaucoma (PACG) in Indian and Asian eyes.
- There is an increased risk of Uveal melanoma in light color eye population [18].
- Location: The iridotomy specially if large can affect the vision and causes major discomfort for the patient.

There are many references on the best location for the peripheral iridotomy. The most practical is to use a small hole around 0.2–0.3 mm in size and locate it between 11 and 1 o'clock to be covered by the upper eyelid to prevent extra image on the retina through the newly induced hole. There are suggestions of other locations for the iridotomy, but each has their benefits and disadvantages. In a recent review article it was suggested that the location of iridotomy did not make any difference on patients post laser visual symptoms (Dysphotopsias) by 6 months follow up of their comparison groups [9].

The iridotomy procedure can be very difficult and not successful if the iris is very thick or the iridotomy is performed at the wrong area. The complications can increase if the patient is at high risk of bleeding. Induced iatrogenic iritis due to excess laser energy to the iris can also result in painful red eye. Another side effect can be from the sudden release of pigment that can clog the fenestrations of the angle structures which can cause the raise in intraocular pressure.

There has been studies on OCT evaluation of the iris that discussed the curvature and thickness of the iris but no reference to the location of the defects and location of the Fuchs crypts on the iris [21]. The OCT equipment that is capable of perform both iris topography and 3D volume calculation would be very helpful in these situations. Recently the iris surface topography has been described [4].

The laser iridotomy is also indicated for the patients with narrow iridocorneal angle and pigmentary glaucoma as a preventative procedure to protect them against the angle closure glaucoma attack.

The standard evaluation of the angle of the eye is a part of standard examination by the ophthalmologist and is called Gonioscopy. This is done by placing a contact lens with angled mirrors (Gonio-lens) on the cornea to provide view of the angular structures of the eye.

Recently there have been a great improvement in anterior chamber viewing with OCT of anterior segment to evaluate and measure the angular degree and structure.

Dynamics of iris before and after iridotomy has been discussed by Zheng [19].

Iris parameters also has been studied by the iris curvature, area and thickness that was associated with narrow angles [20].

Iris OCT angiography (OCTA) can be a used tool to identify a vascular free zone for laser iridotomy which prevents the accidental hitting of the blood vessels that can complicate the procedure [11]. Iris Angiography can also identify the location of the major blood vessels and the evidence of iris rubeosis [2, 12] and iris micro-hemangioma [3] which can be avoided during laser procedure [1].

The specific anatomical structure of the surface of the iris, the lack of anterior surface epithelium, the fenestration of the surface area and its submergence in the aqueous humor make the iris susceptible to manipulations and interventions by various Sources.

A new specific and precise iris optical coherence tomography system to give 3-dimensional topography of the iris for assessing desired location on the iris for placement of an iridotomy would be very desirable and practical of iris specific OCT equipment.

Applications of tissue transplantation, nanoparticles, artificial implants, chemicals, dyes, small molecules and tissue adhesives can be possible via entering the anterior chamber of the eye under direct observation and with the aid. There are further discussions on the OCT of the iris in the following chapters.

Bibliography

1. Kang AS, et al. Optical coherence tomography angiography of iris microhemangiomatosis. Am J Ophthalmol Case Rep. 2017;6:24–6.
2. Ang M, et al. Optical coherence tomography angiography for anterior segment vasculature imaging. Ophthalmology. 2015;122:1740–7.
3. Bakke EF, Drolsum L. Iris microhaemangiomas and idiopathic juxtafoveolar retinal telangiectasis. Acta Ophthalmol Scand. 2006;84:818–22.
4. Benalcazar DP, et al. A 3D iris scanner from multiple 2D visible light images. IEEE Xplore. 2019;7:61461–72.
5. Cedrone C, et al. Epidemiology of primary glaucoma: prevalence, incidence, and blinding effects. Prog Brain Res. 2008;173:3–14.
6. Edwards M, et al. Analysis of iris surface features in populations of diverse ancestry. R Soc Open Sci. 2016;3:150424.
7. Friedmman DS. Who needs an iridotomy. Br J Ophthalmol. 2001;85:1019–21.
8. Gazzard G, et al. A prospective ultrasound biomicroscopy evaluation of changes in anterior segment morphology after laser iridotomy in Asian eyes. Ophthalmology. 2003;110:630–8.
9. Kavitha S, et al. Resolution of visual dysphotopsias after laser iridotomy: six-month follow-up. Ophthalmology. 2019;126:469–71.
10. Kashiwagi K. Angle-closure glaucoma: iridotomy. In: Pearls of glaucoma management. Berlin, Heidelberg: Springer; 2016. p. 511–6.
11. Di Lee W, et al. Optical coherence tomography angiography for the anterior segment. Eye Vis. 2019;6:4.
12. Moazed K. Rubeosis iridis in "pseudogliomas". Surv Ophthalmol. 1980;25:85–90.
13. Okafor K, et al. Update on pigment dispersion syndrome and pigmentary glaucoma. Curr Opin Ophthalmol. 2017;28:154–60.

14. Sheth V, et al. Diagnostic potential of iris cross-sectional imaging in albinism using optical coherence tomography. Ophthalmology. 2013;120:2082–90.
15. Reibaldi A, et al. Iris receptors of fresh human eyes. Europe PMC. Ann Ophthalmol. 1984;16:746–8.
16. Rudhakrishnan S, et al. Comparison of optical coherence tomography and ultrasound biomicroscopy for detection of narrow anterior chamber angles. JAMA Ophthal. 2005;123:1053–9.
17. Schwab C. Iris freckles a potential biomarker for chronic sun exposure. Invest Ophthalmol Vis Sci. 2017;58(6):BIO174–9.
18. Vajdic CM, et al. Eye color and cutaneous nevi predict risk of ocular melanoma in Australia. Int J Cancer. 2001;92:906–12.
19. Zheng C, et al. Analysis of anterior segment dynamics using anterior segment optical coherence tomography before and after laser peripheral iridotomy. JAMA Ophthalmol. 2013;131:44–9.
20. Wang B, Lisandro M. Sakata, David S. Friedman, Yiong-Huak Chan, Mingguang He, Raghavan Lavanya, Tien-Yin Wong, Tin Aung. Quantitative Iris Parameters and Association with Narrow Angles. Ophthalmology. 2010;117(1):11–7.
21. Wang B-S, Narayanaswamy A, Amerasinghe N, Zheng C, He M, Chan Y-H, Nongpiur ME, Friedman DS, Aung T. Increased iris thickness and association with primary angle closure glaucoma. British Journal of Ophthalmology. 2010;95(1):46–50.

Chapter 3
Iris Histology

Abstract The histology of iris is considered to be very specific and unique in general and varies in different individuals according to their inheritance. These cellular composition and distribution in the iris tissue are very variable according to the iris color. The unusual and specific characteristics of iris histology is also very different from other organs.

The anterior surface/border of the iris is a thin layer of fibroblasts and collagen, without being covered by endothelium or epithelium which make the iris float and be exposed to the Aqueous Humor and its contents. This effect also participates in the light reflection and the emerging observable color of the iris. It also facilitates the constant movement of the iris due to light and accommodation and the constant exposure to the molecules and signaling pathways and the immune privilege condition in the anterior chamber.

The layer beneath the fibroblasts composed of melanocytes with variable pigment which is different in different color eyes. These melanocytes have very specific characteristics that make them very different from other types of melanocytes such as skin melanocytes. For example, the iris melanocytes do not respond to UV exposure (No tanning) due to lack of, or nonfunctioning specific Melanocortin receptor (MC1R). Iris melanocytes do not transfer as many pigment organelles (melanosomes) into neighboring cells as in the skin.

The stroma is very loose with specific acid Mucopolysaccharide and collagen components to also facilitate its constant motility. The iris does not heal or form scar tissue due to many factors. The lack of collagen VII in stroma and the Lack of bleeding during or after surgical intervention which is necessary for scar formation, causes lack of healing and scar formation after injury or surgery. The lack of blood clot at the insult area and the immune privilege environment also contribute to this process. The iris usually does not bleed by surgical incision or laser penetration due to specific blood vessel structure which carry an elastic band around the arterioles.

The specific receptors of the iris melanocytes and their signaling pathways are very specific and are discussed elsewhere. For more details please refer to chapters on this book on Iris molecular biology and Iris wound healing.

Histologic differences that contributes to the reflected eye color is discussed in this chapter.

© Springer Nature Switzerland AG 2020
K. T. Moazed, *The Iris*, https://doi.org/10.1007/978-3-030-45756-3_3

Discussion

Iris can be considered an internal organ because it composed of connective tissue, pigment epithelium, muscles (Dilator and Sphincter), vascular tissue such as arteries and veins and nerve supply with sensory, vasomotor, motor, sympathetic and parasympathetic origins.

The Iris is completely submerged in aqueous humor which constantly flow from posterior chamber as it secreted by ciliary processes through the pupil to get absorbed at the angle of the eye via trabecular meshwork and Schlemm's canal.

The important feature about the iris is that it the only internal organ that is directly observable with the naked eye and can be examined in a noninvasive manner by slit lamp, without the need for endoscopy. In recent years the iris histology can be evaluated with more advanced technologies like optical coherence tomography (OCT) without the need for invasive procedures or biopsy. This make Iris a valuable source of information for research and development to evaluate the physiologic anomalies and/or systemic or ocular diseases and/or malignant conditions.

There are specific histological characteristics that are unique to iris tissue which needs to be addressed:

The melanocytes of the iris unlike the skin melanocytes, are not very active and transfer minimal pigment to their surrounding tissues. As the result they have short cytoplasmic projections extended to the neighboring cells.

The iris has little or no capacity to heal after being incised, ruptured or cut by laser as in standard laser iridotomy or standard surgical iridectomy. Exceptions to this rule are complicating factors like rubeosis, inflammation, infections and neoplasms. This phenomenon is complex, and many factors are involved.

- Lack of healing process in the iris can be partly explained by the lack of Collagen VII in the stroma of the iris that is responsible to promoting the healing and scar formation after injury [5].
- Decreased inflammatory response due to natural immune compromised anterior chamber environment is also another factor responsible for lack of healing process due to suppressed inflammatory stage of normal wound healing process.
- The lack of bleeding after incision is another factor in preventing the normal healing process [16].
- The iris also will not bleed after surgical or laser incision, due to unusual elastic layer around the iris blood vessels (Fig. 3.1) which prevent bleeding. Minimal bleeding can on occasion occur if the blood vessels are directly hit by laser beam, but usually it is self-limiting. Exceptions includes the patients on anticoagulant medications or other coagulation anomalies and existence of abnormal blood vessels like iris neovascularization (rubeosis Irides) or hemangiomas [15].
- The iris melanocytes do not respond and change color by exposure to UV light except for pigmented iris freckles which increase by sun exposure. In other word the iris will not tan by sun exposure [14].

Fig. 3.1 Light microscopy ×40, central full thickness iris. Iris blood vessels with their specific elastic band around them. Surface pigmented melanocytes on the right and dilator muscle and iris pigment epithelium on the left

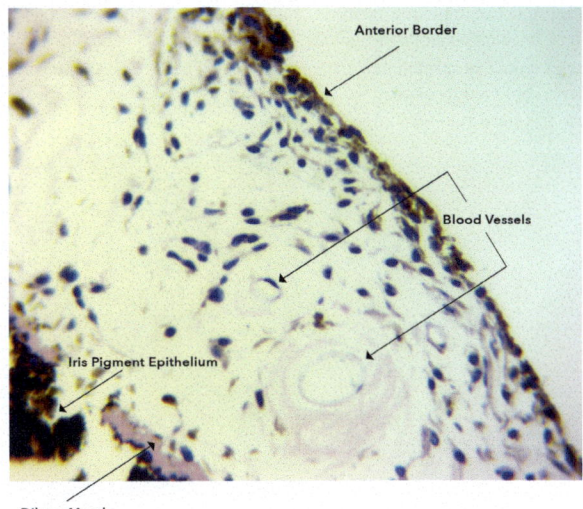

- The Iris melanocytes do not respond directly and change color by hormones such as MCH, or MSH due to lack or non-functioning of specific receptors MC1R [9].
- The topography, the color and the shape of the iris is very specific in each individual and it will not change by aging to the point that it is used as an identity tool by many banks and security device manufacturers [10].

The Iris contains different distinctive layers that are originating from different embryonic origins: neural ectoderm, Neural Crest, and mesoderm. Each layer can be subdivided into more specific parts according to their histological specifications and their cellular structure and morphology.

To understand the histology of the iris it is essential to review the embryology chapter of this book.

Histologic Specifications of the Iris Color Variation

There are many factors involved in the process of the reflection of light from the iris that stablishes the color of the eye.

The variation in the histology of the iris that is inherited and contribute to its color are being discussed here.

In order to appreciate different components that attributes to the reflected iris color, the role of cornea and the anterior chamber Aqueous Humor (AH) was evaluated. The cornea was removed surgically from 3 different color fresh postmortem eyes from the eye bank (dark brown, light brown and blue eye) and external photography was obtained. Surprisingly the reflected iris colors were not as vivid as seen when the iris is observed through the AH and cornea.

Fig. 3.2 Fresh postmortem dark brown eye from the eye bank. The cornea has been removed to expose the iris for direct viewing

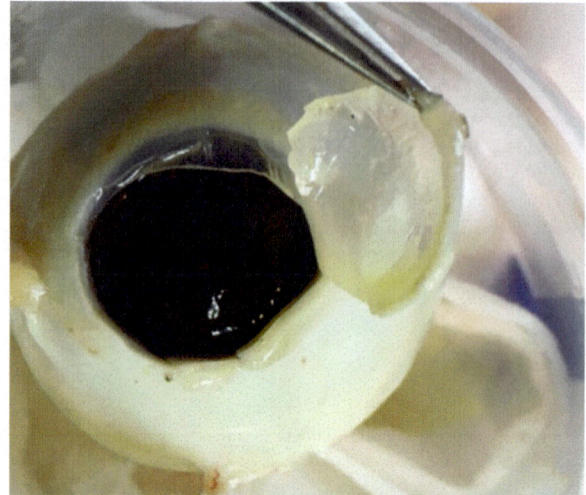

Fig. 3.3 Fresh postmortem light brown eye from the eye bank. The cornea has been removed to expose the iris for direct viewing

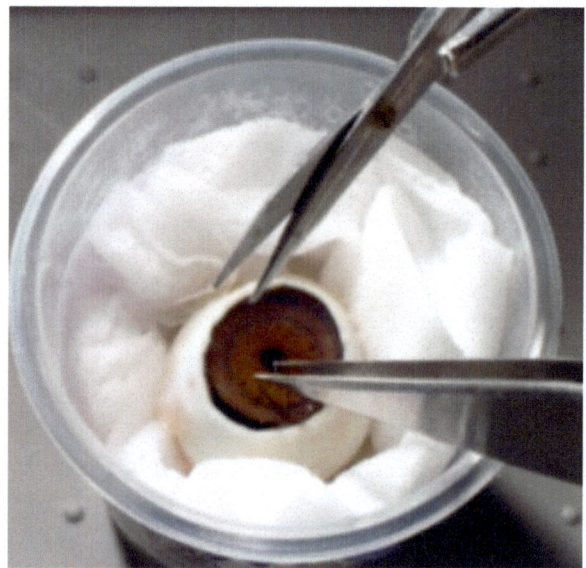

The picture of 3 colors of the iris after removal of the cornea is being presented in attached figures (Figs. 3.2, 3.3, and 3.4).

The histological iris color contributors from the front to the back:

1. Collagen content of the cornea.
2. Aqueous Humor light scattering.
3. Anatomical variation of structure of the anterior border of the Iris.

Fig. 3.4 Fresh postmortem light blue eye from the eye bank. The cornea has been removed to expose the iris for direct viewing

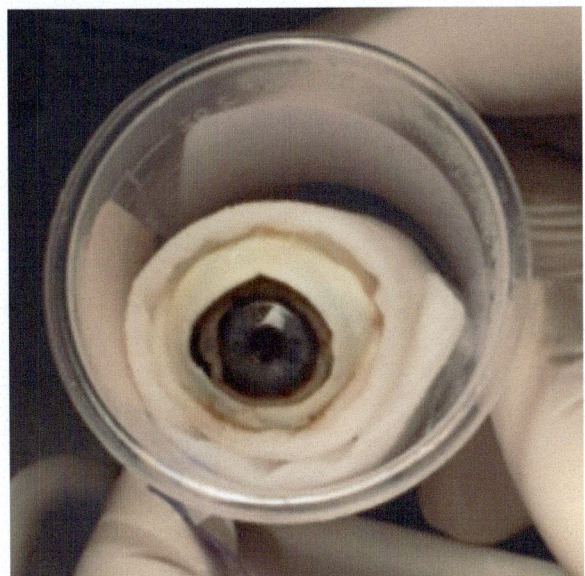

4. The number of fibroblasts on the anterior surface.
5. Amount of collagen produced by fibroblasts on the anterior border.
6. The amount of intercellular matrix in anterior border and stroma.
7. The number of melanocytes of the anterior surface of the Iris.
8. Variation of melanosomes location in the melanocyte cytoplasm.
9. Number, size & melanin content of Melanosomes.
10. The stages of melanosomes in melanocytes.
11. The nature of melanin contents and ratio of Eumelanin to Pheomelanin.
12. Perinuclear position of melanosomes in the melanocyte cytoplasm.
13. The number of melanocytes in the stroma.
14. Number of melanin contained macrophages in the stroma.
15. The amount of melanin in macrophages of the stroma.
16. Anatomical variations in the structure of the stroma.
17. The amount of intercellular matrix in the stroma.
18. Posterior double layers of iris pigment epithelium.
19. Blue shift spectrum absorption of reflected light through the soft tissue proteins, Collagen, Melanin and air interface.
20. Tindal effect = light scattering in colloidal particles
21. Rayleigh Effect = light scattering by particles.

The melanocytes of the iris also have different characteristics that has been described in Table 3.1.

Different types of pigment with different ratio can be detected in different individuals (Table 3.2).

Table 3.1 Iris pigment epithelium vs. stroma melanocytes

Characteristic differences of iris pigment epithelium (IPE)
1. Basement membrane is present
2. Dilator muscle is attached to IPE
3. IPE has large melonine granules
4. Packed melanocytes with tight junction
5. Structure is independent of the iris color
6. Embryonic origin from nueroectoderm
Charachteristic differences of stromal melanocytevs
1. Basement membrane is not present
2. Fibroblasts attached to melanocytes
3. Stroma melanocytes have smaller melanine granules
4. Dispersed melanocytes
5. Structure is completely dependent on the iris color
6. Embryonic origin from neural crest

Table 3.2 Eumelanin/pheomelanin ratio in human uveal melanocytes

Ratio from light colored irides = 1.31
Ratio from dark colored irides = 7.32
Ratio in malignent melanoma cells = 0.41

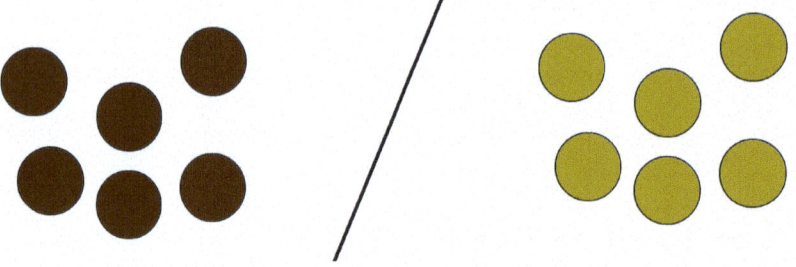

The melanoctes of the iris are considered as a non-Classical melanocytes, the different types of melanocytes and their classifications are summarized in Table 3.3.

The layers of Iris from anterior to the posterior are composed of:

- The anterior border, the stroma, the Iris dilator and sphincter muscles and the double layers of Iris pigment epithelium located on the very posterior surface of the iris next to the lens (Fig. 3.5).

Table 3.3 Non-classical melanocytes vs. classical melanocytes

Non-Classical Melanocytes

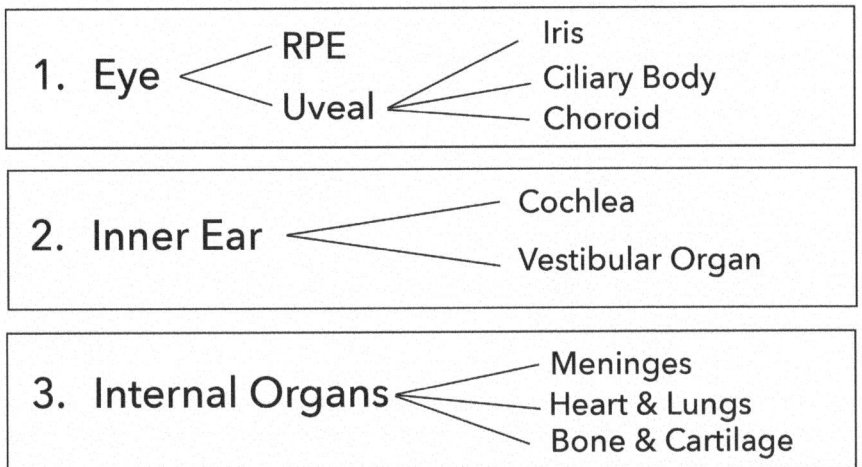

Classical Melanocytes

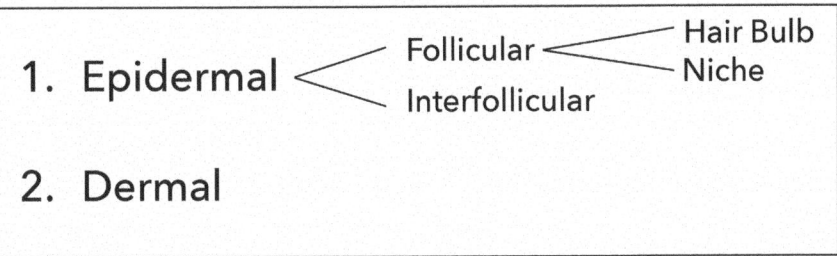

The Anterior Border

This layer is of mesoderm origin and has a sponge like texture. It can be divided into two components (Fig. 3.5):

– Single surface layer of fibroblasts with branching processes that interconnect with each other. This is not a real layer and is non-continuous and missing in certain areas exposing the stroma directly to the aqueous humor (AH). This layer has variable thickness and is missing at certain areas called Iris crypts or crypts of Fuchs. The fibroblasts have micro villi on the anterior surface exposed to the Aqueous Humor (Fig. 3.6).

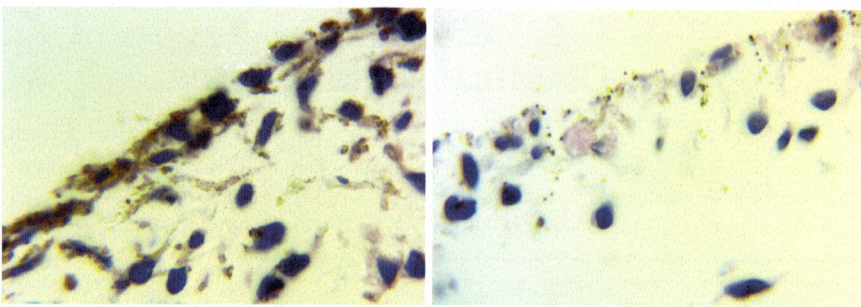

Fig. 3.5 Light microscopy ×40, anterior surface of a dark brown iris (left) and a blue iris (right). Displayed as a comparison, the higher density and number of melanocytes in the brown iris and scattered and the low-density melanocytes with minimal pigmentation in the blue iris

– The melanocyte layer has the highest density in dark color irides. This is a compact aggregation of melanocytes located under the surface of single fibroblasts layer and it contains variable population of fibroblasts. In the previous studies there have been conflicting reports regarding the number of melanocytes on different people with different eye colors, studies by Fuchs [4] and Dietrich [3].

Reveals that the number of melanocytes varies in different color eyes [12].

Other studies claim that the number of melanocytes do not contributing to the color of the eye [17].

Imesch et al. reported that the number of stroma melanocytes and cellularity does not have a major contribution to the iris color [7] Our observarion could not confirm their claim.

The Type of melanin components of the melanosomes have been reported to contribute to the variety of human eye colors. The ratio between Eumelanin (Dark Brown) content of melanosomes and Pheomelanin (yellow-red) content of melanosomes also affects the reflected color of the iris [8].

However, the amount of pigment and accordingly the stages of melanosomes in these melanocytes and the location of the melanosomes in the cytoplasmofthe melanocytes varies in different people with different eye colors and races. These variations in melanosomes have not been addressed before. The density of melanocytes and their pigment contents in different eye colors can be appreciated in attached figure (Fig. 3.5).

The majority of pigment is located at the anterior surface area of the brown Iris. There are minimal or no pigment on the anterior surface of a very blue eyes or in Albinism.

There are many direct and indirect cellular hormonal and molecular interaction between the fibroblasts and the melanocytes that will be discussed in molecular biology chapter.

Anterior border cells are not overlying iris crypts and are more condense in brown eyes. Contraction furrows are more prominent also in darker irides.

Fig. 3.6 Light microscopy
×100. Layers of
melanocytes on the brown
iris surface on the top,
fibroblasts, and loose
stroma with a macrophage
in the center

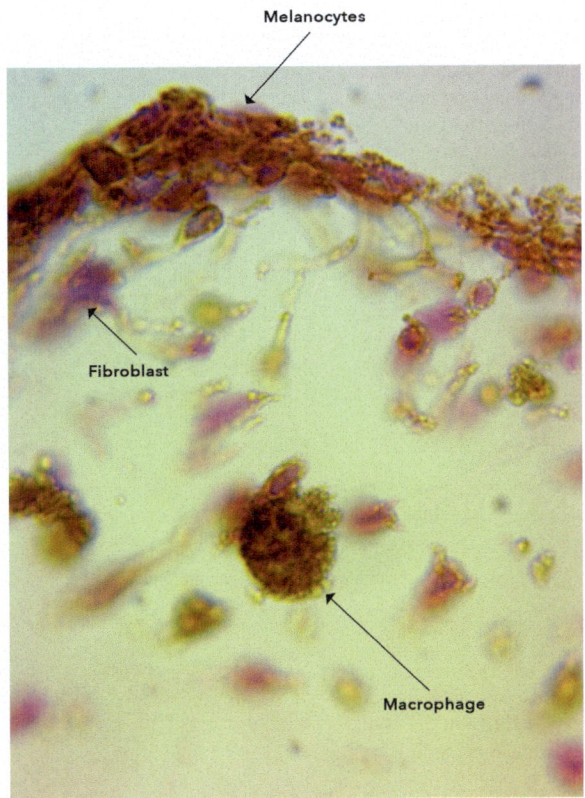

The anterior border layer ends at the iris root but may extend outward in a spoke-like fashion (Fig. 3.7).

The collagen components of the cornea and the anterior border of the iris does indeed absorb the red component of the reflected light spectrum which contribute to the blue appearance of the irides with minimal melanin pigment on their anterior surface.

Similar situation can be observed in the viewing of the blood vessels on the skin which looks blue, but in reality the blood is red, also as the viewing of the blue nevus that is made of melanin but deep in the dermis looks blue to the obsurver. In all these instances the blue reflected color is due to absorption of the red portion of the light spectrum from the reflected light by the collagen layer of the skin and light scattering in the matrix of the surrounding tissues.

The anterior border of the iris is fairly thick near the pupillary border where it is firmly attached to the two layers of pigment epithelium that form the pupillary ruff. Because the thickness of the anterior border layer varies over the surface of the iris, it is helpful to identify the thinnest area of the iris when performing the laser iridotomy (Fig. 3.8).

Fig. 3.7 Light microscopy ×10. Iris base. The thinnest part of the iris as it attaches to the ciliary processes on the bottme right and trabecular meshwork on the top right

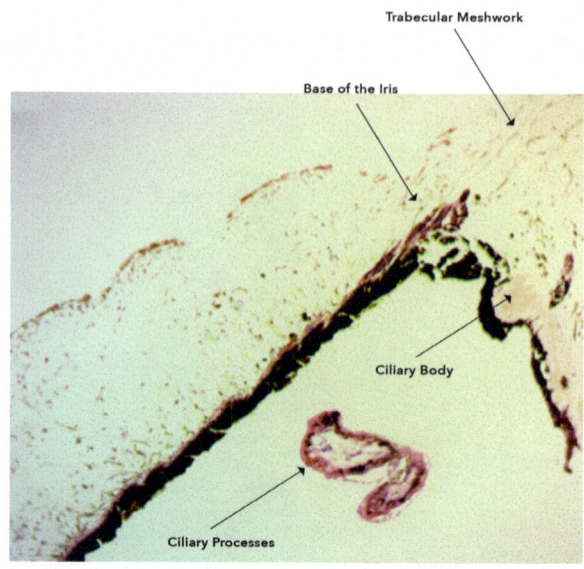

Fig. 3.8 The average diameters of iris thickness vary in different individuals according to the eye color

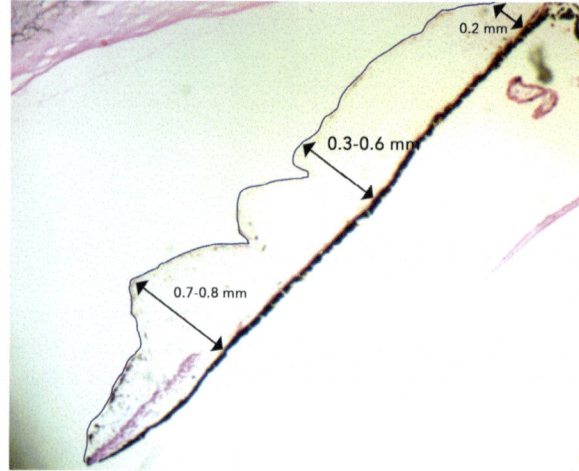

The Stroma

- The stroma is from mesoderm origin and is composed of connective tissue, blood vessels, nerves, muscles, and migrated pigmented cells (Fig. 3.9):
- The loose connective tissue of the iris with high content of Acid mucopolysaccharide and collagen specially around the radially oriented blood vessels, which permits the sudden movements of dilation and constriction (mydriasis and miosis) of the iris by neuronal stimulation due such as light/accommodation and chemicals and medications (Fig. 3.10a, b).

  The specifications of the collagen diversity and its components in iris has an important role in the function of this organ as change or damage to it has severe consequences as has been reported in Glaucoma patients [1].

Fig. 3.9 (**a**) Light microscopy ×100. Iris stroma with loose connective tissue, one small capillary, and fibroblasts. (**b**) Light microscopy ×40. Full thickness blue iris with loose stroma matrix with a scattered fibroblast

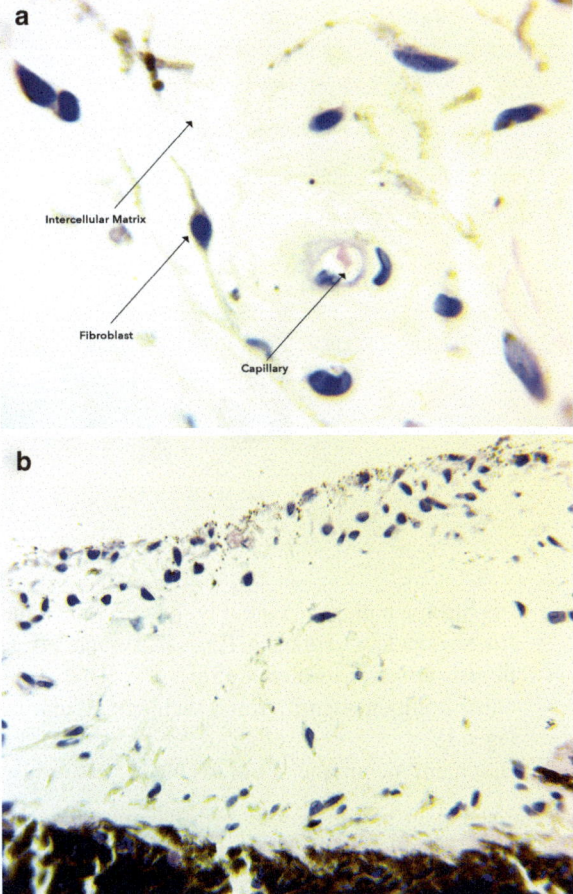

Fig. 3.10 (**a**) Light microscopy ×100, typical iris blood vessel with endothelial cells and elastic cuffing. (**b**) Light microscopy ×40, central full thickness iris. Iris blood vessels with their specific elastic band around them. Surface pigmented melanocytes on the right and dilator muscle and iris pigment epithelium on the left

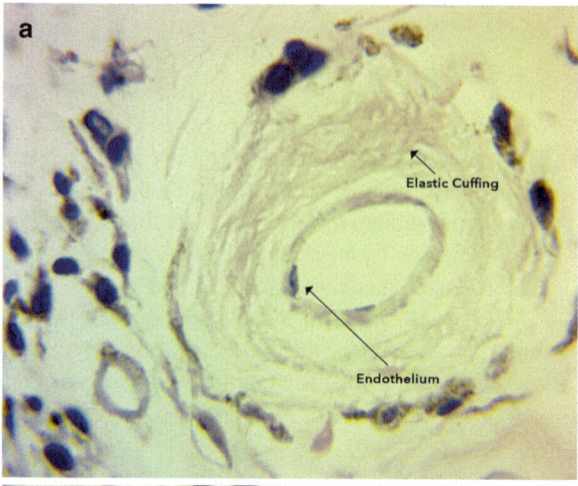

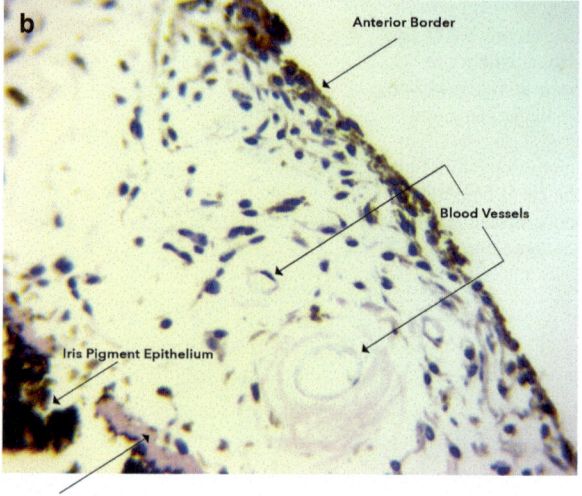

- Iris Stroma collagen content is specific and contain Type I and Type III.
- Iris Stroma lacks collagen Types II, IV and VII which the latter is involved in fibrosis and scar formation [5].
- Other components of stroma such as vascular cells, fibroblasts contain collagen IV.
- Basement membrane of the iris blood vessels also contains collagen type I.

• The abundant blood vessels form the substantial volume of the iris. They are radially oriented and locate in different depths with multiple anastomosis which form the minor vascular circle of iris. The iris blood vessels are very unique due to their specific characteristics that makes them very different from the rest of the body (Fig. 3.10). The thick endothelial lining and the thick collagen fibril collar that located in the adventitia of the iris vessels accounts for:

(a) low permeability of iris blood vessels
(b) limited or no bleeding during trauma or surgical procedures or laser iris surgery
     (Iridectomy & iridotomy procedures)
(c) Fenestration in iris vessels endothelium permits the movement of inflammatory cells into the anterior chamber during certain conditions like Iritis or Uveitis.

- Other cellular components that occupy the stromal connective tissue are macrophages that contain pigment (Clump cells of Koganei Type 1), multinucleated pigment cells that have surrounding basement membrane (Clump cells of Koganei type 2), Mast cells, lymphocytes and plasma cells in varying distributions.
- Nerve endings are from autonomic and sensory, vasomotor and motor nerves and their supporting cells such as Schwann cells are spread and scattered all throughout the stroma, they form neuromuscular synapses with the dilator and sphincter muscles and also have direct synapses to the melanocytes. Disruption of sympathetic neural stimulation known as Horner's syndrome is associated with decreased pigment formation in the iris [2].

The Dilator and the Sphincter Muscles of the Iris

These muscles are of Neural Ectoderm origin.

- The dilator muscle is a smooth muscle. It extends from the region of the sphincter muscle to the base of the iris and is continuous with the anterior Iris pigment epithelium.

- This muscle is a very thin layer and composed of only five muscular processes thick and is separated from stroma by a thin layer of basement membrane (Fig. 3.11).

- The dilator muscle is fused to the sphincter muscle by projections in the midportion called Fuchs Spur the same projections at the peripheral edge of the sphincter muscle is called Michel's Spur, and the projections to the ciliary body is called Grunert spur (Fig. 3.11).

Fig. 3.11 Light
microscopy ×40. Posterior
view of the iris. Dilator
muscle adjacent to the iris
pigment epithelium

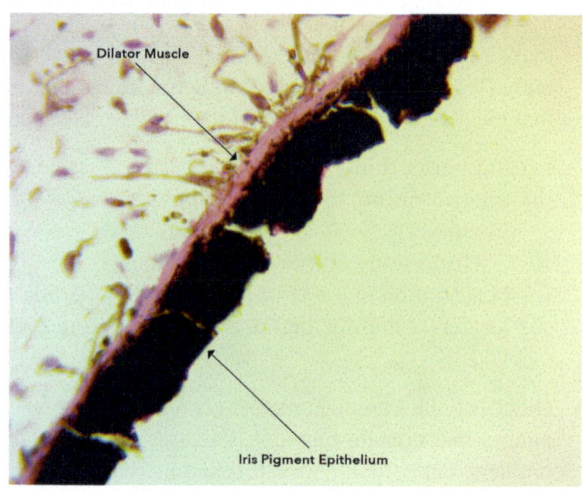

The Effect of Prostate Medication on Iris

Changes in function of dilator muscle due to trauma, chronic inflammation, laser ablation, malignancies, and certain medications can cause visual impairment due to lack of iris motility.

Intraoperative floppy iris syndrome (IFIS) is a recent issue due to the use of the most commonly prescribed alpha-1 adrenergic blocker for the treatment of benign prostatic hyperplasia (BPH).

The IFIS increases the chance of complications during cataract surgery by lack of dilation and as a result small pupil or iris prolapse or tear during the operation. Other complications can follow during or after surgery due to lack of visibility or the vitreous loss during surgery, vitreous hemorrhage, uveitis and macular edema.

Long term use of alpha-1 adrenergic blockers can also cause permanent disuse atrophy of dilator muscle which can be observed by AS-OCT (Anterior segment optical coherence tomography) [13]

- The sphincter muscle is a 1 mm wide band circling the pupil and located at the tip of the iris. It is continuous with the anterior border layer of the iris by a thin layer of connective tissue. It has a close proximity to the Iris pigment epithelium (IPE) and It can curve at the pupillary margin (Fig. 3.12). It may follow the double layer of IPE curvature towards the anterior surface. In extreme conditions such as Rubeosis Irides the IPE can curve over the sphincter and can be visible in the condition known as Ectropion Uveae.

- The sphincter muscle also can be affected by hypertension and diabetes as a result of induced rubeosis irides (Fig. 3.13).

Light microscopic examination shows that the sphincter muscle is composed of spindle-shaped cells that are oriented parallel to the pupillary margin. These cells are arranged in bundles separated by collagenous septae. Melanocytes are also

Fig. 3.12 Light microscopy ×10, tip of the iris. Disrupted anterior surface with melanocytes. Loose stromal connective tissue. Sphincter muscle and posterior iris pigment epithelium

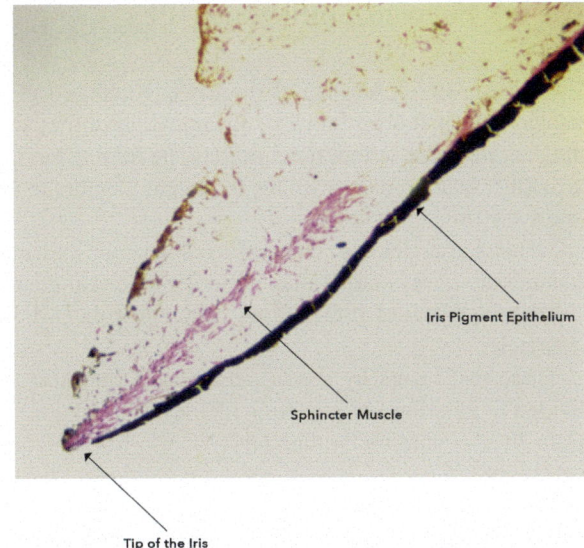

Fig. 3.13 Light microscopy ×40. Rubeosis iridis. Fibrovascular membrane on the surface of the iris. Ectropion uveae and zipping of the angle structure due to retraction of the fibrovcasular membrane

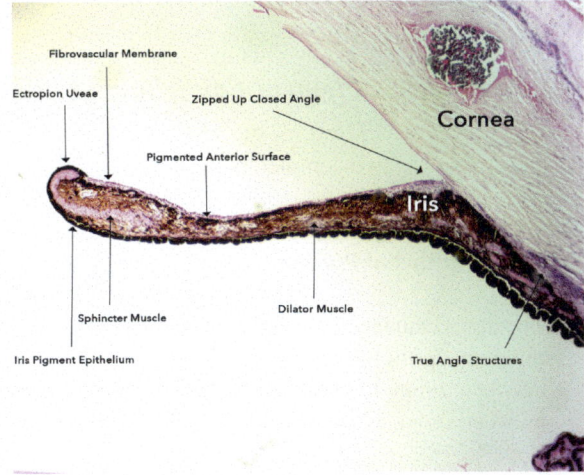

found in association with muscle bundles. The sphincter muscle is surrounded posteriorly by a layer of dense connective tissue that separates it from the dilator muscle and the pigment epithelium. Several pigmented projections or "spurs" extend from the dilator muscle toward the sphincter muscle in the adult iris.

These "spurs" have different names as to their locations:

- Fuchs' spurs in the region posterior to the iris muscle.
- Michel's spurs at the peripheral edge of the sphincter muscle.
- Grunter's spurs at the iris root.

The Iris Pigment Epithelium (IPE)

The most posterior surface of the iris is composed of two layers of heavily pigmented cells that are formed by invagination of the embryonic optic cup on itself and thus are neuro-ectoderm in origin. The folding has caused these layers to lay on each other head to head with the basement membrane located at the outer cell surface away from each other.

Melanin granules are neuroepithelial in origin and are large and spherical. These granules are always larger than mesodermal Uveal granules in the stroma.

The two layers of IPE are very different from each other and will be discussed separately.

These two layers by their orientation in the most posterior of the iris can be divided to anterior and posterior IPE layers. The anterior IPE should not be mistaken by the anterior border layer of the iris that can be pigmented in darker eye colors.

The tip of the fold of the embryonic optic cup forms the pupil which is a very active and constantly moving due to light, accommodation and neural and chemical stimulation.

The Anterior Iris Pigment Epithelium (AIPE)

This layer also has two completely different morphological characteristics.

An Apical Epithelial Portion

(a) The apical surface of this layer is contiguous with that of the posterior iris pigment epithelium (PIPE), These cells have tight junction desmosomes between them however there are some areas of separation can be seen between them. These spaces are filled with microvilli with occasional cilium (Fig. 3.14).

This section contains cell organelles, melanin granules, mitochondria cell nucleus and bundles of myofilaments.

(b) A basal muscular portion located anteriorly forms amelanotic cytoplasmic processes with smooth muscle differentiation that forms the dilator muscle (Fig. 3.14a, b).

The cytoplasm is filled with myofibrils and moderate number of melanosomes. There are 3–5 layers of muscular processes that overlapping each other. There are tight junctions between the cells and are mainly occludentes with few desmosomes. The muscle cells do not have desmosomes. As mentioned earlier the basement membrane surrounds the muscular processes.

Unmyelinated nerve endings with their Schwann cells and also some naked axons are innervating these muscles.

Fig. 3.14 (**a**) Light microscopy ×10, full thickness central iris. Lightly pigmented anterior surface melanocytes, loose stromal connective tissue with typical cuffed blood vessels. Dilator muscle can be observed adjacent to the double layers od iris pigment epithelium. (**b**) Light microscopy ×100, posterior surface of the iris with double layer of the anterior and posterior iris pigment epithelium (IPE). Dilator muscle is located on the anterior border of IPE

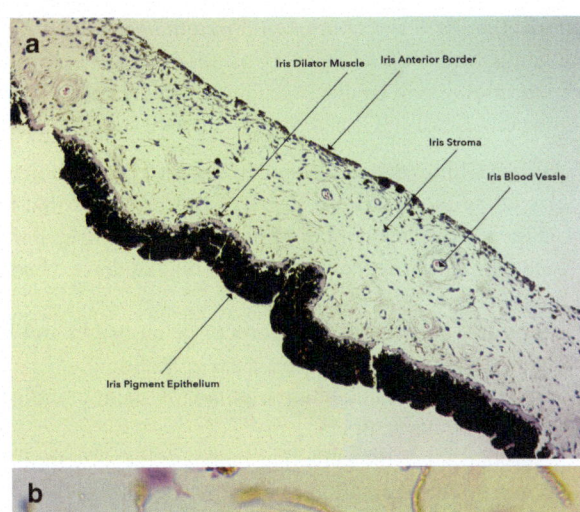

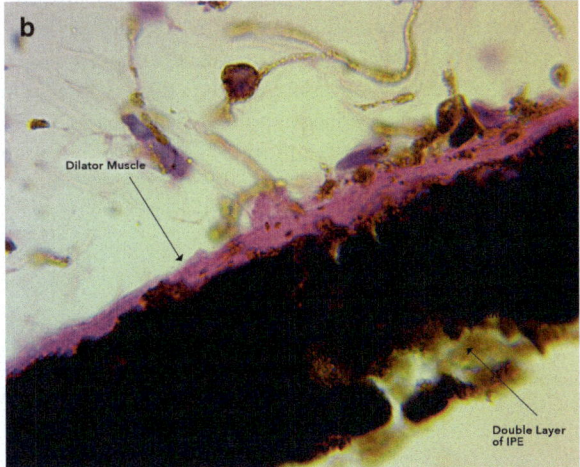

The Posterior Iris Pigment Epithelium (PIPE) (Fig. 3.14a, b)

This layer is the most posterior layer of the iris which has a very dense pigment content. The melanin pigment granules are measuring around 0.8–2.5 nm in size.

There are many tight junctions and desmosomes on the lateral and apical walls.

The basement membrane is located at the basal side at the most posterior part next to the lens [11].

Other Cellular Components of Iris

The pigmented cells (Melanocytes) of the iris stroma. They have different types and origins. In previous studies it was claimed that he stromal melanocyte numbers are almost the same in different eye color, but their melanosome pigment content and pigment granule sizes varies in different eye colors. We could not confirm this and by comparing the melanocytes of different eye colors we noticed many structural variations that will be discussed in the next chapter. These pigment cells originate at the Neural Crest (NC) and migrates via mesoderm to the iris stroma (Fig. 3.15).

- Type I Clump cells of Koganei: These cells do not have basement membrane surrounding them and are migrated macrophages that have phagocytosed pigment (Fig. 3.16). They contain different size and irregular pigment granules and have mulberry-like appearance. They do not have basement membrane surrounding them.
- Type II Clump cells are neuroepithelial origin and have surrounding basement membrane with uniform pigment granules.
- Schwann cells that contain minimal pigment granules and are the supporting tissue for the nerve fibers.
- Fibroblasts are the cells that make up the structural framework or stroma composed of the extracellular matrix and collagen. Fibroblasts are the most common cells in of connective tissue and are important for wound healing. Fibroblast transfection is a commonly used method in molecular and cell biology research. Fibroblast cells are large and flat, with elongated processes protruding from the body of each cell, creating the spindle-like appearance of the cell, with an oval nucleus (Figs. 3.15 and 3.16).

Fig. 3.15 Light microscopy ×40. Anterior surface of the iris. Melanocytes and fibroblasts are scattered on top of the loose connective tissue of the iris stroma

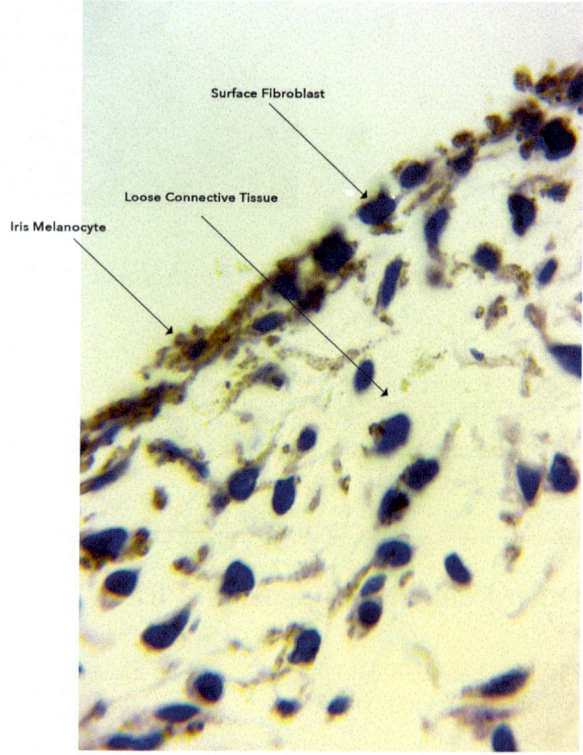

Fig. 3.16 Light microscopy ×100. Macrophages containing pigment in the iris loose stroma. Fibroblasts and melanocytes can be observed

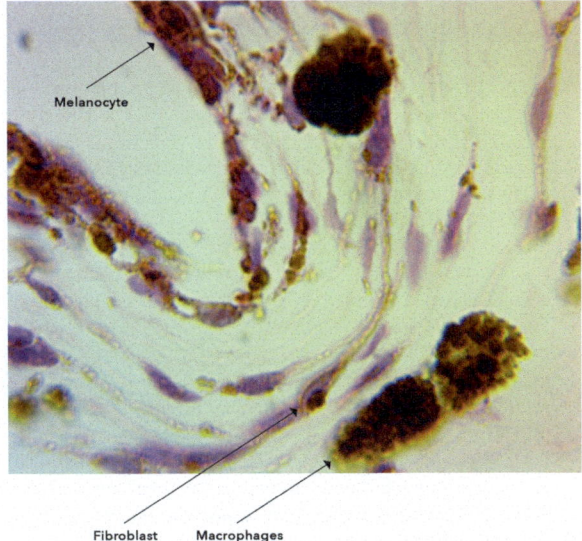

- Fibroblasts are derived from primitive mesenchyme, like all connective tissue cells, which explain their ability to express filament protein vimentin.
- The tissue matrix is made almost entirely of collagen, which is the most abundant protein in mammals. In Iris, fibroblasts are scattered between the collagen fibers of loose connective tissue, which produces collagen subunits. Fibroblasts also produce glycoproteins and polysaccharides for the ground substances, a gel-like material that surrounds collagen fibers of connective tissue, forming an "extracellular matrix" (Fig. 3.9a, b).
- In addition, fibroblasts have a tissue repair function, and wounds stimulate fibroblast production through the complex process of wound healing, however the healing ability in the iris is under influence of many other factors that will be discussed in Chap. 6 of this book. Fibroblasts are the most common cells of connective tissue in iris. The location and concentration of the fibroblasts on the anterior surface of the Iris plays a significant role in the color appearance of the iris. As we will discuss in the electron microscopy chapter, the melanocytes density and melanin content of melanosomes are scares in blue eyes and fibroblasts are abundant. As the result there is more collagen formation at the surface of the blue eyes.

Bibliography

1. Chua J, Seet LF, Jiang Y, Su R, Htoon HM, Charlton A, Aung T, Wong TT. Increased SPARC expression in primary angle closure glaucoma iris. Mol Vis. 2008;14:1886. [Online]. Available at: https://www.ncbi.nlm.nih.gov/pmc/articles/PMC2571946/.
2. Diesenhouse MC, Palay DA, Newman NJ, To K, Albert DM. Acquired heterochromia with Homer syndrome in two adults. Ophthalmology. 1992;99(12):1815–7. [Online]. Available at: https://www.sciencedirect.com/science/article/pii/S0161642092317208.

3. Dieterich DE. The fine structure of the melanocytes of the human iris. Albrecht Von Graefes Arch Klin Exp Ophthalmol. 1972;183(4):317–33. [Online]. Available at: https://ci.nii.ac.jp/naid/30013309698/.

4. Fuchs E. Normal pigmentierte und albinotische Iris. Albrecht von Graefes Archiv für Ophthalmologie. 1913;84(3):521–9. [Online] Available at: https://link.springer.com/article/1 0.1007%2FBF02080373?LI=true.

5. Guerra L, Odorisio T, Zambruno G, Castiglia D. Stromal microenvironment in type VII collagen-deficient skin: The ground for squamous cell carcinoma development. Matrix Biol. 2017;63:1–10. [Online]. Available at: https://www.sciencedirect.com/science/article/pii/S0945053X16303250. Accessed 28 July 2019.

6. Hu DN, Wakamatsu K, Ito S, McCormick SA. Comparison of eumelanin and pheomelanin content between cultured uveal melanoma cells and normal uveal melanocytes. Melanoma Res. 2009;19(2):75–9. [Online].

7. Imesch PD, Wallow IH, Albert DM. The color of the human eye: a review of morphologic correlates and of some conditions that affect iridial pigmentation. Surv Ophthalmol. 1997;41:S117–23. [Online]. Available at: https://www.sciencedirect.com/science/article/abs/pii/S0039625797800185.

8. Ito S, Wakamatsu K. Quantitative analysis of eumelanin and pheomelanin in humans, mice, and other animals: a comparative review. Pigment Cell Res. 2003;16(5):523–31. [Online]. Available at: https://www.ncbi.nlm.nih.gov/pubmed/12950732.

9. Li L, Hu DN, Zhao H, McCormick SA, Nordlund JJ, Boissy RE. Uveal melanocytes do not respond to or express receptors for α-melanocyte-stimulating hormone. Invest Ophthalmol Vis Sci. 2006;47(10):4507–12. [Online]. Available at: https://iovs.arvojournals.org/article.aspx?articleid=2124882.

10. Polash PP, Monwar MM. Human iris recognition for biometric identification. 2007. [Online]. Available at: https://ieeexplore.ieee.org/abstract/document/4579354/authors#authors.

11. Pozzi A, Yurchenco PD, Iozzo RV. The nature and biology of basement membranes. Matrix Biol. 2017;57:1–11. [Online]. Available at: https://www.sciencedirect.com/science/article/pii/S0945053X16303262.

12. Rennie IG. Don't it make my blue eyes brown: heterochromia and other abnormalities of the iris. Eye. 2012;26(1):29–50. [Online]. Available at: https://www.nature.com/articles/eye2011228.

13. Sallam A, El-Defrawy H, Ross A, Bashir SJ, Towler HM. Review and update of intraoperative floppy iris syndrome. Exp Rev Ophthalmol. 2011;6(4):469–76. [Online]. Available at: https://www.medscape.com/viewarticle/748742_5.

14. Schwab C, Mayer C, Zalaudek I, Riedl R, Richtig M, Wackernagel W, Hofmann-Wellenhof R, Richtig G, Langmann G, Tarmann L, Wedrich A. Iris freckles a potential biomarker for chronic sun damage. Invest Ophthalmol Vis Sci. 2017;58(6):BIO174–9. [Online]. Available at: https://iovs.arvojournals.org/article.aspx?articleid=2644236.

15. Shields JA, Bianciotto C, Kligman BE, Shields CL. Vascular tumors of the iris in 45 patients: the 2009 Helen Keller Lecture. Arch Ophthalmol. 2010;128(9):1107–13. [Online]. Available at: https://www.ncbi.nlm.nih.gov/pubmed/20837792.

16. Smith PC, Martínez C, Martínez J, McCulloch CA. Role of fibroblast populations in periodontal wound healing and tissue remodeling. Front Physiol. 2019;10:270. [Online]. Available at: https://www.ncbi.nlm.nih.gov/pmc/articles/PMC6491628/.

17. Wilkerson CL, Syed NA, Fisher MR, Robinson NL, Albert DM. Melanocytes and iris color: light microscopic findings. Arch Ophthalmol. 1996;114(4):437–42. [Online]. Available at: https://jamanetwork.com/journals/jamaophthalmology/article-abstract/641593.

Chapter 4
Iris Electron Microscopy

Abstract Examination of the ultrastructure of the iris is essential for recognizing the structural specifications and differences in human irides. The vast range of structural differences represent themselves as a variety of different color eyes as it is seen in human populations.

Here for the first time the ultrastructural comparison of light microscopy and electron microscopy of 3 color eyes (Blue, hazel/green and dark brown) has been described and the images presented side by side.

These essential ultra-structure characteristics are identified and described as they play an important role in the reflected variety of iris structures and colors.

There are multiple factors that are involved in the iris structural differences and it is the sum of all these factors, not an individual factor, that represent the final appearance of the iris color.

Population of melanocytes on the anterior surface of the Iris. Population of melanosomes in the cytoplasm of melanocytes. Melanosomes location and distance from nucleus. Stages of maturation of melanosomes. The type of melanin and its ratio in the melanosomes. Population of fibroblasts on the iris surface. Amount of collagen in between and on the surface of the Iris. Number of Lysosomes in melanocytes. Number of cytoplasmic vacuoles in melanocytes. Number of mitochondria. Finger like projections in fibroblasts. Number of Stromal melanocytes. Number of Stromal macrophages. Stromal collagen content and intercellular matrix.

An interesting observation while reviewing our EM database collection was that in blue iris there was evidence of new incomplete pigment formation process in progress but at the same time the shedding of these incomplete melanosomes into the extra cellular matrix could be seen. This phenomenon brings up the notion that melanocytes follow their natural behavior of transferring pigment to their surroundings but there are no keratinocytes to adopt the melanin pigment as in the skin. In the iris, fibroblasts and macrophages play the role of keratinocytes in the skin and endocytose the transferred melanosomes. However, unlike the keratinocytes, fibroblasts do not keep the melanosomes but digest and destroy them. This process explains the evidence of pigment in surrounding fibroblasts and macrophages in the iris stroma.

Another important observation was that the iris is a dynamic cellular structure with the constant interaction between the fibroblasts and melanocytes. These interactions occur in many different pathways, from surface receptors, to collagen coating, to basement membrane (BM) like properties of fibroblasts. Through these pathways the fibroblasts affect the function and maturation of the melanocytes and their melanosomes and their pigment transfering process.

Many of these observations have never been addressed in the literature and are presented in this book for the first time. We hope these findings and new information would stimulate other academic, scientific institutions and pharmaceutical companies and encourage them to look deeper into these concepts by further evaluation and future studies.

Note: All of the electron microscopy images presented in this chapter are from our own personal database and protected by copyright as our own intellectual property.

Note: We divided the iris colors into 3 categories for simplification:

1. The very dark brown Iris melanocyte/melanosome as Black.
2. The brown and hazel Iris melanocyte/melanosome we refer as Brown.
3. The green and blue and gray Iris melanocyte/melanosome we refer as Blue.

New Concepts presented here are based on meticulous observation and interpretation of our database EM images and their relevant supporting articles:

1. The role of fibroblasts in controlling and limiting the pigment production of the iris melanocytes.
2. The role of laminin and Fibronectin produced by fibroblasts on iris melanocytes.
3. Collagen coating of melanocytes by iris fibroblasts.
4. The dynamic and ongoing interaction and pigment exchange between iris melanocytes and fibroblasts and macrophages.
5. The different modes of pigment exchange.
6. The location of melanosomes in cytoplasm in different iris colors.
7. The stages of melanosomes in different iris colors.
8. Phagocytosis of iris melanocytes by fibroblasts and macrophages.

Sample Preparation

The iris tissue was collected from fresh postmortem eyes immediately removed after death that was delivered in ice from the eye bank of New York. The cornea was removed immediately, and the entire iris was removed with forceps and scissors. The iris disc was then cut in half. One half of the iris was placed in a mixture of 4% paraformaldehyde for processing and staining for light microscope. The slides were prepared in standard manner micro-cutting and stained and then they were photographed by digital camera attached to the light microscope.

Note: All of the electron microscopy images presented in this chapter are from our own personal database and protected by copyright as our own intellectual property.

Preparation of iris tissue

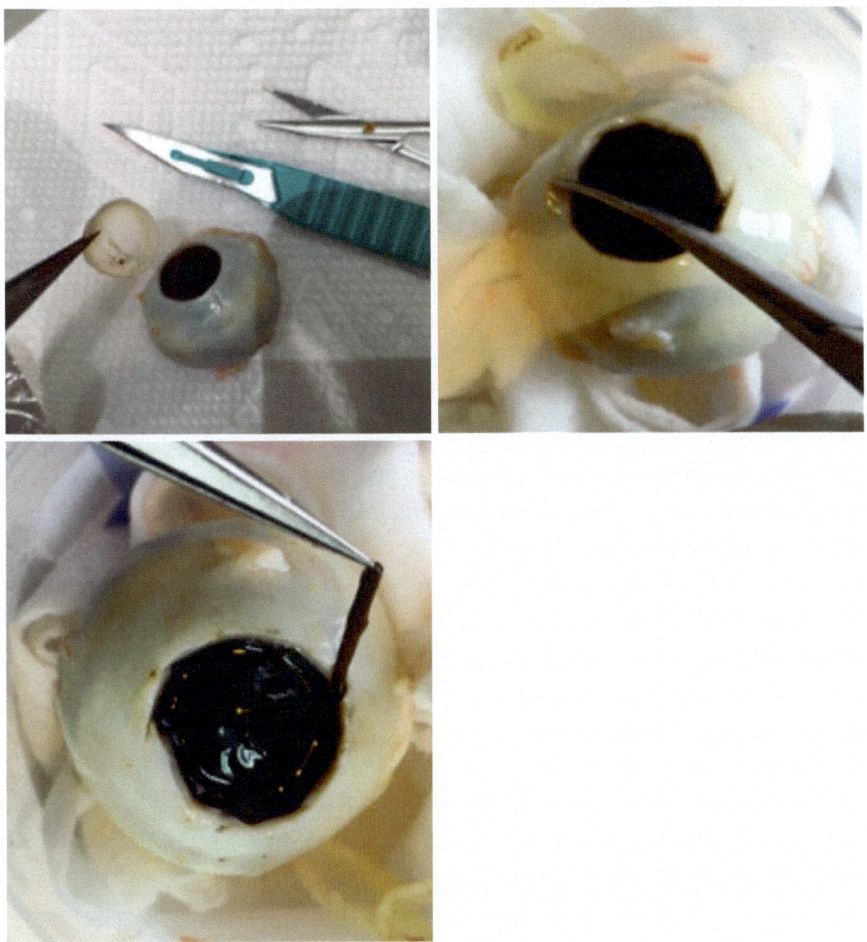

Fig. 4.1 Dissection of the iris from a fresh post-mortem eye, from the eye bank

The other half of the iris was placed in 2% glutaraldehyde solution for process-ing for electron microscopy. After post-fixation with 2% osmium tetroxide for 2 hours it was dehydrated in ethanol and embedded in EPON resin. A 300-nm sec-tions of sample, stained with 2% uranyl acetate and lead citrate, was examined in a transmission electron microscope (Fig. 4.1).

Discussion

Electron microscopy enable us to have a closer look at the ultra-structure of the iris to recognize the vast structural difference that represents itself as different color iris.

In another word, the differences in iris color in human is nothing but variation in ultra-structure components and that necessitates an emphasize in iris color presentation in this chapter.

These structural differences mainly present at the anterior border and stroma of the iris.

The posterior double layer of the Iris Pigment Epithelium (IPE) is constant in all different eye colors and does not show any structural variations in different eye colors.

Low magnification (×200) electron microscopy of the three different color eyes are shown here with the black iris on the top, brown iris in the middle and the blue eye on the bottom.

Each trio images represent the different layers of the iris (Fig. 4.2a–c).

First picture on the top is the anterior border (surface) of the iris, then the middle portion (Stroma) followed by the posterior segment on the bottom.

Melanocytes, fibroblasts and microphages are all playing an important role in the structural variety of different irides. There is constant interaction between these cellular residents of the iris. We discuss these cellular components first, followed by discussions on anterior surface (border) of the iris, then the stroma, and finally the posterior iris pigment epithelium (IPE).

Melanocytes

Melanocytes are Neural Crest origin cells that are specialized in pigment (Melanin) production.

They are divided in classic and non-classic categories as seen in (Fig. 4.3).

Melanocytes synthesize melanin in a complex process of melanogenesis which is summarized in (Fig. 4.4a).

The melanin is synthesized and stored in the special organelles called melanosomes (Fig. 4.4b).

Melanin can be in a dark Eumelanin or orange/yellow Pheomelanin. In the skin melanocytes are anchored to the basement membrane and their activity is harnessed by anchoring proteins Laminin and Fibronectin and have no direct contact with fibroblasts. In Iris anterior surface and stroma, the melanocytes are not attached to basement membrane but are located in direct contact with fibroblasts and are being controlled by the fibroblasts production of laminin, fibronectin and collagen, which behave in a similar way, mimicking the basement membrane of the skin (Fig. 4.17).

In addition, melanocytes contain multiple receptor and signaling pathways to communicate with fibroblasts that will be discussed in the next chapter on molecular biology of the iris.

The double layered melanocytes of the iris pigment epithelium on the posterior surface of the iris are attached to the basement membrane as described and shown in Chap. 1, on embryology of the iris and related figures.

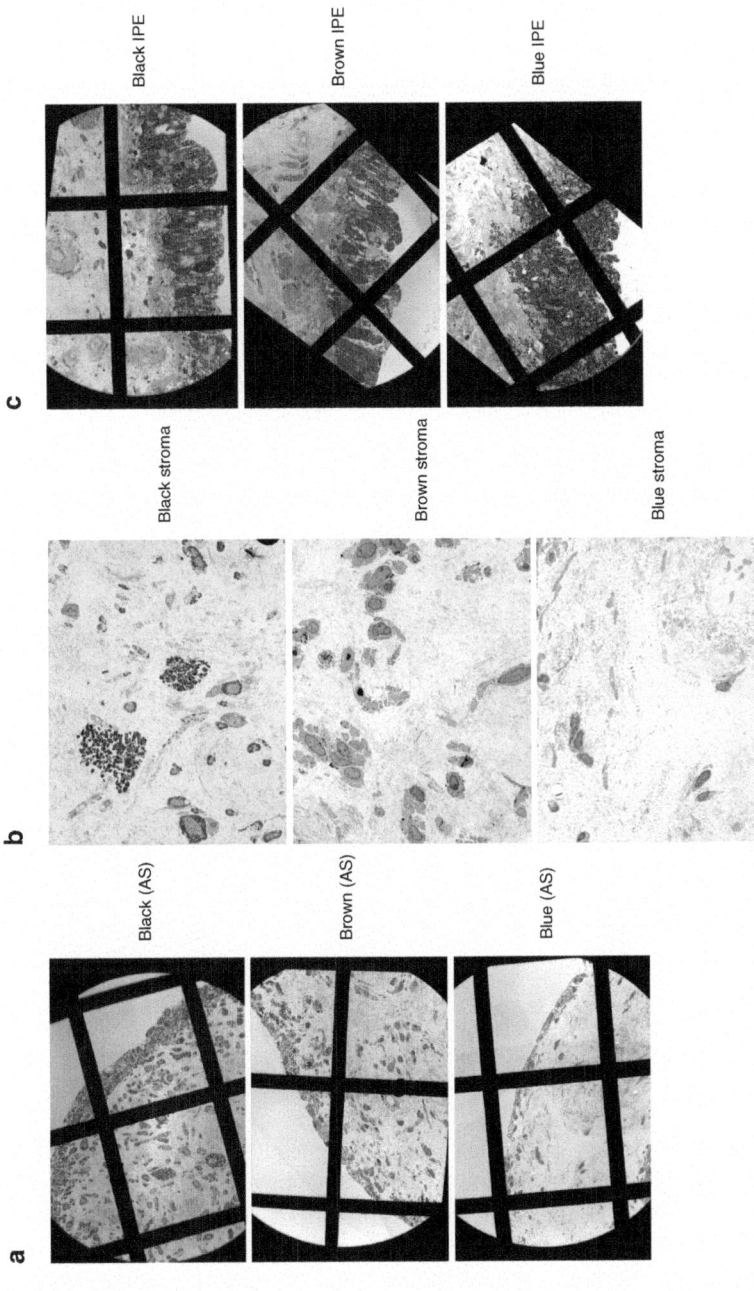

Fig. 4.2 (**a**) Comparison of black, brown, and blue iris and anterior surface. Electro microscopy ×200, comparison of anterior surface of different color irides. (**b**) Comparison of black, brown, and blue iris stroma. Electro microscopy ×200, comparison of stroma of different colored irides. (**c**) Comparison of black, brown, and blue iris pigment epithelium (IPE). Electron microscopy ×200. Iris pigment epithelium are similar in their pigmentation regardless of the color of the irides, as shown in these images

Non-Classical Melanocytes

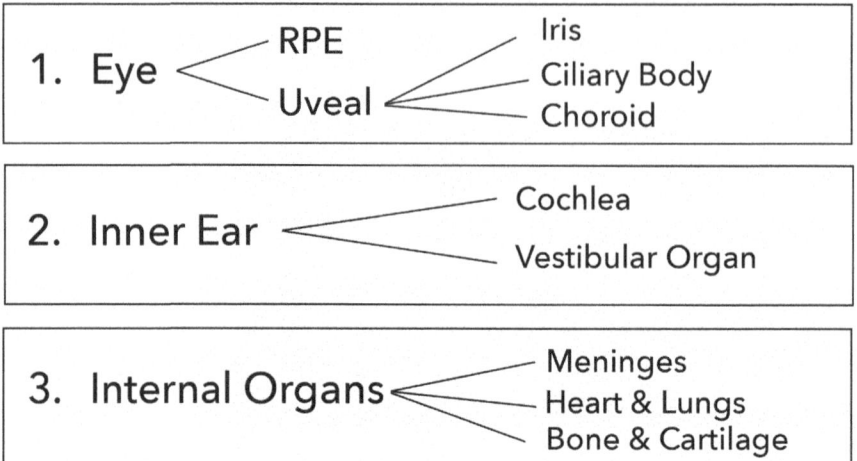

Classical Melanocytes

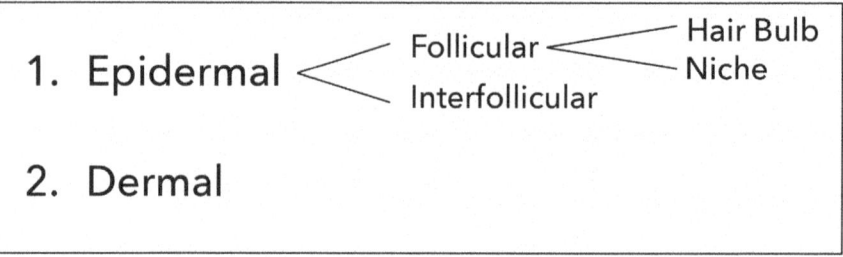

Fig. 4.3 Melanocyte classification

Melanocytes are dendritic cells, but the dendrites are much longer in black iris melanocytes as compared to blue iris melanocytes. They also have the ability for phagocytic, antigen expression, and proinflammatory cytokines expression (Fig. 4.5a, b).

In the iris, melanocytes are most often found just beneath fibroblasts at the anterior surface and stroma, and contain mitochondria, smooth and rough endoplasmic reticula, free ribosomes, and melanin granules in various stages of development depending the color of the eye. The lighter eye colors have melanosomes mainly in stages I, II, III, and the dark eye colors have mainly stage IV melanosomes (Fig. 4.6a).

In brown iris, melanocytes contain melanosomes that mimic both blue and black melanocytes but has fewer numbers of melanosomes as compared to the black iris and contain more early stage melanosomes (Fig. 4.6b).

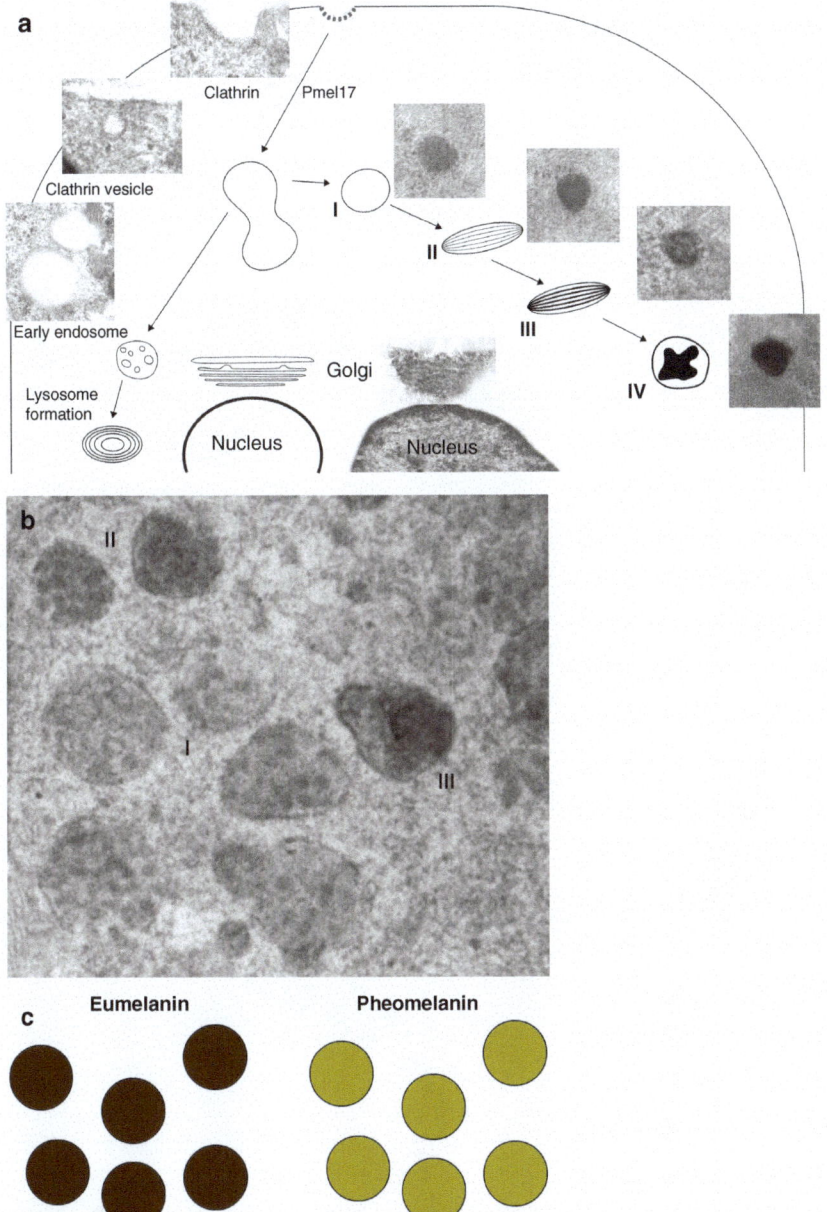

Fig. 4.4 The process of melanogenesis. (**a**) The schematic process of melanogenesis with its matching electronmicroscopy images are presented here. The process begins with clathrin formation of early vesicle, which then progresses to early endosome, and then it because melanosome by formation of the four stages of maturation, or it can become lysosome. Information from the nucleus goes to the golgi apparatus to be processed and transported to melanosomes for proper melanine deposition. (**b**) Blue iris stages of melanosomes. Electron microscopy ×50,000. Blue iris. Incomplete maturation of the melanosomes from stages I to III. (**c**) Eumelanin/pheomelanin in human uveal melanocytes. Comparison of the different colors of melanin derivatives, as shown above

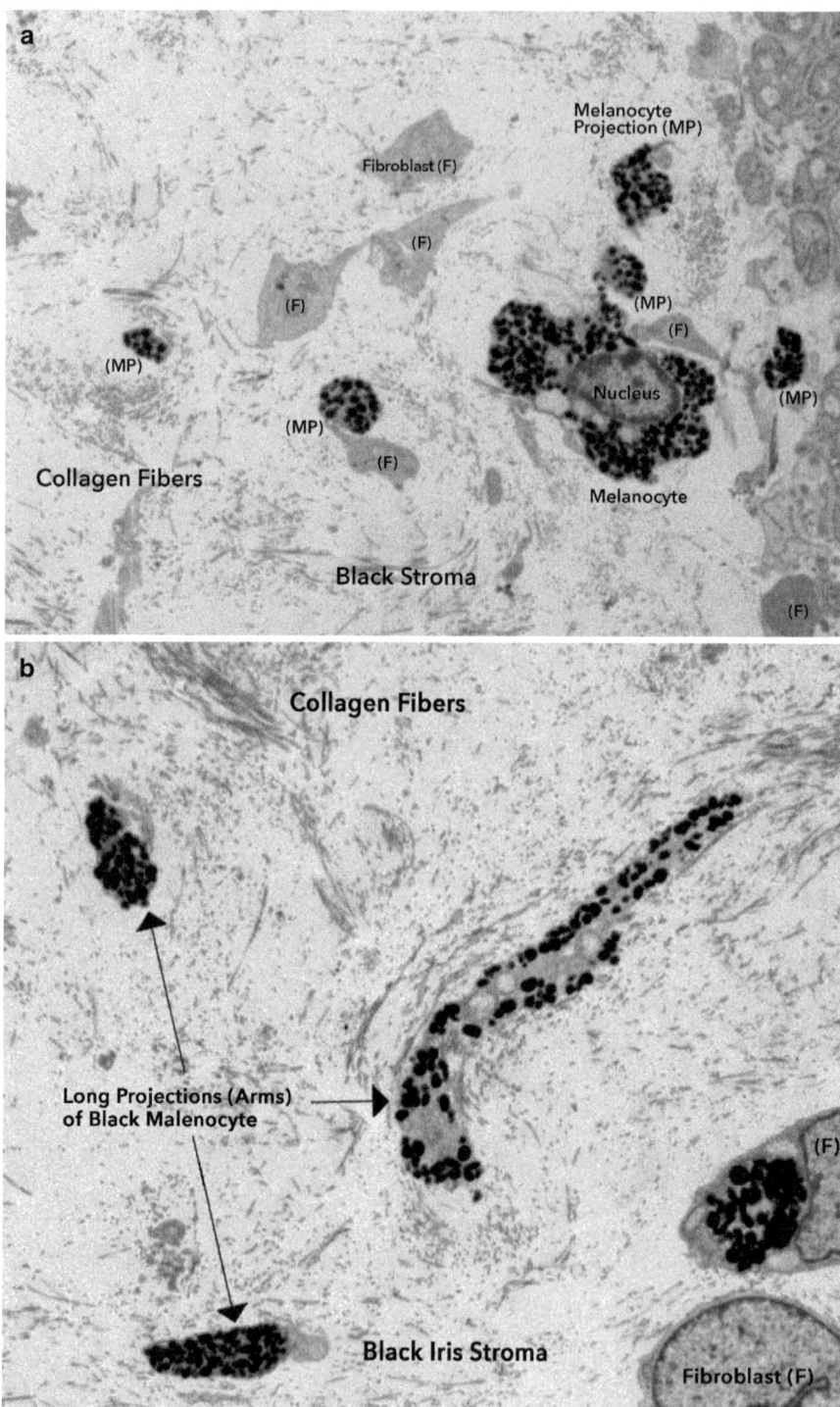

Fig. 4.5 (**a, b**) Black iris stroma melanocyte long projections. Electron microscopy ×500. Black iris melanocytes have long projections that can be seen in the image above

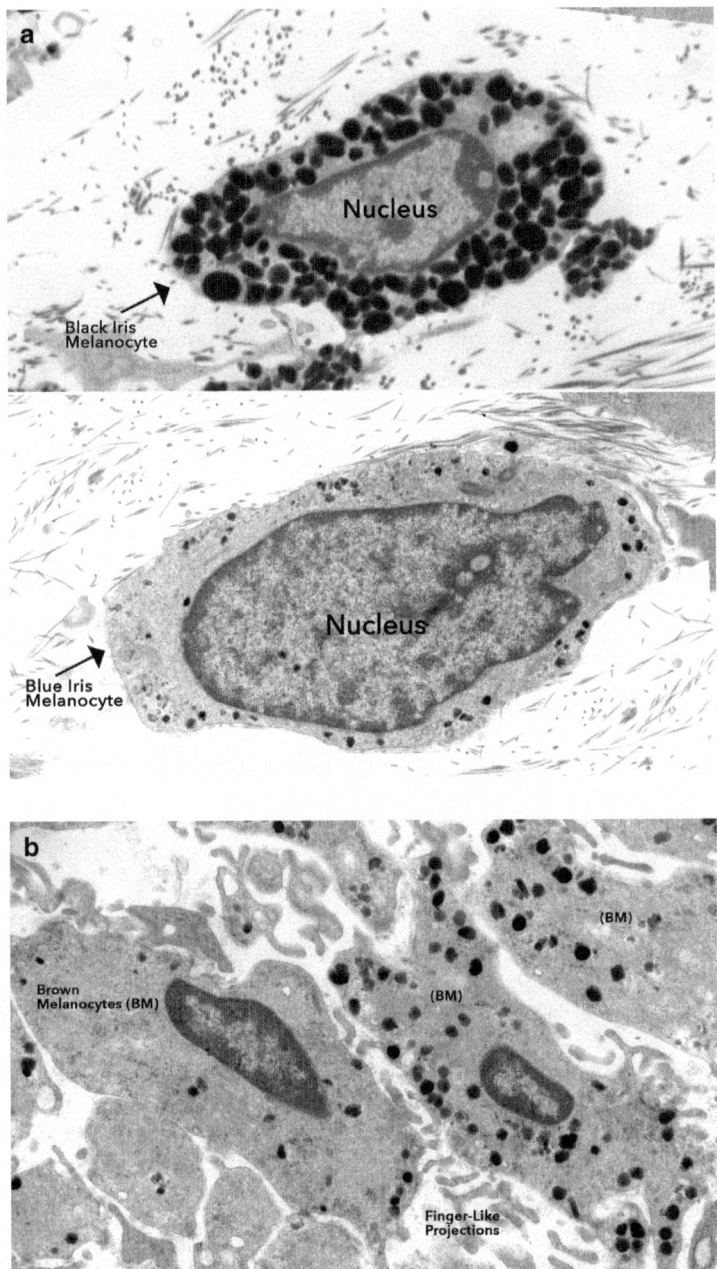

Fig. 4.6 (**a**) Electron microscopy ×4000. Black and blue iris melanocytes presented for comparison. Black melanocyte cytoplasm is filled with stage IV melanosomes. The blue iris melanocyte cytoplasm contains scattered immature melasnosomes at all four stages located at the periphery. (**b**) Brown iris melanosome characteristics. Electron microscopy ×6000. Brown iri scattered melanosomes in all stages, but primarily in stage IV. Some close to the nucleus, some at the periphery. Cellular projections containing clusters of melanosomes can be seen in the middle towards the top. Multiple finger-like projects can also be observed

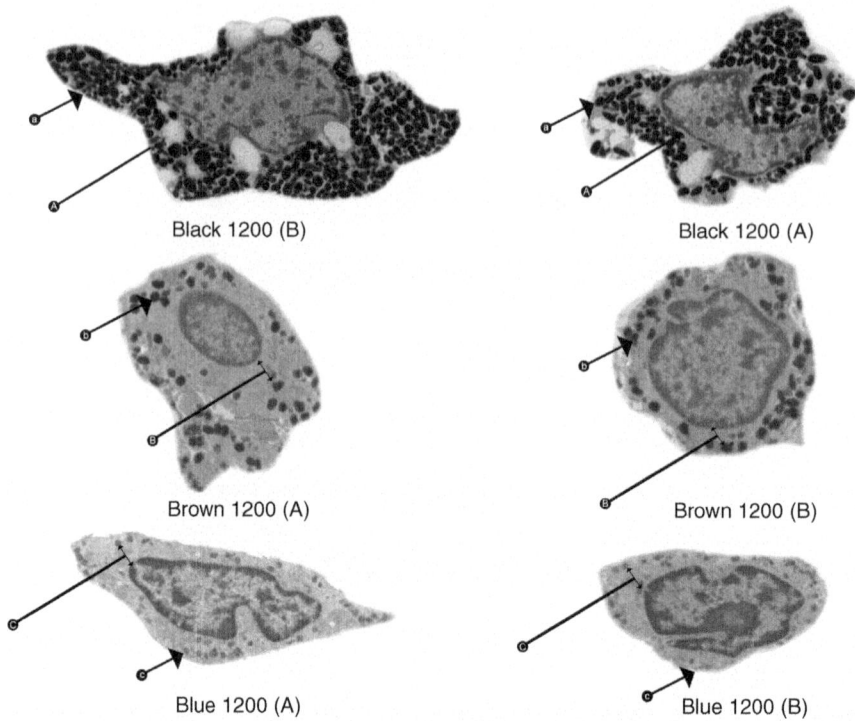

Fig. 4.7 Melanocyte cellular comparison. Electron microscopy ×1200, malancocyte comparison of three different color irides; black, brown, and blue

There are conflicting reports on the structure of anterior surface of iris and the number of melanocytes in previous publications, these controversies include the content of melanocytes, and iris stromal cellularity and their contributions to the iris color [1, 2].

There are very few comparative electron microscopy <u>illustrations</u> in any of the previous publications and in the literature, other than statistic numbers to prove these concepts.

Authors in one study [3] described EM study of human iris in a patient with Horner's syndrome.

Their reported EM results are very similar to our normal blue eye postmortem specimen, confirming the ongoing process of melanogenesis and interplay of different hormonal and neural signaling processes between these cells in the iris.

In this chapter, there is a comparative EM and related histology pictures of 3 eyes (Blue, Hazel, and dark Brown) next to each other and the differences can be easily recognized even by non-scientific background readers (Fig. 4.7).

Light microscopy and Electron microscopy slides that are discussed here are used as an example that represent each iris color microstructures:

As was described in the embryology chapter, the anterior surface of the iris is covered with a continuous layer of endothelium during embryonic development, this layer will disappear at birth or soon after birth. The anterior border layer is then become a modification of the stroma composed of combination of melanocytes and fibroblasts with associated collagen fibers. By studying the comparative electron microscopy of three different color eyes (Blue, Hazel /brown and black eyes) the previous controversial claims about density and the number of melanocytes on the anterior border layer of iris with different colors will be discussed.

The above comparison study has revealed different structural components. In our observation there was more melanocyte population on the iris surface of the darker iris as compared to the blue iris. The lighter the color of the eye, the more population of fibroblasts exist on the anterior surface of the iris (Figs. 4.8 and 4.9).

Our study confirms that the darker irides have more abundant melanocytes, contains larger melanin granules, and the cytoplasmic volume of melanocytes is increased. However, in previous studies there was no mentioning of the location and the stages of the melanocytes in regard to their distance from the nucleus. As we observed here, the melanosomes in light color eyes are located at the periphery of the cytoplasm of the melanocytes away from the nucleus (Fig. 4.10a, b).

This condition mimics the concept of changing surface color in animals by moving the melanosomes (inward and outward) from the nucleus in their cytoplasm to change and adjust their color according to the environment as a camouflage technique for survival or social interaction and mating. The melanosomes in lighter eye colors are located away from the nucleus mimicking the lighter color transformation in certain reptiles such as Chameleons [4] and fish such as Flounder (Fig. 4.11) [5].

The darker irides have the melanosomes around the nucleus mimicking the darkening adaptation in color changing animals. Human Iris melanocytes do not have the ability to move their melanosomes back and forth towards and away from the nucleus instantaneously as those animal's melanosomes can.

In Human melanocytes, the melanosome aggregation and dispersion are mediated by three families of motor proteins: Myosin V, Heterotrimeric Kinesin-2 and cytoplasmic Dynein.

Kural et al. [6]

Reilein et al. [7]

Lighter color Iris fibroblasts have delicate cytoplasmic processes, and at the anterior iris surface have a complex interdigitation and abundant collection of collagen fibers that cover the surface (Wolfflin nodules).

Darker irides have minimal or no fibroblasts at the anterior iris surface and have shorter cytoplasmic processes, minimal or no collagen on the surface.

The interesting observation is that the melanocytes of blue eyes have short projections with immature melanosomes accumulated at their tip, whereas the black eye's melanocytes have very long cytoplasmic projections filled with mature melanosomes, as can be seen in the related images (Figs. 4.12 and 4.13).

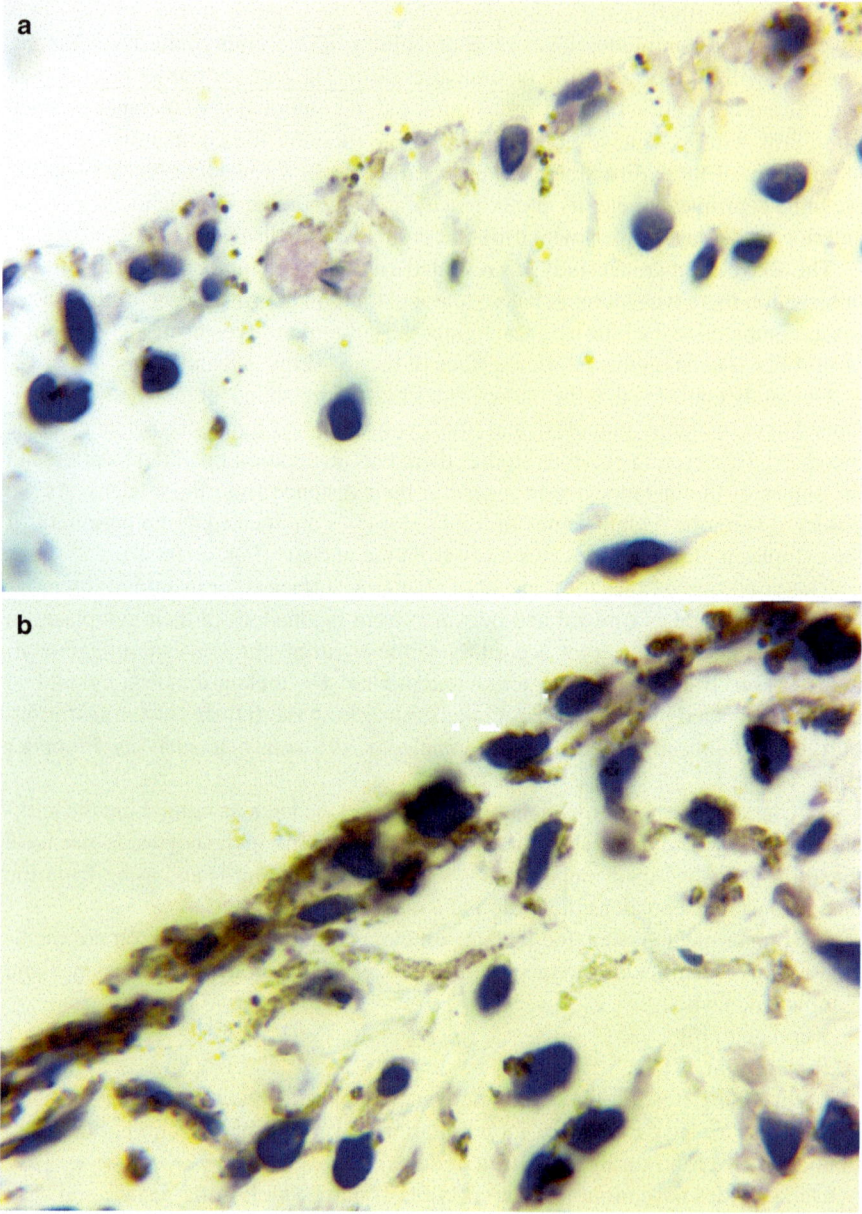

Fig. 4.8 Iris anterior surface of different color irides. Light microscopy ×40, anterior surface of a blue iris (top) and a brown iris (bottom). Displayed as a comparison, the higher density and number of melanocytes in the brown iris and scattered and the low-density melanocytes with minimal pigmentation in the blue iris

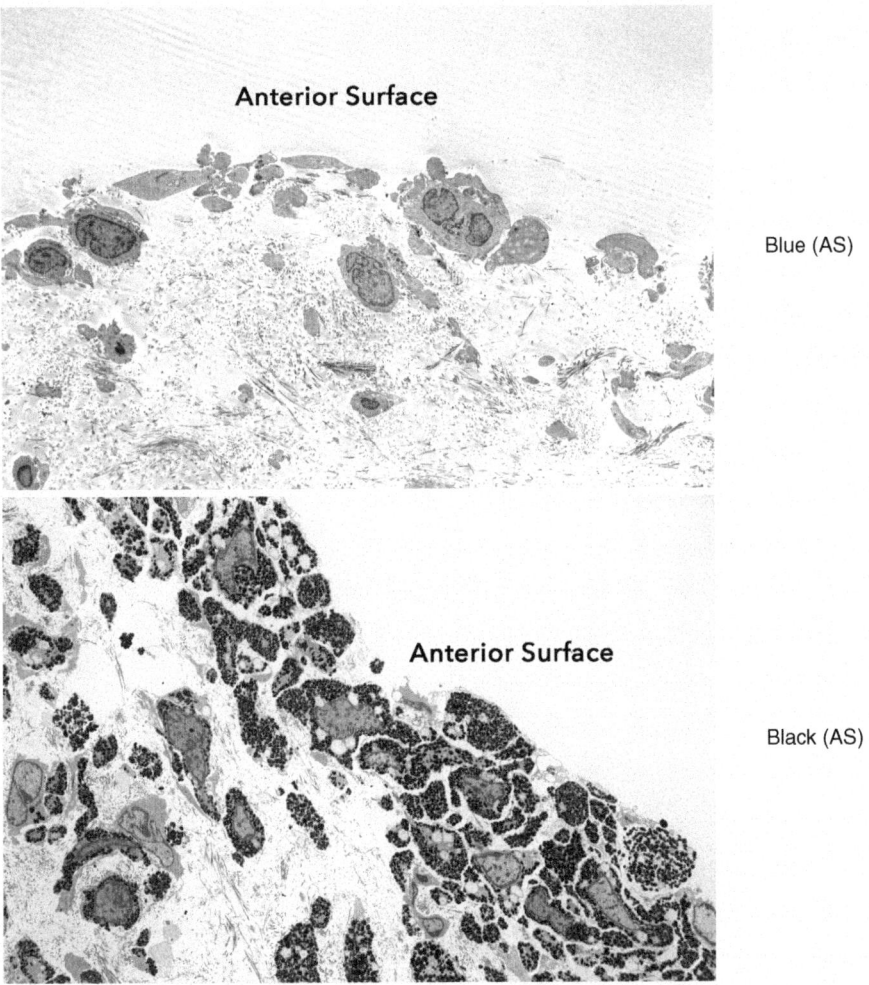

Fig. 4.9 Blue and black iris anterior surface (AS). Electron microscopy ×7000. The blue iris has few scattered melanocytes with fibroblasts. The black iris has a condensed population of melanocytes with rare fibroblasts

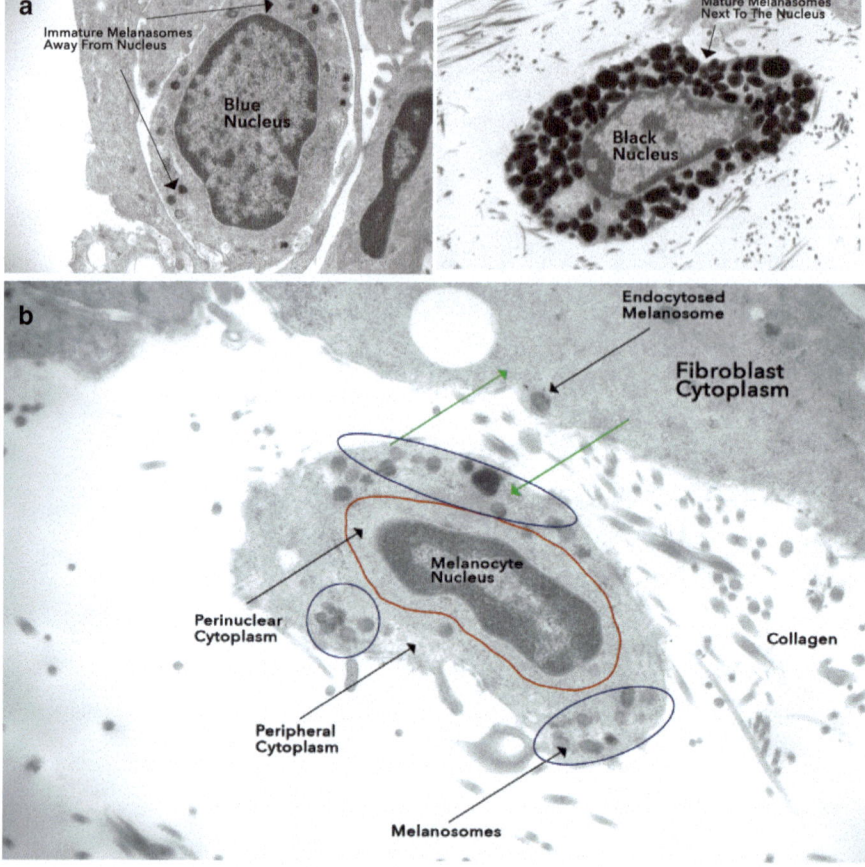

Fig. 4.10 (**a**) Melanosome location in melanocytes. Electron microscopy ×8000. Blue and black melanocytes. Different orientation and location of melanosomes can be observed. (**b**) Blue eye melanocyte. Electron microscopy ×8000, blue eye melanocyte with red line dividing cytoplasm into perinuclear area and periphery. The clustered immature melanosomes (blue circles) located mostly at the periphery away from the nucleus. The exocytosis of melanosomes by the melanocyte and their endocitosis by fibroblast can be observed in this image

Fibroblasts

Fibroblasts are typically Spindle-shaped cells with an oval nucleus that are the most prominent cellular structure of the iris. Fibroblasts are the primary source of extracellular matrix production. Fibroblasts have a major role in homeostasis of connective tissue including wound repair, immune response, antigen presenting, and phagocytosis.

The precise role of <u>dermal</u> fibroblasts on melanocytes have been described elegantly in a publication by Wang et al [8] but there is no reference to the iris.

Fibroblasts are prominent on the iris surface of the light color (Blue) eyes/irides.

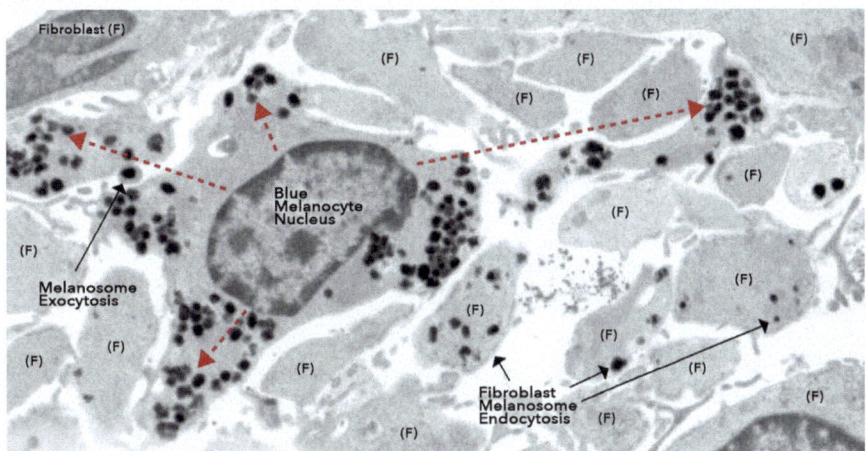

Fig. 4.11 Blue iris melanosome transfer. Electron microscopy ×25,000. Blue iris. The process of melanosome transport through the projections to the periphery, in preparation for exocytosis

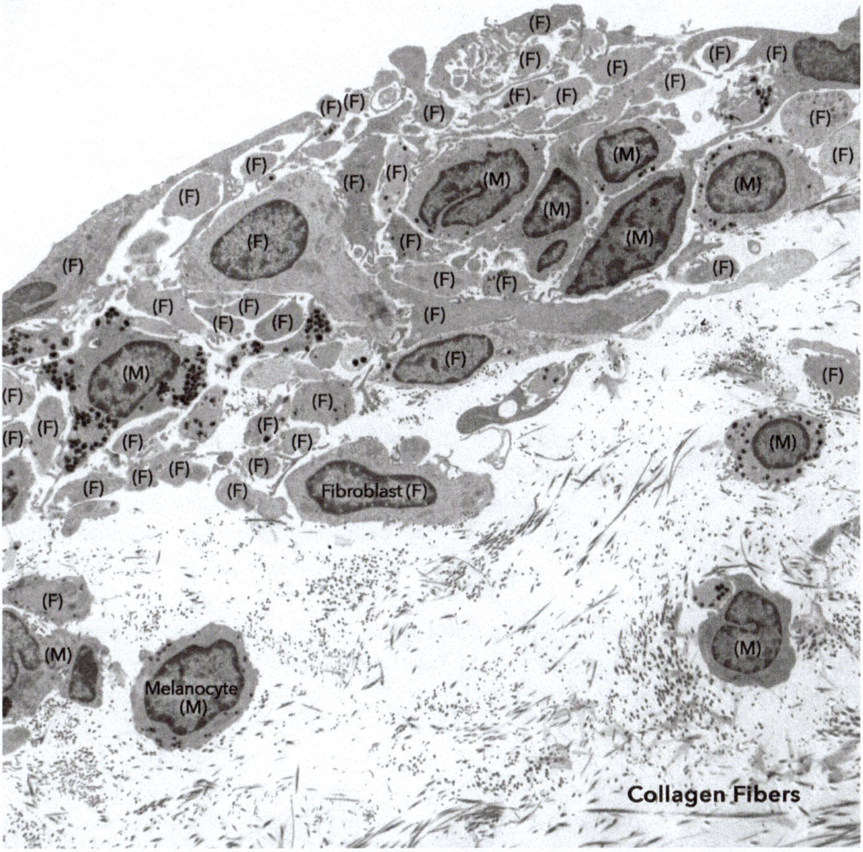

Fig. 4.12 Blue iris anterior surface. Electron microscopy ×1000. Blue iris. Anterior surface melanocytes are surrounded and engulfed by numerous fibroblasts. As a result, collagen production is at its maximum

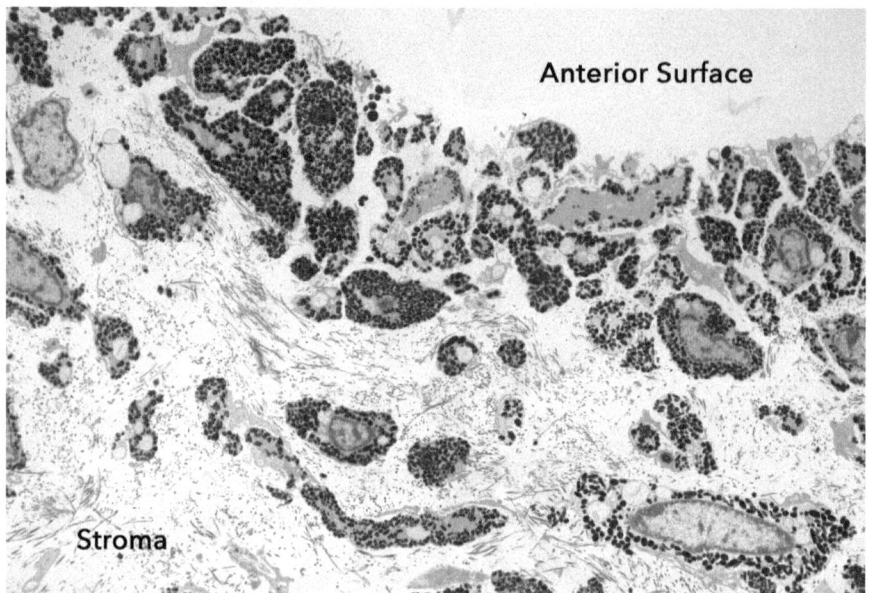

Fig. 4.13 Black iris anterior surface and stroma. Electron microscopy ×1000. Black iris. Anterior surface and stroma with highly pigemented melanocytes. Very few fibroblasts and collagen on the surface. Crowded stroma with highly pigmented melanocytes with stage IV melanosomes

These fibroblasts have abundant mitochondria, rough endoplasmic reticula, free ribosomes, and bundles of filaments. Some fibroblasts have basal bodies in their cytoplasm with associated cilia projecting into the anterior chamber (Fig. 4.14a).

Fibroblasts control melanin production of melanocytes by many different pathways. In theory, in black iris, due to minimal population of fibroblasts on the anterior surface and stroma, the melanocytes produce large amount of melanin as they are programmed to do so. In blue iris the large number of fibroblasts on the anterior surface and stroma control and limit the production of melanin by melanocytes (Fig. 4.14b, c). In one study on the skin melanocytes [9], when they removed the basement membrane, the melanocytes migrate and proliferate. By adding the fibroblasts, the process of migration and proliferation was halted. The condition that makes the environment similar to the anterior surface of the iris that does not have BM. As we mentioned before, Iris BM is located in the posterior surface anchoring the two layers of the iris pigment epithelium head to head (Fig. 4.17).

There is no Basement Membrane (BM) on the anterior surface of the iris for that reason, the melanocytes are wondering free from BM and occupy the stroma and anterior surface of the iris.

In the above mentioned experiment the conclusion was that the BM proteins are necessary for anchoring the Melanocytes, and affect their response to hormonal

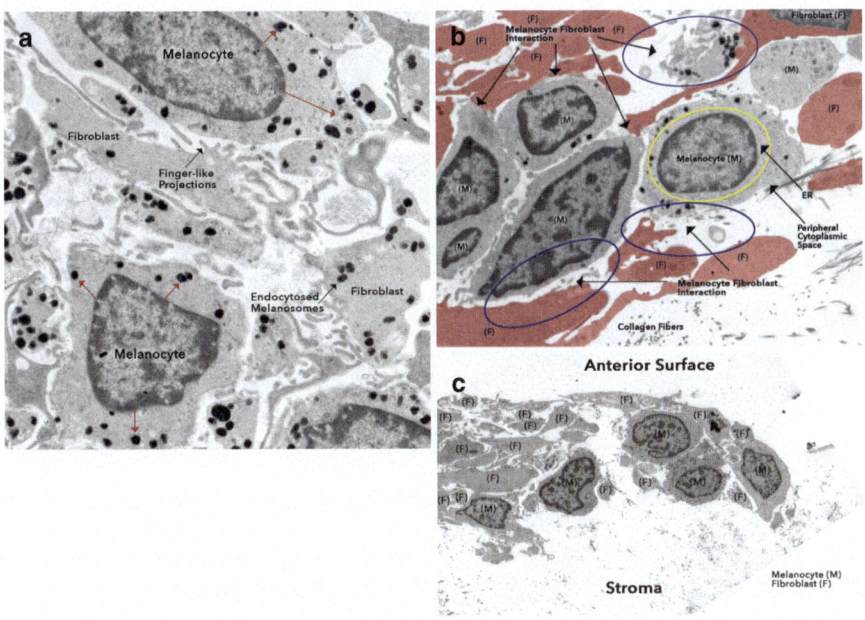

Fig. 4.14 (a) Electron microscopy ×1500, fibroblast finger-like projections (arrow) adjacent to blue eye melanocyte. Melanosome transfer from melanocytes to fibroblasts can be observed. Peripheral location of melanosomes in cytoplasma indicated by red arrows. (b) Electron microscopy ×25,000. Blue iris. Fibroblast (tinted red) in direct contact interacting with melanocytes. This image illustrates the numerous fibroblasts surrounding of the melanocytes. (c) Blue iris anterior surface with multi-layered fibroblasts. Electron microscopy ×1500. Blue iris. Multiple laters of fibroblasts on the anterior surface. Coarting of the melanocytes

response such as alpha-Melanocyte-Stimulating Hormone (Alpha-MSH) and Adrenocorticotropin Hormone (ACTH) to produce melanin.

As we mentioned earlier when the BM was removed, the melanocytes moved freely and produced melanin. Adding the fibroblasts to the melanocytes stopped melanin production, even adding the MSH and other melanogenic hormones could not trigger melanin production.

This also explain why the iris melanosomes do not respond to hormonal stimulation such as alpha-Melanocyte-Stimulating Hormone (Alpha-MSH) and adrenocorticotropin hormone (ACTH) probably due to influence of fibroblasts on melanocytes [9].

As we mentioned earlier, the main function of melanocyte is pigment formation in their specific organelles called melanosomes and transferring them to the neighboring cells as to keratinocytes in the skin and or extracellular matrix as in Iris.

In the iris the process of pigment transfer has not been elucidated in the past. We have many images of this process in all different forms, Cytophagocytosis, Membrane Fusion, Shedding-Phagocytosis and Exocytosis-Endocytosis as was described in the skin melanocytes [10] (Fig. 4.15a–c).

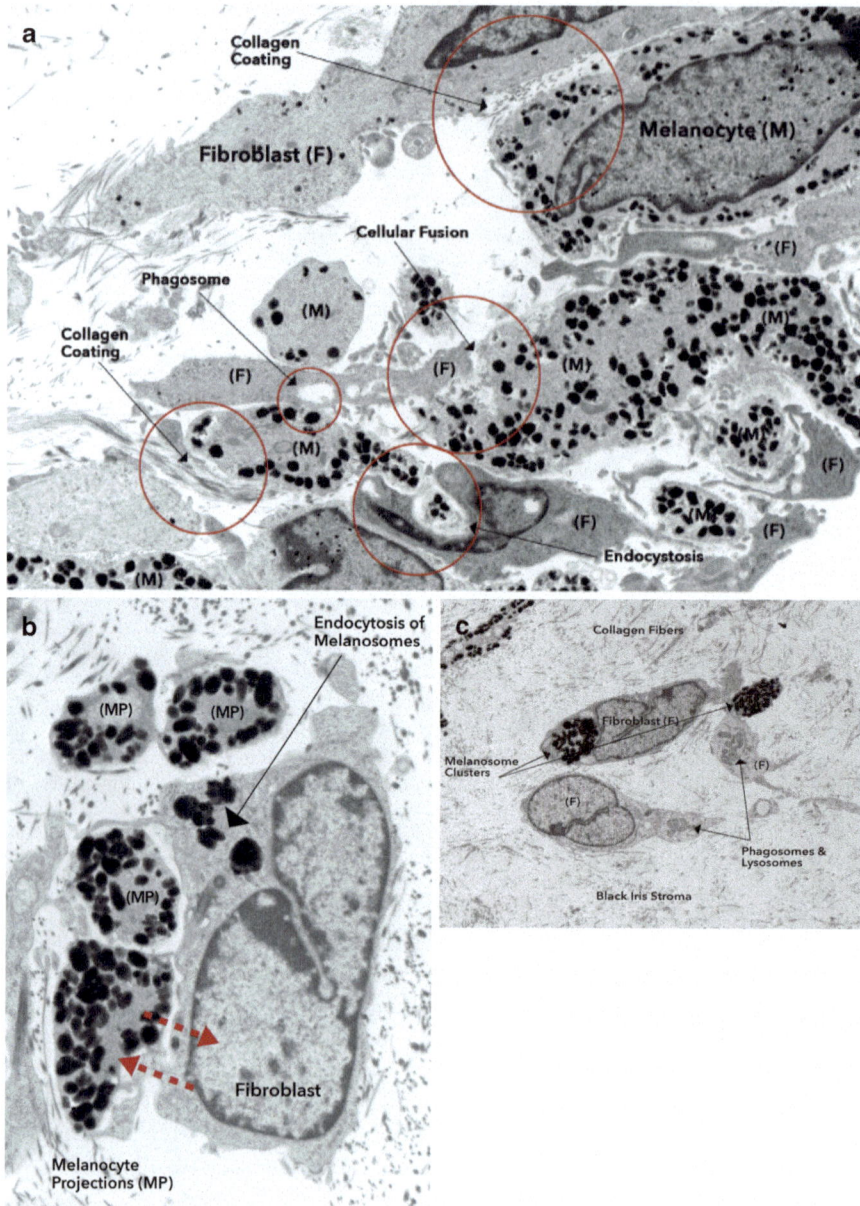

Fig. 4.15 (**a**) Electron microscopy ×2500. Blue iris. Multiple interactions between fibroblasts and melanocytes are depicted within the red circles. (**b**) Electron microscopy ×500. Black iris. Fibroblast engulfing melanosomes by endocytosis. Interaction between fibroblast and melanocyte as indicated by opposite red arrows. (**c**) Electron microscopy ×500. Black iris. Melanosome cluster endocytosis by iris fibroblasts in the stroma of black iris

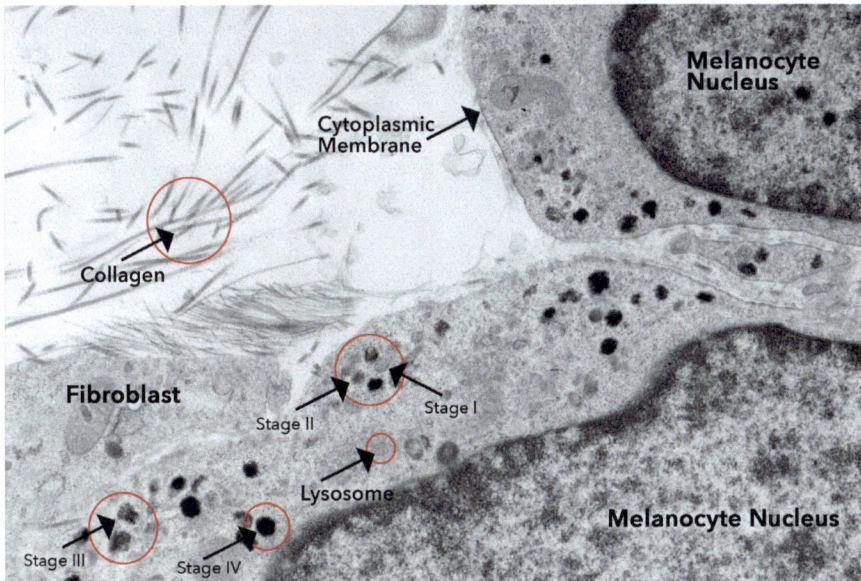

Fig. 4.16 Electron microscopy ×7000. Blue iris. Fibroblast on the left interaction with melanocyte and coating it with collagen fibers

Therefore, the combination of exocytosis and shedding of the melanosomes and inhibition of melanin production by collagen coating and production of Laminin and Fibronectin makes the fibroblasts an essential contributor and participant in the melanogenesis process of the surface of the iris and as the result the color of the iris (Fig. 4.16).

Paracrine effect of fibroblasts on the skin has been described well in the articles by Xu et al [11].

While dermal fibroblasts are not in direct contact with melanocytes, the iris melanocytes have a direct contact with the melanocytes which increases their influence on melanocytes (Fig. 4.17).

The close and direct contact between fibroblasts and melanocytes in the iris not only control and decrease the melanin production by collagen coating and laminin and Fibronectin, but also by depleting the melanosomes by endocytosis-exocytosis of melanosomes in different pathways and by degradation of ingested melanosomes by phagosomes and lysosomes (Fig. 4.18a, b).

Laminins

Laminins are glycoproteins molecules of extracellular matrix and are the major components of basal lamina portion of the basement membrane. Laminins are the active components of basement membrane and are influencing the differentiation, adhesion and migration of adjacent cellular structures including melanocytes. Laminin molecules are trimeric proteins in a cross-like shape. They contain three

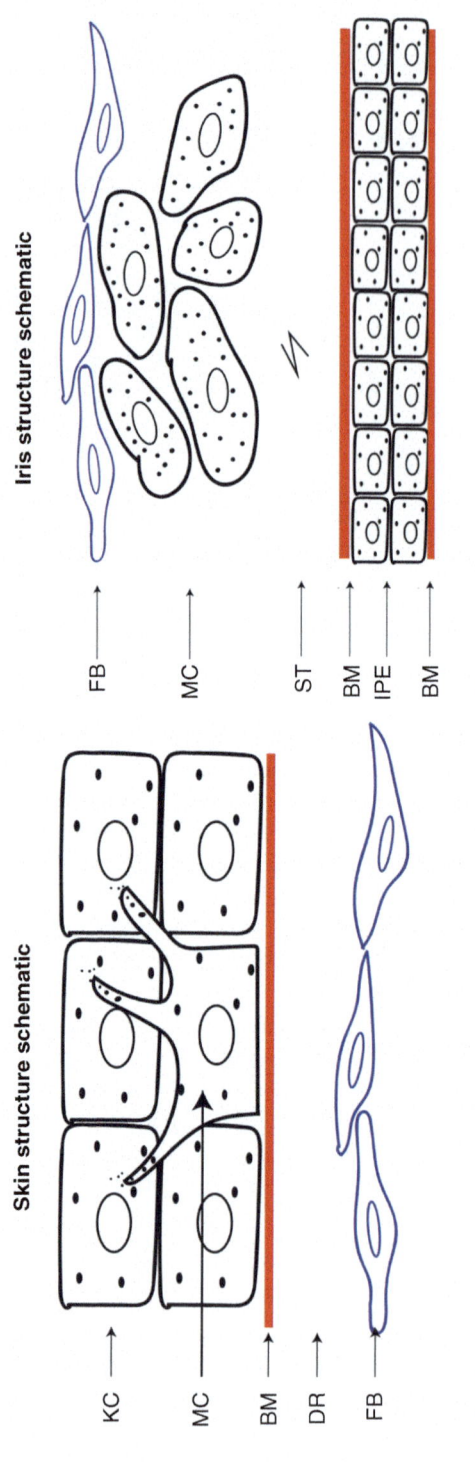

Fig. 4.17   Skin versus iris schematic structures

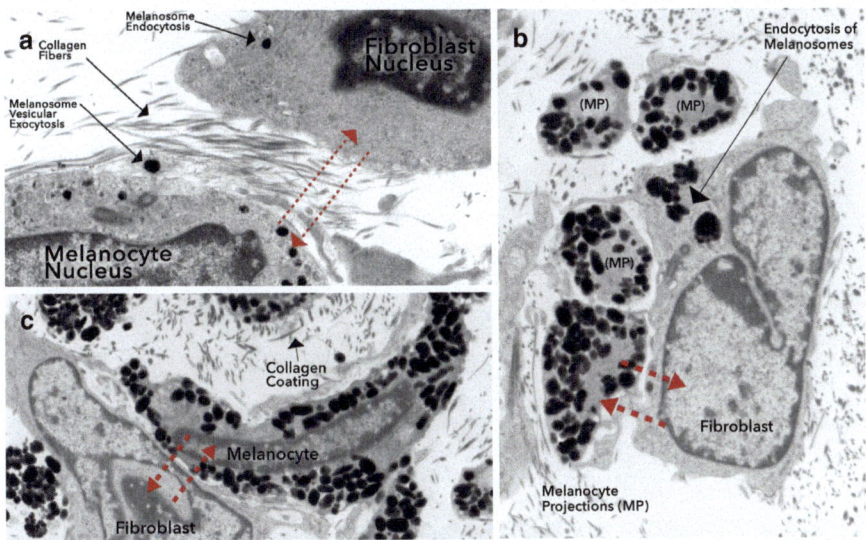

Fig. 4.18 (**a**) Electron microscopy ×20,000. Blue iris melanocytes adjacent to fibroblast with collagent fibers in between. The fibroblast, as shown, is producing collagen fibers and simultaneously coating the melanocyte adjacent to it. Also, the shedded melanosomes are being endocytosed by the fibroblast. (**b**) Electron microscopy ×500. Black iris. Fibroblast engulfing melanosomes by endocytosis. Interaction between fibroblast and melanocyte as indicated by opposite red arrows. (**c**) Electron microscopy ×500. Black iris. Fibroblast-melanosome interaction indicated by opposite red dashed arrows. The coating of the melanocyte is indicated by the black arrow

short arms and a long arm. The short arms can attach to the proteins in extracellular matrix and/or to each other and form a sheet and the long arm attaches to the cell membrane to anchor [12].

Laminins are also can be produced by fibroblasts that mimics the function of basement membrane in the iris stroma.

Laminins have a major role in harnessing and controlling the melanocytes, as the damage or the removal of the basement membrane have a direct influence of uncontrolled migration, differentiation and pigment production as seen in Epidermolysis Bullosa [13] and dermal Melasma [14].

Fibronectin

Fibronectin is a glycoprotein that has a wide variety of cellular interaction with the extracellular matrix and is secreted mainly by fibroblasts [15].

Fibronectin has an important role in melanocytes adhesion, migration, growth and differentiation. It binds to extracellular matrix proteins such as collagen, fibrin and heparan sulfate proteoglycans. It has a major role in wound healing process and fetal development (Fig. 4.18a–c).

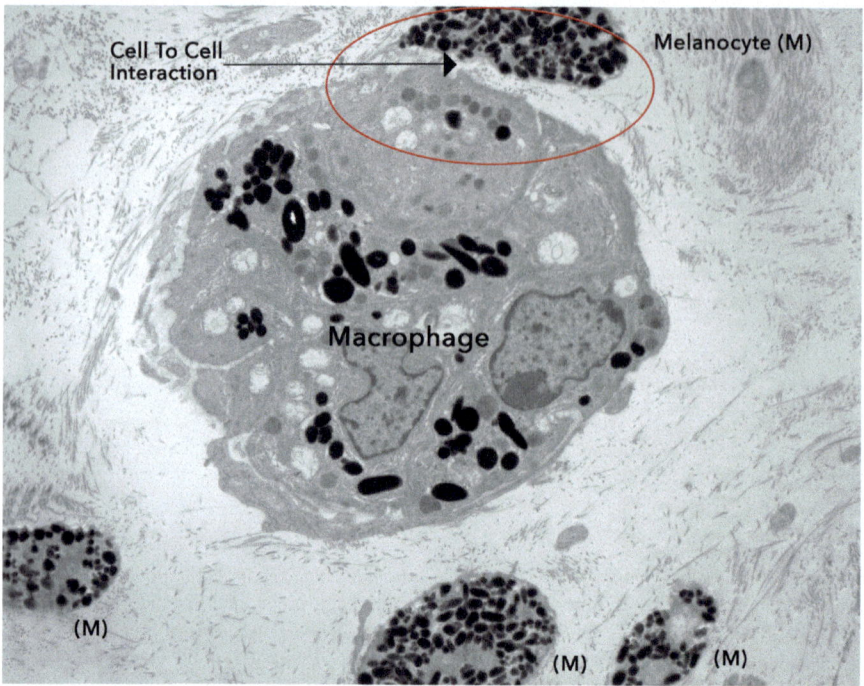

Fig. 4.19 Electron microscopy ×2000. Black iris. Macrophage in the stroma of the black iris digesting the melanosomes and surrounded by highly pigmented melanocytes. The macrophage approaching the melanocyte is circled in red

Macrophages

Macrophages are produced by differentiation of monocytes in the tissue. They have many functions including phagocytosis of pathogens, antigen presenting to T-cells, cytokines production, and secretin of many immune response proteins (Fig. 4.19).

The process of phagocytosis starts with the ameboid movement of macrophage towards the pathogen followed by engulfing the pathogen and formation of phagosome. The lysosomes will then join and fuse with phagosome and form a phagolysosome. The highly acidic components, multiple enzymes and toxic peroxides of lysosomes digest the pathogen in phagosome and the residue is expelled out by exocytosis process by the macrophage (Fig. 4.20).

Macrophages in the stroma of the dark iris carry melanosomes and melanin particles, most likely from the dead melanocytes or other macrophages at the end of their physiologic life span. Detail of this process has never been reported in the Iris. There is a resemblance between the pigment in the stroma of the dark iris to the tattoo process in the dermis layer of the skin (Fig. 4.21).

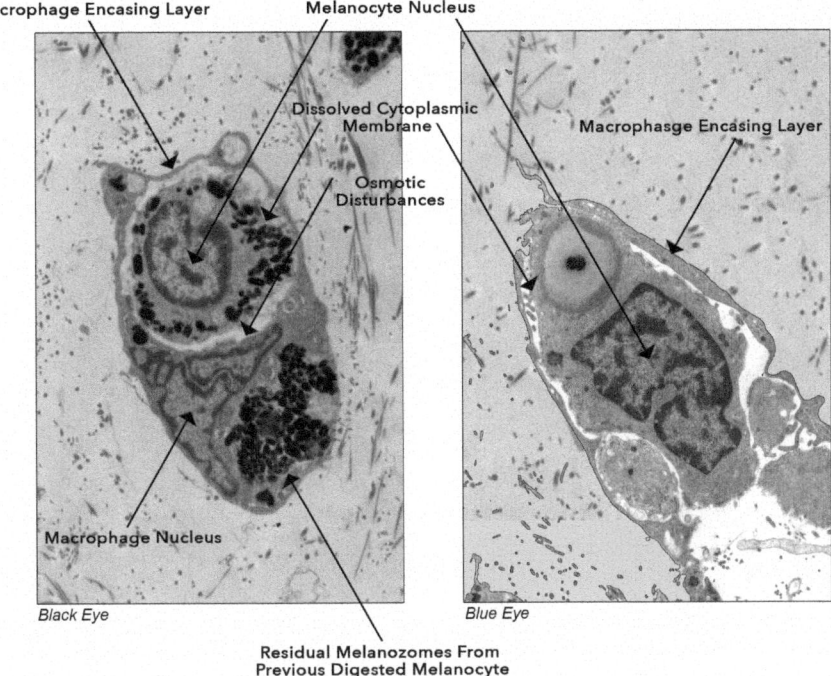

Fig. 4.20 Electron microscopy ×4000. Macrophage engulfing a melanocyte in a black iris (left) and a blue iris (right). The cytoplasmic membrane of the engulfed dying melanocytes are dissolved in certain areas, and the melanosomes are pulled away from their nuclei. The clear area surrounding the melanocytes resembles osmotic disturbance

There are recent articles regarding the mechanism of tattoo pigment particles storage in the dermis. These studies revealed that the tattoo pigment is picked up by macrophages by endocytosis in a capture-release-capture fashion and will be replaced in the new macrophages at the end of their physiologic life span of the old ones. This makes the pigment remain in place for years to come [16].

We serendipitously observed a macrophage engulfing a melanocyte in a dark iris. There is a remaining melanosome from the previous phagocytosis on the lower part of the picture and a new engulfed melanocyte on the top of the figure. There is a light layer of osmolarity disturbance around the melanocyte. The cytoplasmic membrane of the engulfed dying melanocyte is dissolved in certain areas and the melanosomes are pulled away from its nucleus (Fig. 4.20).

We can assume that the dying melanosomes are phagocytosed by macrophages and stay in place like a tattoo pigment and will be transferred to the next generation of macrophages which makes the color of the eye permanent as in tattooing process.

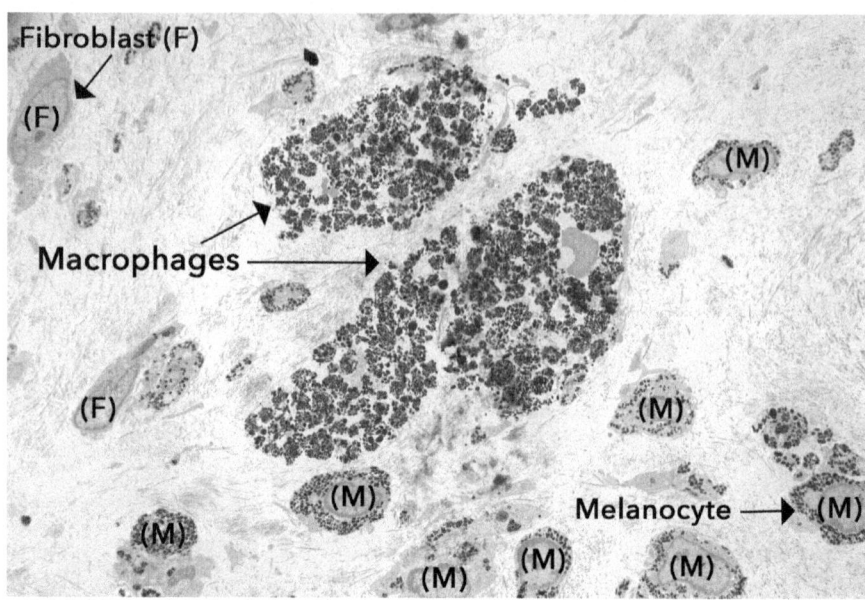

Fig. 4.21 Electron microscopy ×700. Black iris. Macrophages in the stroma of the black iris. Multiple pigmented melanocytes can be seen in the surrounding space

Iris Blood Vessels

The blood vessels and nerve fibers of the anterior border layer are similar to those in the deeper stroma (Fig. 4.22a–c).

There are large number of blood vessels in the stroma that form the substantial volume of the iris. They are radially oriented and located in different depths with multiple anastomosis which form the minor vascular circle of iris. The iris blood vessels are very unique due to their specific characteristics that makes them very different from the rest of the body. The thick endothelial lining and the thick collagen fibril color that are located in the adventitia of the iris vessels account for:

- low permeability of iris blood vessels
- limited or no bleeding during trauma or surgical procedures or laser iris surgery (Iridectomy & iridotomy procedures)

Iris vessels include arterioles, venules, and capillaries. Iris arterioles are lined with endothelium and surrounded by pericytes (Fig. 4.23).

Melanocytes and fibroblasts are also found in the stroma. Iris venules have very thin walls consisting of endothelium surrounded by a thin layer of collagen. Capillaries are formed by a single layer of non-fenestrated epithelium.

Nerves may be present along larger blood vessels, in the anterior border layer, in the stroma, or among the muscles. Iris nerves are generally unmyelinated, although some may have Schwann cells.

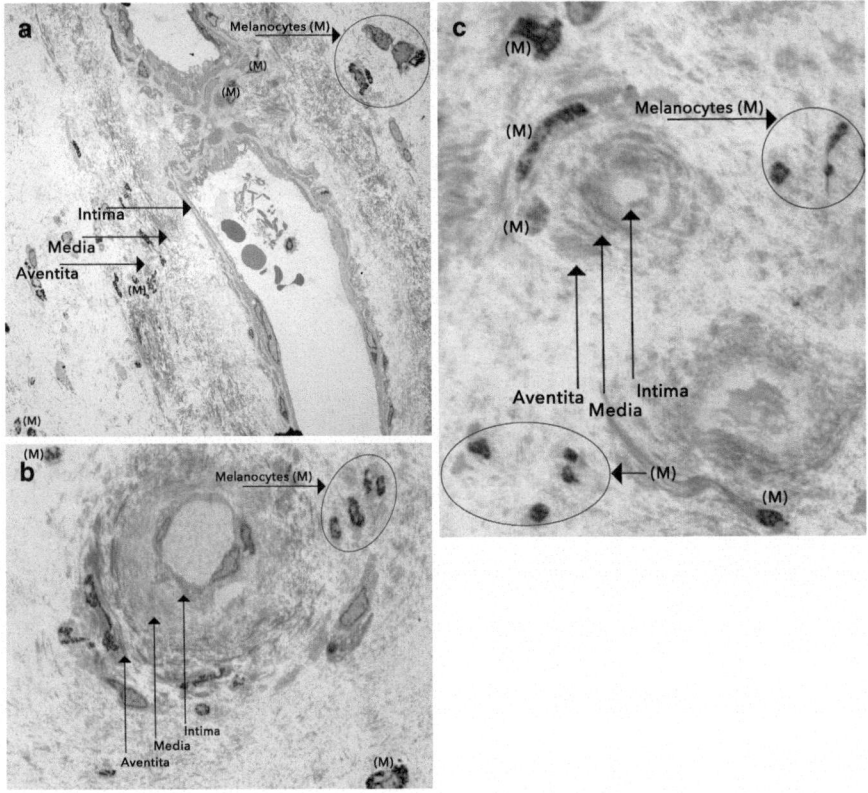

Fig. 4.22 (**a**) Electron microscopy ×10,000. Black iris blood vessel. Pigmented melanocytes can be observed around the blood vessel. (**b**) Electron microscopy ×10,000. Black iris mid-size blood vessel. Pigmented melanocytes can be observed around the blood vessel. (**c**) Electron microscopy ×10,000. Black iris capillary. Pigemented melanocytes can be observed in the vicinity of the capillary

- Other cellular components that occupy the stromal connective tissue are macrophages that contain pigment (Clump cells of Koganei Type 1), multinucleated pigment cells that have surrounding basement membrane (Clump cells of Koganei type 2), Mast cells, lymphocytes and plasma cells in varying distributions (Fig. 4.24).
- Nerve endings are from sensory, vasomotor, and motor nerves, as well as supporting cells such as Schwann cells are spread throughout the stroma. They form neuromuscular synapses with the dilator and sphincter muscles and also have direct synapses to the melanocytes.
- Disruption of sympathetic neural stimulation known as Horner's syndrome is associated with decreased pigmentation of the iris due to decreased anterior border cells and stromal melanocytes and lack of sympathetic nerve endings [3].

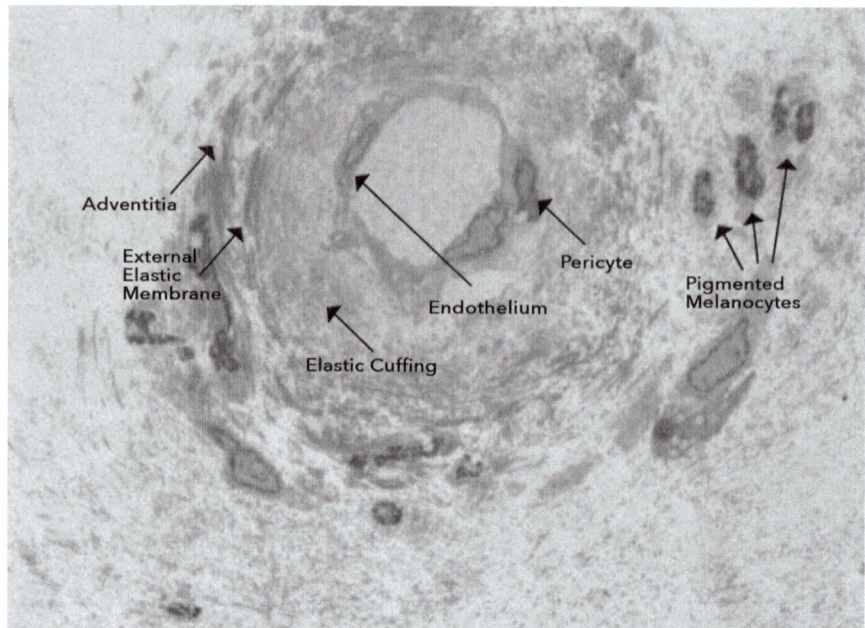

Fig. 4.23 Electron microscopy ×25,000. Black iris blood vessel. Pigemented melanocytes surrounding the blood vessel

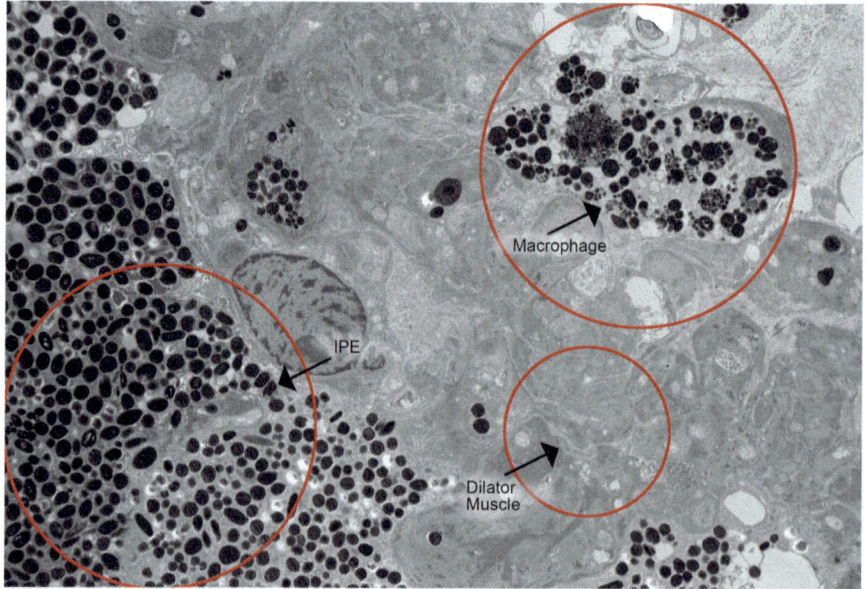

Fig. 4.24 Electron microscopy ×1500. Dilator muscle in a dark brown iris. In the center is pigement epithelium on the left and the macrophage on the top right

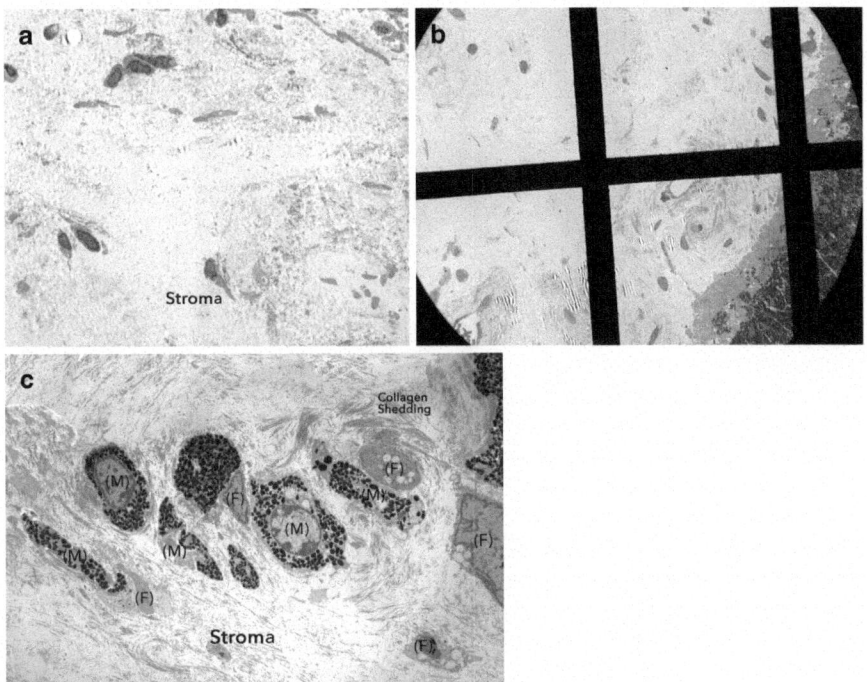

Fig. 4.25 (**a**) Electron microscopy ×200. Blue iris stroma. Scattered fibroblasts in a loose connective tissue. (**b**) Electron microscopy ×200. Blue iris. Posterior segment. Loose connective tissue with scattered fibroblasts and blood vessels. (**c**) Electron microscopy ×1200. Black iris. Stroma with highly pigmented melanocytes. Melanosomes are at stage IV

The loose connective tissue of the iris with high content of Acid mucopolysaccharide and collagen specially around the radially oriented blood vessels, which permits the sudden movements of dilation and constriction (mydriasis and miosis) of the iris by neuronal stimulation by light/accommodation and chemicals and medications (Fig. 4.25a–c).

The specifics of the collagen diversity and components has an important role in the function of this organ, as the change or damage to the iris has severe consequences evident in Glaucoma patients.

– Stroma collagen content of the iris is specific and contain Type I and Type III. They are produced by fibroblasts (Fig. 4.26).
– Iris Stroma lacks collagen Types II, IV and VII which the latter is involved in fibrosis and scar formation [17].
– Other components of stroma such as vascular cells and fibroblasts contain collagen IV
– Basement membrane of the iris blood vessels also contains collagen type I.

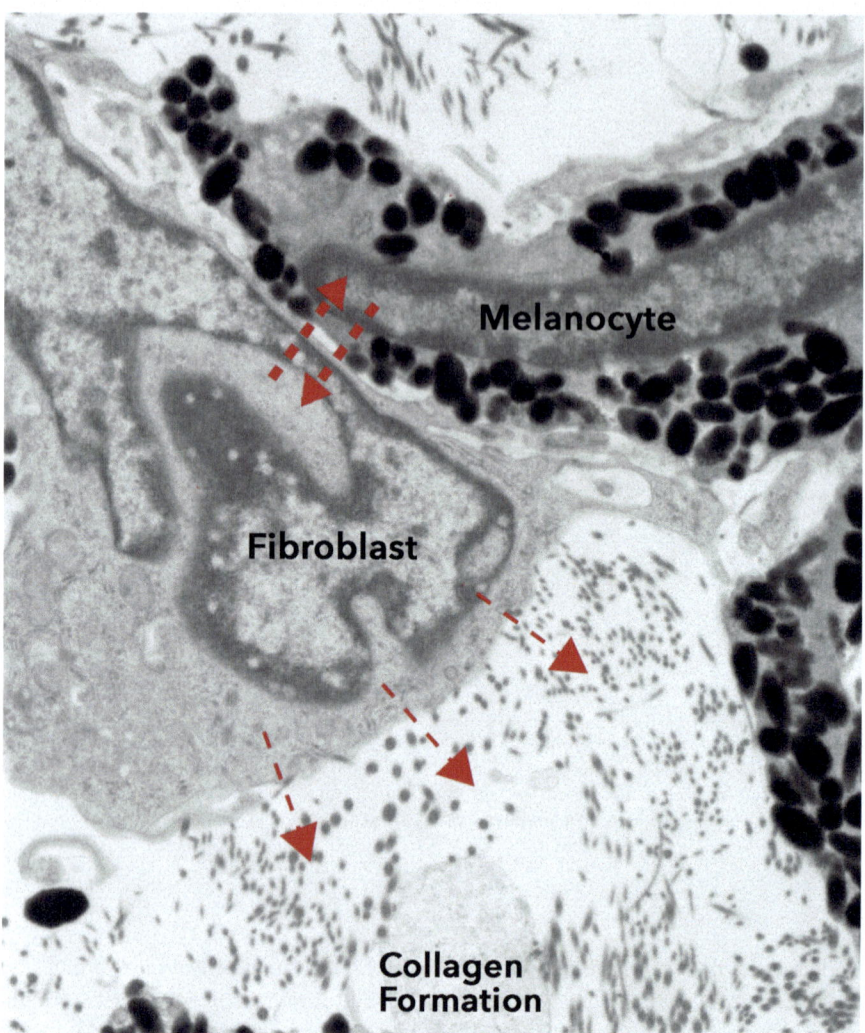

Fig. 4.26 Electron microscopy ×25,000. Black iris. Collagen production by fibroblast as indicated by three red arrows. Intimate contact between fibroblast and melanocyte indicating their interaction, as shown by the opposite double red arrows

Blood vessels, nerves, and a mixture of pigmented and nonpigmented cells occupy this connective tissue framework. The stroma extends from the anterior border layer to the anterior surface of the dilator muscle. The collagen fibrils measure approximately 600 angstroms in width and are arranged in large and small bundles forming spaces of variable size (Fig. 4.16).

Collagen is most abundant around blood vessels and nerves, in iris base, and between the bundles of the sphincter muscle. The stroma is freely permeable to aqueous humor.

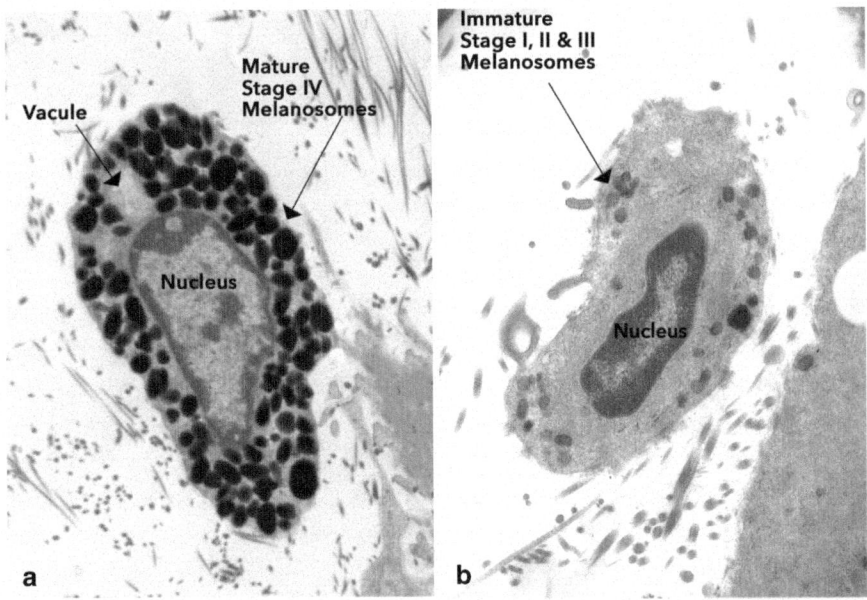

Fig. 4.27 (a) Electron microscopy ×25,000. Classic black iris melanocyte with vacule and mature stage IV melanosomes. The melanocyte cytoplasm is filled with melanosomes obscuring other elements of cytoplasm. (b) Electron microscopy ×25,000. Classic blue iris melanocyte and immature stage I, II, and III melanosomes. The melanocyte cytoplasm is not filled with melanosomes. The melanosomes are located at the periphery of the cytoplasm

Several cell types have been described in the stroma of the iris. These include fibroblasts, melanocytes, mast cells, clump cells, macrophages, and lymphocytes.

Fibroblasts are the most prominent cell type and are often found in close association with blood vessels, muscles, and nerves. Their ultrastructure is similar to that described for fibroblasts of the anterior border layer. Melanocytes can be found around the adventitia of blood vessels and form plexuses with fibroblasts and other adjacent melanocytes. The characteristics of melanosomes varies among irides of different colors (Fig. 4.27a, b).

It is also similar to that described above for anterior border melanocytes (Fig. 4.28a, b).

An unusual type of macro-melanosome has been identified in the cytoplasm of stromal melanocytes in patients with melanosis oculi. These abnormal melanosomes are not seen in the posterior pigment epithelium of these patients, suggesting that melanosis oculi are considered a disorder of neural crest-derived melanocytes.

Clump cells of Koganei are most commonly found just anterior to the pupillary sphincter muscle and in the anterior ciliary body near the iris root, although these cells can be seen elsewhere in the iris stroma. These cells appear as heavily pigmented, round cells on light microscopic examination. It is now generally accepted that the term "clump cell" actually includes two distinct populations of cells. Type I clump cells are probably macrophages. Transmission electron microscopic

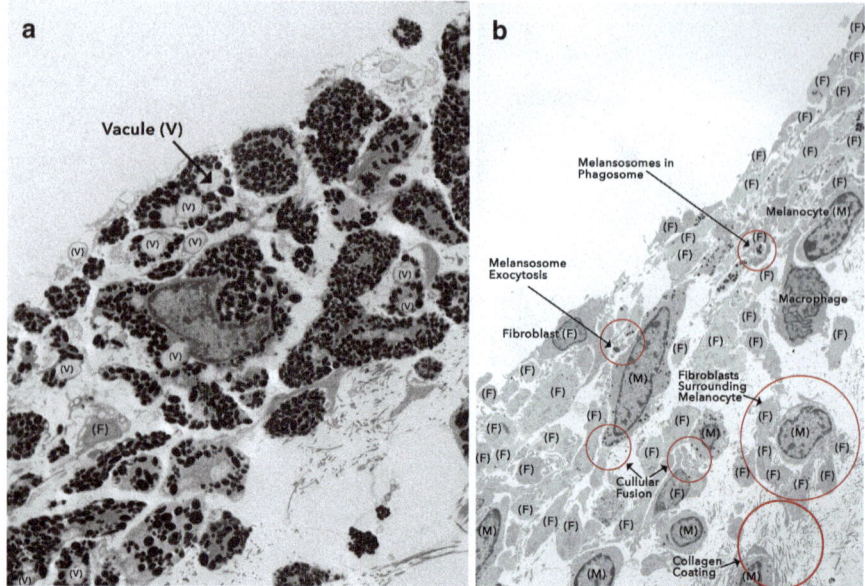

Fig. 4.28 (**a**) Electron microscopy ×1200. Black iris anterior surface. Highly pigmented melano-cytes with multiple vacules and stage IV melanosomes. There are rare fibroblasts (F), with no cellular interaction with melanosomes detected. (**b**) Electron microscopy ×1000. Blue iris. Cellular fusion between the fibroblast and melanocyte projection, and pigment transfer is circled in red and indicated by the arrow

examination reveals that type I clump cells have delicate villi projecting from their surface, and their cytoplasm is filled with clusters of melanin granules of varying shapes and sizes. The nucleus is often eccentrically located, and the cells typically contain round or irregular bodies that are thought to contain either lipid or lipofus-cin. These cells have no basement membrane. Type I clump cells are difficult to find in the irides of children and are more common in older individuals. These macro-phages are probably responsible to engulfing melanin shedding from melanosomes and also the entire melanocytes.

To the best of our knowledge, pigment shedding of the iris melanocytes has not previously been reported in the literature.

The peripheral distribution of melanosomes and their exocytosis by shedding, as we see in our EM, can be translated as all stroma melanocytes transfer pigments out as part of their physiologic process (Figs. 4.29 and 4.30).

There are different mechanisms of pigment transport in skin melanocytes, as described in the literature. These modes of pigment transfer can also be seen in the iris as shown in these relevant electron microscopy images (Fig. 4.32c):

- Cytophagocytosis (Fig. 4.32a).
- Membrane Fusion (Fig. 4.31a),
- Shedding-Phagocytosis (Fig. 4.31a),
- Exocytosis-Endocytosis (Fig. 4.31b). Wu and Hammer [10].

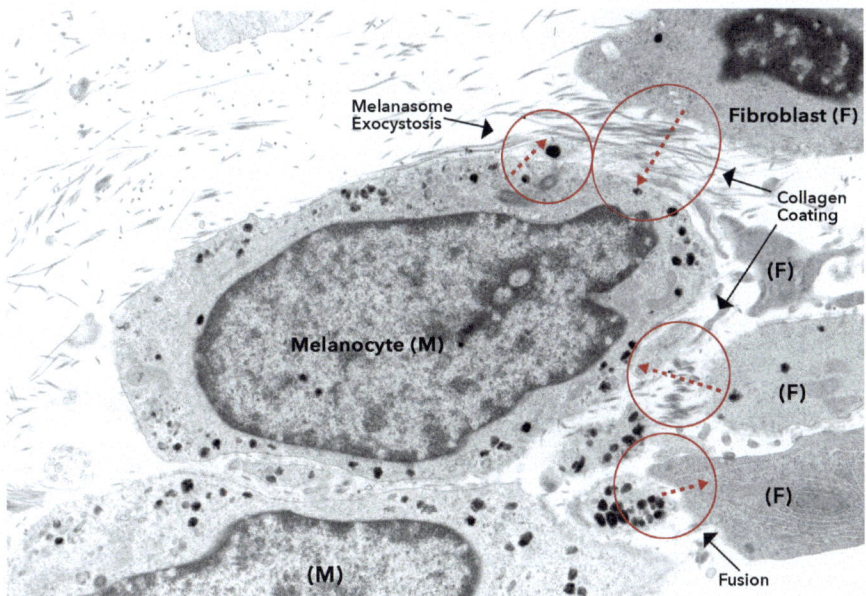

Fig. 4.29 Electron microscopy ×4000. Blue iris. The collagen coating of melanocyte by fibroblasts are circled in red and contain red arrows. Melanosome exocytosis and cellular fusion between melanocyte and fibroblast are also circled in red and contain red arrows

Pigment transport and shedding in iris melanocytes have not been addressed in the past and is a very important phenomena to explore (Figs. 4.15a and 4.32a, b).

In our database EM collection, it was observed that in black color iris the entire melanocytes can be phagocytosed by macrophages while the pigment shedding was not detected.

We also observed the phagocytosis of melanocytes by macrophages and fibroblasts in blue iris (Fig. 4.15a–c).

Blue Iris surface melanocytes have scattered melanosomes in different stages of maturation and they are located away from the nucleus and located closer to the cytoplasmic membrane and their cytoplasmic projections contain melanosomes for shedding. Blue iris fibroblasts have abundant amount of collagen formation on their surface (Fig. 4.33).

Internalization of melanosomes by fibroblast can be observed in our EM images (Fig. 4.11).

We did not observe pigment shedding in black irides.

The shedding can have a significant effect on the process of pigment exocytosis on blue eyes and is part of the reason why these cells do not retain pigment in their cytoplasm. Also, it indicates that this process is fast enough which does not give the melanosomes the chance to accumulate enough melanin to get to their mature form as stage IV melanosomes, and that is the reason we rarely see any stage IV melanosomes in the cytoplasm of blue iris melanocytes. This also explains the reason the

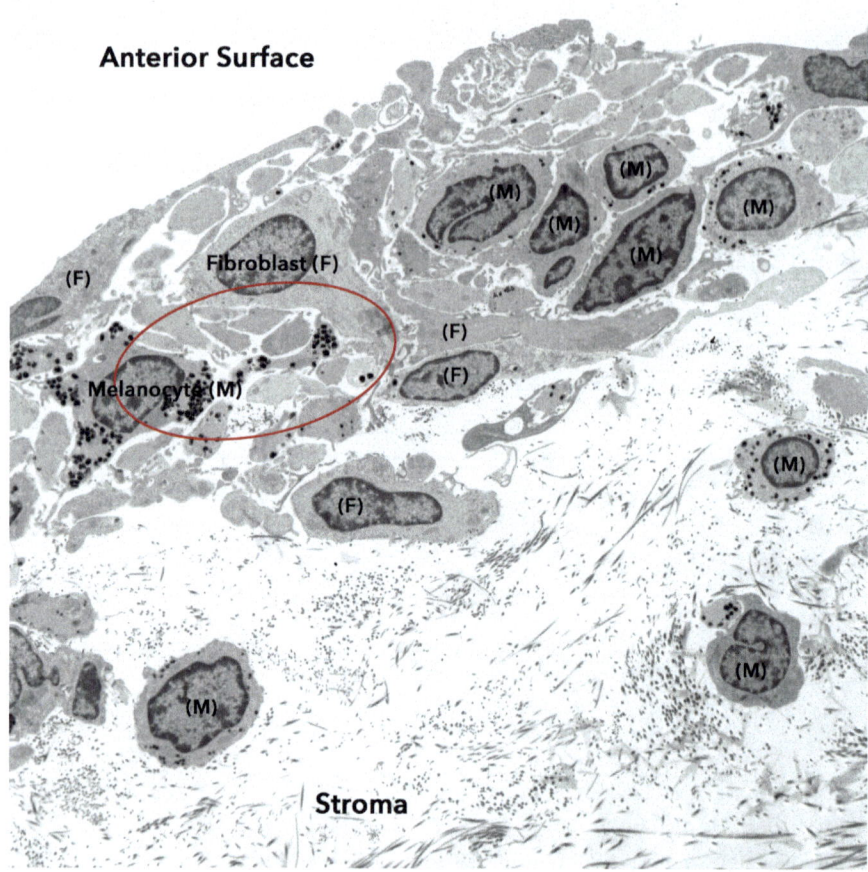

Fig. 4.30 Electron microscopy ×1000. Blue iris. Blue melanocytes on the left transferring its melanosomes toward the projections. There are multiple stages of shedding from bulging of the cell membrane to separation/shedding of the melanosome that can be seen in this picture

cytoplasm of melanocytes contains few melanosomes and in certain areas lack of melanosomes in their cytoplasm (Fig. 4.27b).

Iris macrophages resemble type I clump cells, differing only in their more elongated shape and in the contents of their residual bodies that may contain substances other than melanin.

Type II clump cells are less common and are thought to represent smooth muscle cells in arrested stages of development. Light microscopic examination shows that type II clump cells have a more regular outline with more homogeneously distributed pigment granules than type I clump cells. Examination by transmission electron microscopy shows that type II clump cells are a group of cells that contain pigment granules identical to those found in the iris pigment epithelium. These cells may form clusters surrounded by a continuous basement membrane and bordered by apical villi that extend into cleft-like spaces. These cells are attached to each other by desmosomes and contain intracytoplasmic filaments and vesicles (Fig. 4.34).

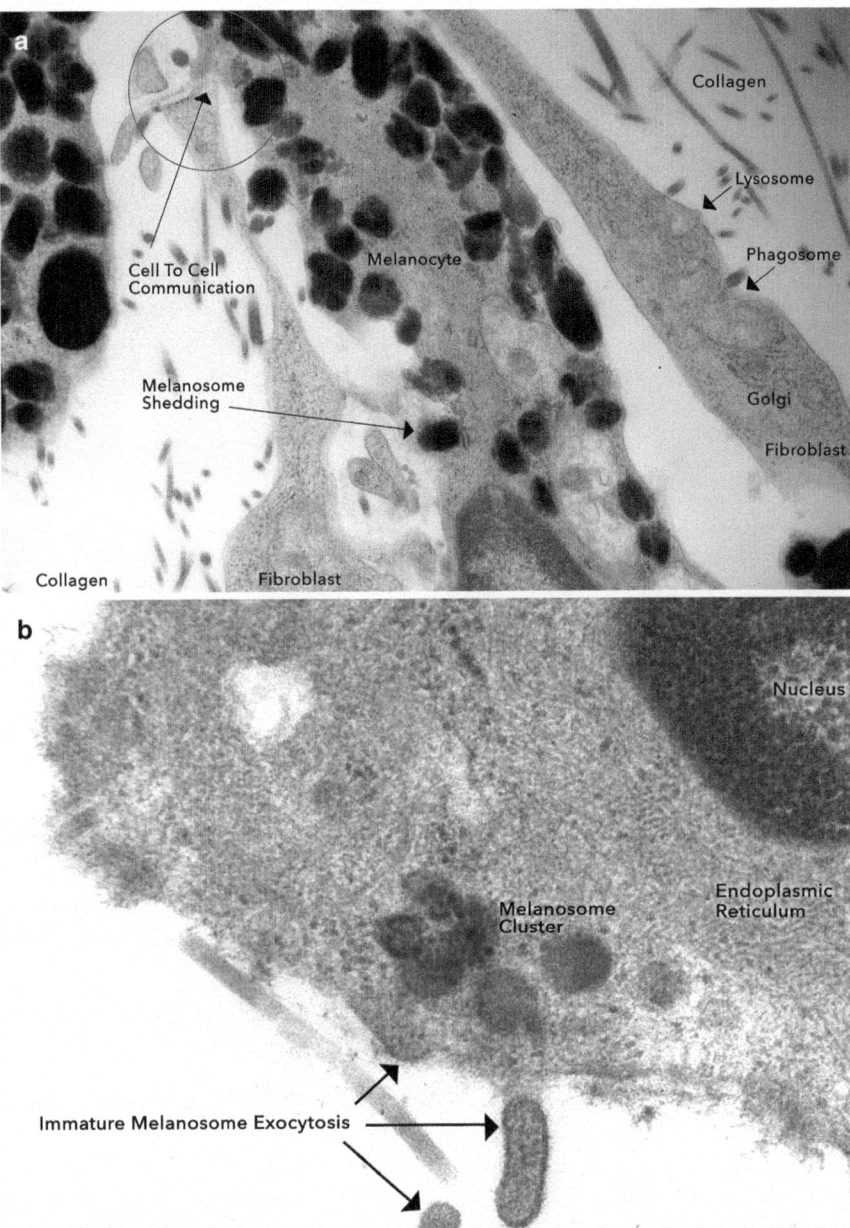

Fig. 4.31 (**a**) Electron microscopy ×25,000. Blue iris. Different modes of pigment transfer can be observed. The cell membrane fusion can be seen at the top, and exocytosis can be seen at the bottom. Both are marked with arrows. (**b**) Electron microscopy ×25,000. Blue iris. The process of exocytosis in different stages can be observed. (**c**) Electron microscopy ×2500. Blue iris. Multiple interactions between fibroblasts and melanocytes are depicted in the red circles

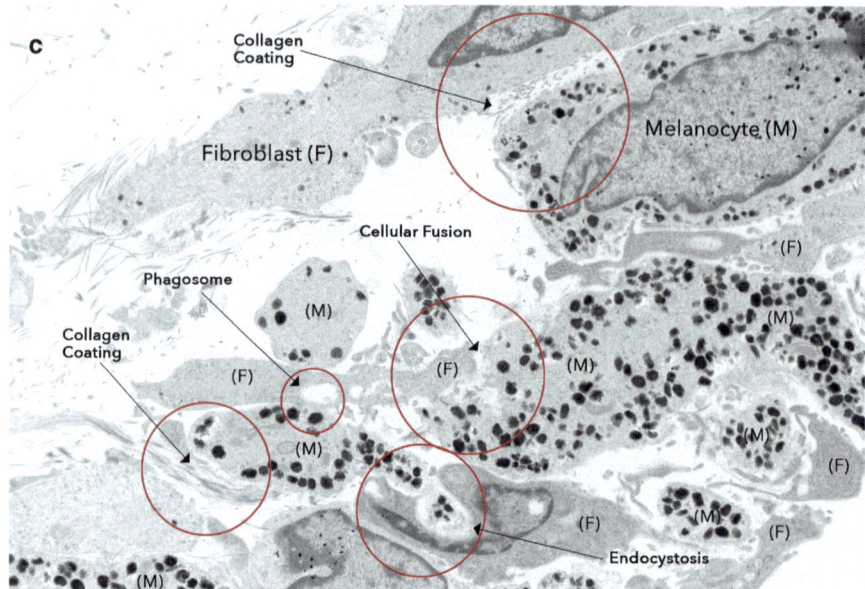

Fig. 4.31 (Continued)

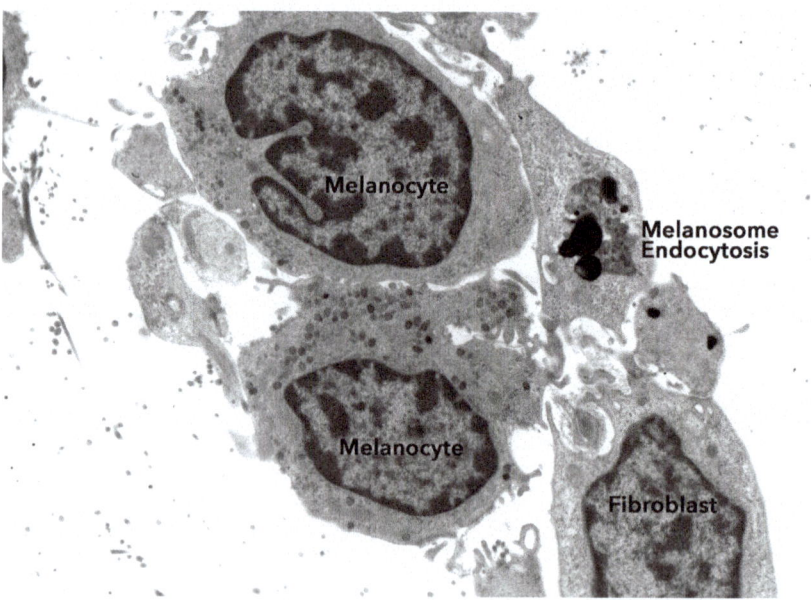

Fig. 4.32 Electron microscopy ×4000. Blue iris. Fibroblast endocytosis of melanosomes by phagocytosis can be observed

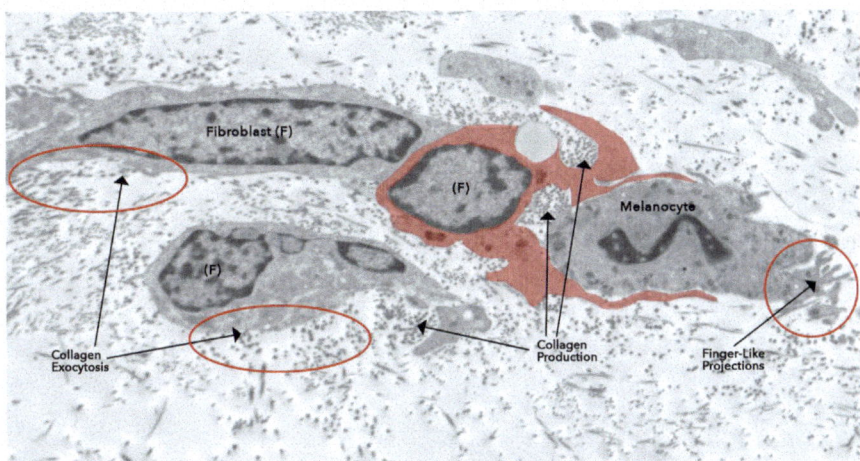

Fig. 4.33 Electron microscopy ×1200. Blue iris. Fibroblast collagen production and coating of melanocyte. The engulfment of melanocyte can be seen shaded in red

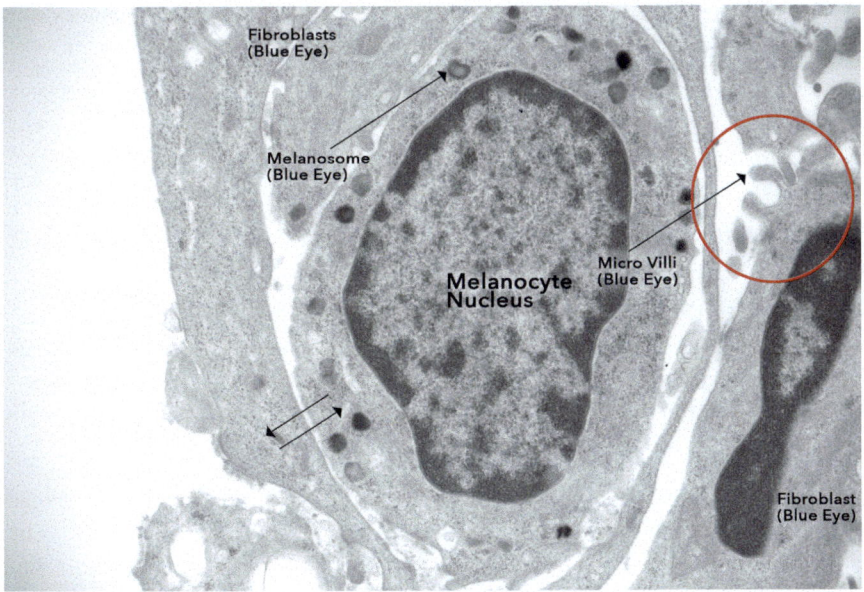

Fig. 4.34 Electron miroscopy ×8000. Blue eye melanocyte (left) with scattered immature melanosomes at the periphery of cytoplasm. Fibroblast (right) with micro villi projections adjacent to each other. The melanocyte is completely engulfed and surrounded by fibroblasts. The parallel arrows indicate the constant molecular interaction between fibroblasts and melanocytes

Iris Muscles

The sphincter and dilator muscles of the iris are of neuroectodermal origin, developing from the anterior epithelial layer of the primitive optic cup. The sphincter cells are originating from the neuroectoderm near the iris edge and develop into smooth muscle bundles around the pupil.

There are other studies that suggests the possibility of Neural crest as an origin of these cells.

The iris sphincter muscle is located in the pupillary portion of the iris stroma. It measures 0.75–1 mm in diameter and 0.1–1.7 mm in thickness.

The Sphincter Muscle

Iris sphincter muscle is composed of five to eight bundles that are connected with tight junctions.

The cytoplasm of sphincter muscle contains standard organelles such as mitochondria, rough endoplasmic reticulum ribosomes and Golgi apparatus.

The sphincter muscle also contains aggregates of myofilaments and pinocytotic vesicles, at the periphery in the muscle cells.

The Dilator Muscle

There is a close relationship between iris fibroblasts and the dilator muscle (Fig. 4.35).

- Iris fibroblasts form a boundary between the dilator muscle and the iris stroma.
- Iris fibroblasts are characteristically accompanied by numerous naked axonal synaptic vesicles on the dilator muscle side.
- The stromal surface of the dilator muscle layer is incompletely covered by a single layer of iris fibroblasts.

It is suggested that iris fibroblasts in the dilator muscle region play some role in the innervation of the dilator muscle [18].

Iris Pigment Epithelium (IPE)

This layer composed of two distinct layers: The anterior and the posterior layers (Fig. 4.35).

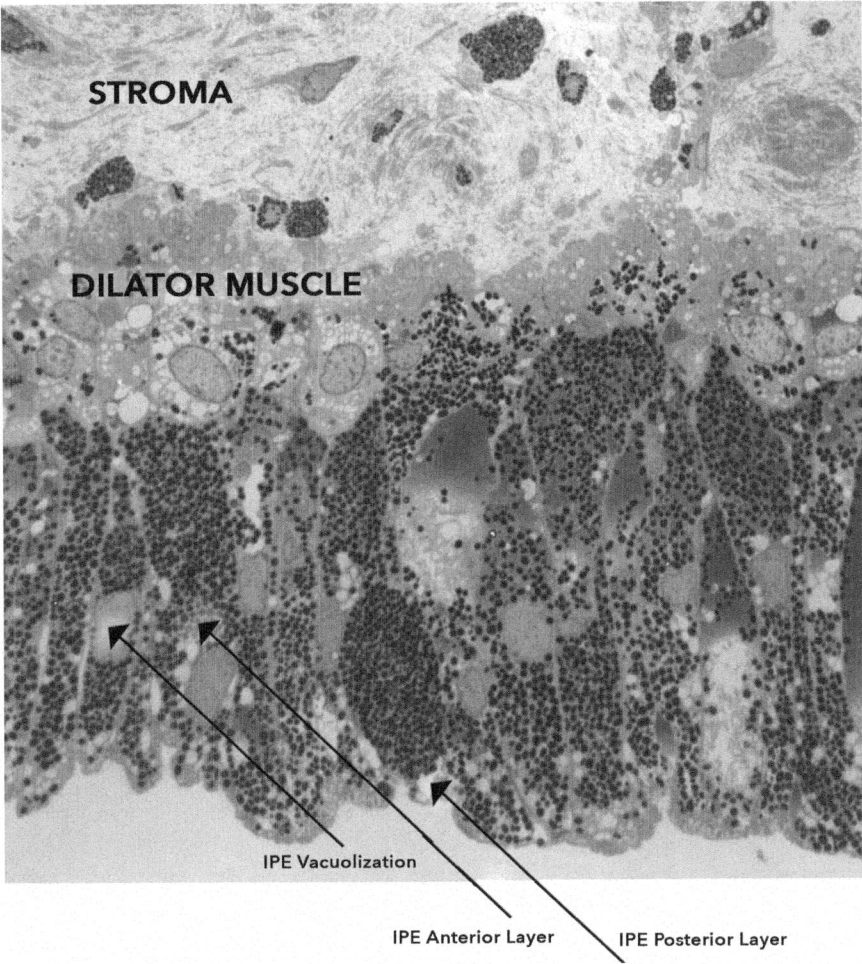

Fig. 4.35 Electron microscopy ×8000. Blue iris. Posterior surface with posterior stroma, dilator muscle, and two layers of iris pigment epithelium (IPE)

The Anterior Iris Pigment Epithelium

The anterior layer of Iris pigment epithelium (IPE) also composed of two distinguishable layers. The muscular basal portion (anteriorly) and the epithelial apical portion (posteriorly). The muscular portion of the cell is adjacent to the iris stroma and makes up the pupillary dilator muscle. The epithelial portion is attached to the posterior pigment epithelium layer this head to head (Tet a Tet) arrangement is similar to that seen between the pigmented and nonpigmented epithelium of the ciliary body and is due to invagination of their common embryologic precursor, the optic cup.

The muscular portion of the cell of the anterior layer measures about 4 µm in thickness. The dilation of the pupil is due to contraction of this muscular tissue. The nucleus of these cells is located in the epithelial apical portion. These cells contain ribbon-like muscular processes surrounded by a basement membrane that terminates at the epithelial apical portion of the cell. The muscle cells are joined by tight junctions.

The cytoplasm of the muscular portion of the cell contains:

- Myofilaments.
- Mitochondria.
- Densities resembling the Z-discs of skeletal muscle.
- Rare pigment granules.
- Pinocytotic vesicles.
- Unmyelinated nerve endings to the muscle processes.

The epithelial apical portion of the cells is similar to the posterior pigment epithelium. The apical surfaces of the anterior and posterior pigment epithelium are separated by intercellular spaces containing numerous microvillous processes projecting from the two cell layers.

- The anterior and posterior layers are joined to each other by tight intercellular junctions and desmosomes.
- The basement membrane of the muscular portion of the anterior iris epithelium is due to generation of dilator muscle from the neural ectoderm.
- Mitochondria, pigment granules, rough endoplasmic reticulum, free ribosomes, smooth endoplasmic reticulum, a Golgi apparatus are present.

Posterior Pigment Epithelium

The characteristics of this layer is summarized as follows:

- The posterior layer of iris pigment epithelium (IPE) is more heavily pigmented than the anterior layer.
- The cells are generally rectangular and contain large and compacted pigment granules.
- A thin basement membrane is present on the posterior surface of these cells facing the lens.
- The basal cell membrane has numerous infoldings.
- The lateral walls of these cells are joined to adjacent cells by maculae adherens and occludens.
- They contain central nucleus and round intra-cytoplasmic pigment granules that measure approximately 0.8 µm in diameter.
- Intercellular junctions are present between these cells.

These granules are much larger than those found in the iris stroma, which range in diameter from 0.1 to 0.5 µm. The posterior pigment epithelium also contains glycogen, mitochondria, rough endoplasmic reticulum, and a Golgi apparatus (Fig. 4.36).

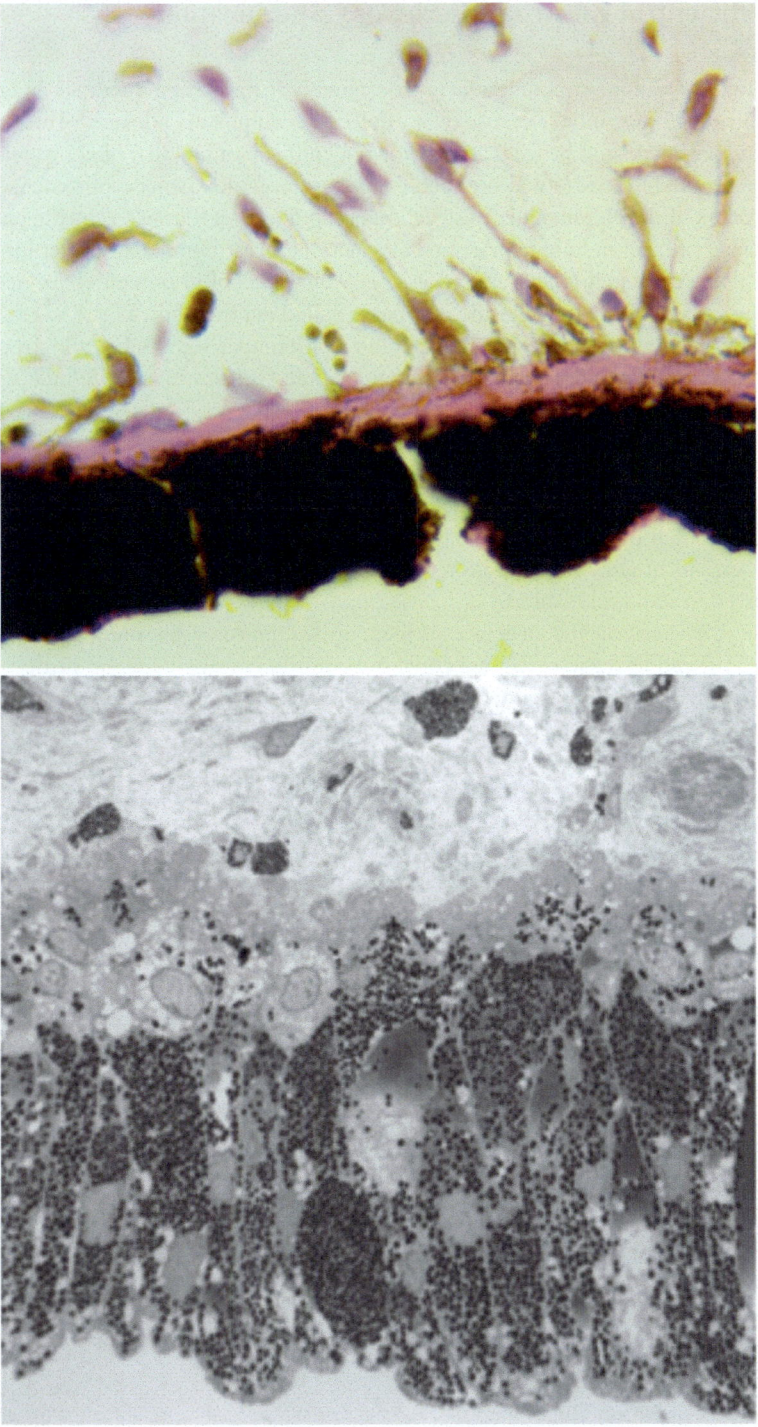

Fig. 4.36 Photo and electron microscopy. Posterior surface with posterior stroma, dilator muscle, and two layers of iris pigment epithelium (IPE)

Iris Structural Electron Microscopy Specifications

Iris has a very unique structure which varies greatly in different individuals and it can be easily identified without the use of any detection equipment or devices. This unique property has made it to be used as individual identification tool like finger printing.

These structural variety is the result of a very complex genetic inheritance and the process of developmental construction and pigment cell transfer during embryonic stage of each individual. As a result, there is a vast number of eye colors and forms that we see in human population. It is even more colorful in other species due to more variety of pigments in the iris that is called chromophores.

There are few references in the literature on comparison studies on structural differences of the iris color and there are no detailed illustrations on cellular definitions to confirm their claims.

We studied 3 immediate postmortem eyes from The New York Eye-bank with 3 different colors, Black (very dark brown), Hazel (light brown) and blue eyes as was explained earlier.

Half of each Iris was removed and placed in formalin for light microscopy and the other half in glutaraldehyde for electron microscopy. The specimens were then processed in standard fashion.

The difference on the structure of these eyes confirmed the older literature by Fuchs [19] and Dieterich [20] and could not confirm newer studies by Eagle [21].

There are other studies on the correlation of melanocytes and the color of the iris with different analysis and results for example:

Wilkerson et al. [2]

Prota et al. [22]

Imesch et al. [23]

It was noticed that there are many cellular and structural differences between the different color irides that has not been referred to in the past.

These significant differences in iris structure of different colors can be appreciated in light and electron microscopy comparison slides (Fig. 4.2a–c).

In the previous chapter the histologic differences in light microscopy was discussed. Here the electron microscopic aspect of the iris variations is being discussed.

These electron microscopy differences can be summarized as follows:

1. Population of melanocytes on the anterior surface of the Iris
2. Population of melanosomes in the cytoplasm of melanocytes
3. Melanosomes location and distance from nucleus
4. Stages of maturation of melanosomes
5. Population of fibroblasts on the iris surface
6. Amount of collagen in between and on the surface of the Iris
7. Number of Lysosomes
8. Number of cytoplasmic vacuoles
9. Number of mitochondria
10. Finger like projections
11. Number of stromal melanocytes

12. Stromal macrophages
13. Stromal collagen content and intercellular matrix

Each issue will be discussed and will be referred to in dark color eyes as dark brown and blue color eyes. It is interesting that there is only one-color source Melanin (Eumelanin/Pheomelanin) (Fig. 4.5) in the melanocytes of the iris yet there are large variety of colors due to different light reflections due to different circumstances.

In our study the population of the melanocytes are varies according to the iris color. The more layers of melanocytes the darker the color of the eye appears (Fig. 4.13).

In the attached figure we can see 5-6 layers of melanocytes on the surface of the dark color iris whereas in light color irides there is barely a single disrupted layer on the surface of the blue eyes (Fig. 4.37).

The melanocytes are packed together on the surface of the dark iris (Fig. 4.27a) and there are very few fibroblasts can be seen in between them. In the contrary on the light color eyes the melanocytes are in a thin layer and are dispersed and there are multiple fibroblasts in between them (Fig. 4.27b).

These findings do not confirm previous studies that claim, "the number of surface melanocytes are the same in all different color eyes, but the only difference is the amount of melanin in the melanocytes".

Number of mature stage IV melanosomes are much higher in dark irides and there are very few or no early stages of lysosomes can be observed. This is in conflict with previous studies that claim the number of melanosomes is equal in all different color irides (Fig. 4.38).

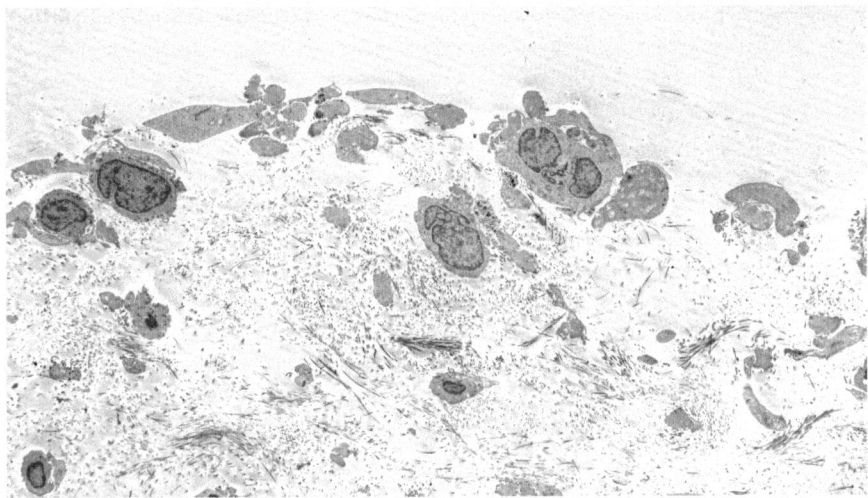

Fig. 4.37 Electron microscopy ×700. Blue iris. Anterior surface. Few scattered melanocytes with minimal immature melanosomes in the cytoplasm. Multiple fibroblasts can be seen at the surface with abundant collagen fibers in the anterior stroma

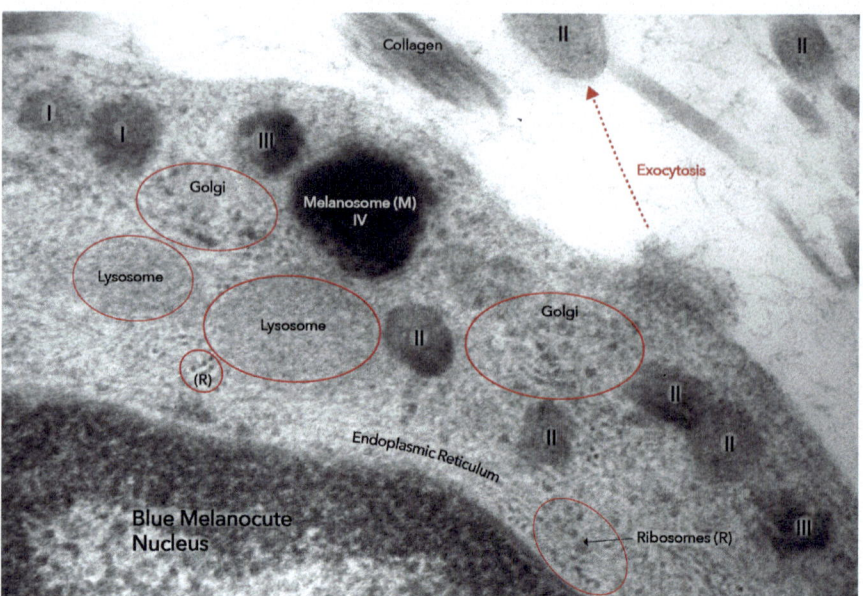

Fig. 4.38 Electron microscopy ×40,000. Blue iris. Maturation of melanosomes and exocytosis of different immature stage II melanosomes

Counting the number of Stage IV melanosomes in the dark color iris melanocyte is very easy. In the blue eye melanocytes however, melanosome counting is very difficult. It is not easy to differentiate between lysosomes and Stage one melanosomes, so by counting all of these incompletely processed multivesicular endosomes one can come to the conclusion of equal number of melanocytes in all eye colors. One can conclude that this can explain the reported result of previous studies of equal number of melanocytes in different eye colors.

We observed many more melanosomes in the dark color eyes melanocytes and fewer melanosomes in the blue eye melanocytes.

The lysosomes and single membrane vesicle structures in melanocytes of the blue irides that resembles multivesicular endosomes (Fig. 4.4a) should not be confused with melanosomes. In melanocytes the process of stage IV melanosome (Fully pigmented) formation is a very complex and requires many signaling pathways and adaptors to be completed. Any disruption of the process could end up with a range of products from retention of multivesicular endosomes to formation of lysosomes and stages of I and II melanosomes with incomplete pigmentation or formation of early or late stages of lysosomes (Fig. 4.39a).

Any disruption in the formation of melanosome at the very early stage also can cause vacuole formation. This process initiates when specialized early endosomes bud off into spherical vacuoles which is to become stage I melanosomes (Fig. 4.39b).

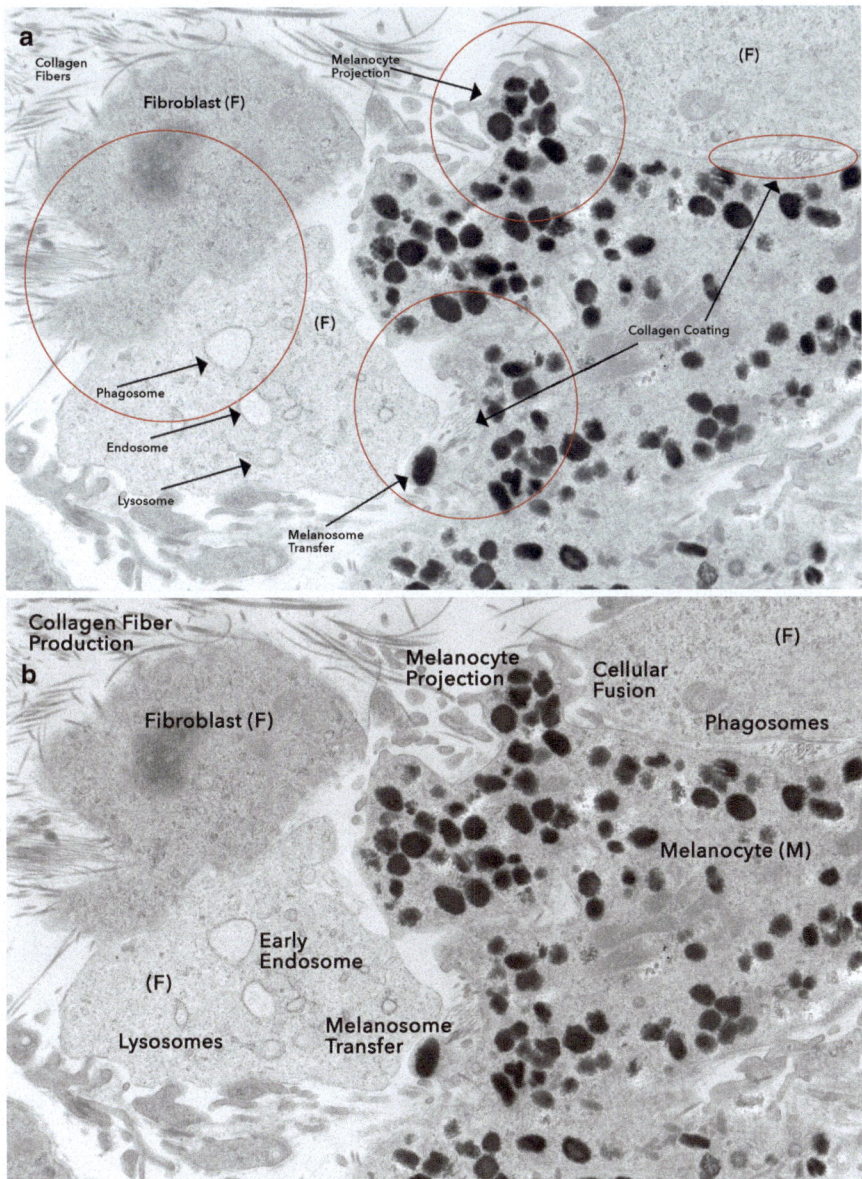

Fig. 4.39 (a) Electron microscopy ×5000. Blue iris. Fibroblast in direct contact interaction with melanocyte. This image illustrates the numerous lysosomes, endosomes, and phagosomes in fibroblasts. Collagen coating of melanocytes by fibroblasts are indicted with arrows. (b) Electron microscopy ×5000. Blue iris. Collagen formation by fibroblast, top left. Multiple stages of early endosome, phibromsome, and lysosome formation can be seen. Cell membrane fusion of fibroblast with melanocyte projections and exocytosis/endocytosis of melanosomes can be observed. (c) Electron microscopy ×15,000. Four stages of melanosome development

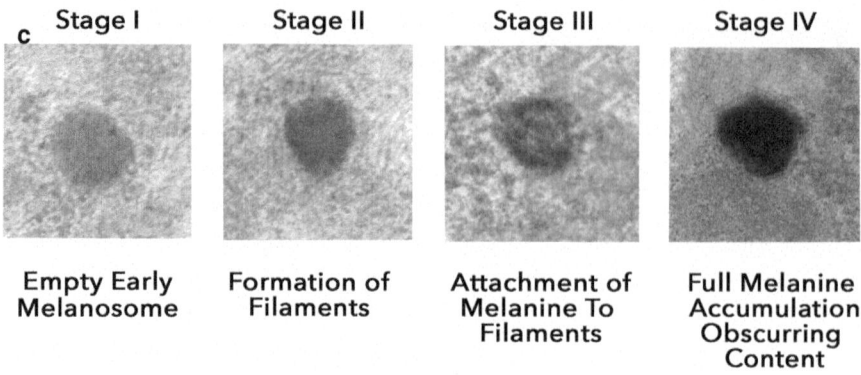

Stage I	Stage II	Stage III	Stage IV
Empty Early Melanosome	Formation of Filaments	Attachment of Melanine To Filaments	Full Melanine Accumulation Obscurring Content

Fig. 4.39 (Continued)

Another theory is that the early melanosomes get discarded by exocytosis and shedding before being able to complete the process of pigment transport and storage in the melanosomes preventing them to become stage IV melanosomes (Fig. 4.39c).

The formation of early coated vesicles starts at the cell membrane with the help of Clathrin protein which is a triskelion shape composed of three heavy chain and three light chain, which together form a polyhedral lattice that surrounds the newly formed vesicle (Fig. 4.40).

These vesicles are involved in multiple physiologic functions, from transport of cargo to endocytosis and exocytosis to formation of lysosomes and melanosomes (Fig. 4.41).

Some viruses and pathogens can use clathrin endocytosis system to enter the cell and transfer their genetic material inside the nucleus to reproduce and cause infection. Hepatitis C virus, for example, uses Clathrin endocytosis as the port of entry to the cell.

Reference: Meertens et al. [24]

By exploring the EM images of the blue irides one can observe that there are many varieties of incompletely processed melanosome/lysosome products exists at the same time in a melanocyte cytoplasm. This includes early and late stages of lysosomes, and all different stages of melanosomes <u>except</u> stage IV melanosomes which is very rare. This will give the impression that there are many genes and signaling pathways and proteins are involved in formation of the eye color and many are defected or mutated in the process of maturation. Other possibility is that the immature melanosomes being discarded by exocytosis and shedding before maturation to stage IV melanosomes being completed.

In molecular biology chapter we will discuss this process in detail [25].

There have been many studies on the ability of camouflage in certain fish and animals by changing the color of their skin according to the environment for example Octopus and Chameleon. It has been shown that by moving the melanosomes in the cytoplasm of the melanocytes, to and from the nucleus, the reflective light ray changes its frequency and results the emitted color to change. The skin gets darker

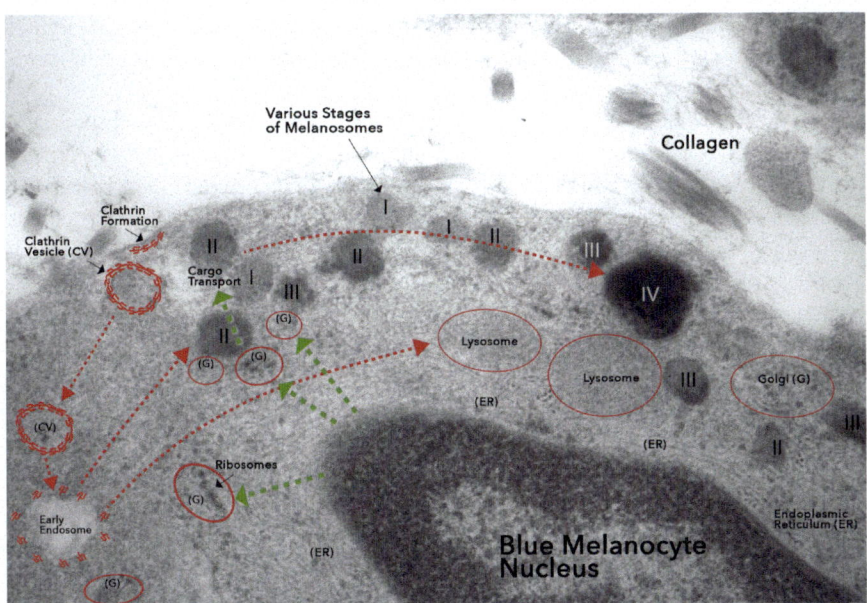

Fig. 4.40 Electron microscopy ×25,000. Blue iris. The process of melanogenesis starting with formation of clathrin to clathrin vesicle to early endosome. The formation of melanosomes and lysosomes can be observed

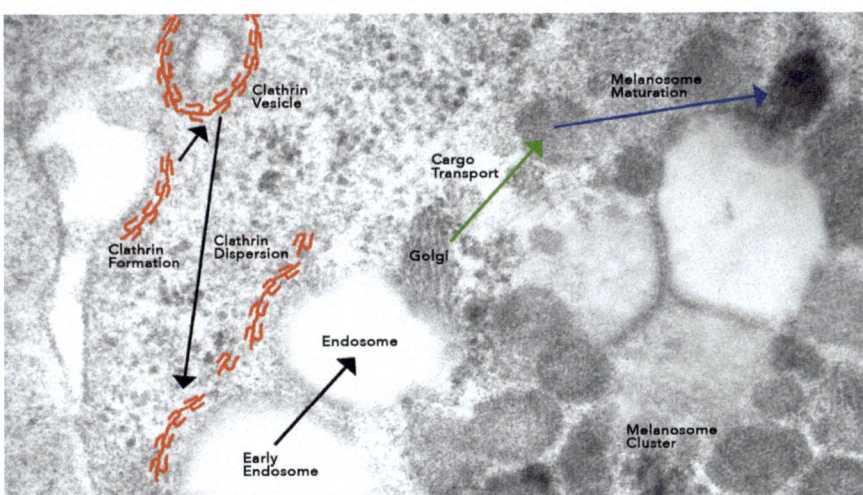

Fig. 4.41 Electron microscopy ×40,000. Blue iris. The whole spectrum of the melanogenesis can be observed in this image. The process from membrane clathrin, vesicle formation to early and late endosome formation, and golgi cargo transport to maturation of melanosomes all have been illustrated

when pigmented melanosomes moves close and around the nucleus and get lighter when pigmented melanosomes spread in the periphery by dispersion in the cytoplasm away from the nucleus.

The melanosomes are carried by intracellular microtubule motor– family to and from the nucleus for camouflage purposes in these animals. Kinesin and Dynein are motor proteins that use microtubules in anterograde and retrograde movements.

It is interesting to see that the location of the melanosomes is closer to the nucleus in melanocytes of the darker irides, and more spread in the cytoplasm and at the periphery of the melanocytes of the light irides. In contrast in human iris these melanosomes are not moving back and forth and are stable or very slowly moving to the periphery as seen in blue irides and as the result the reflected color of the iris is not changing (Fig. 4.27a, b).

In Human skin the melanosomes are transported to the periphery into the cytoplasmic projections in order to be transported to the surrounded keratocytes. Therefore, there is an outward movement of the pigment cargo to the periphery. The Iris melanocytes have cytoplasmic projections and transfer pigment cargo instead into fibroblasts and macrophages.

Interesting observation is that the fully pigmented melanosomes (stage IV) are formed in the cytoplasm of melanocytes of the black/dark brown iris and remain there or maybe transported later on close to the nucleus. This is not a case in the blue eyes, as the incompletely formed melanosomes are transported to the periphery of the cytoplasm where they remain or transfer out by different mechanisms as will be described later.

Melanosome transport is similar to the universal organelle transport system and composed of cytoskeleton motors, adaptors, effectors and microtubule/actin filaments. This process that is called motor/cargo interaction can be summarize as follows:

Cytoskeleton motors (Kinesin, Dynein, Myosin) molecules have the motor section that binds to the microtubule/actin filaments and generates force by ATP hydrolysis to move in cytosol, and cargo binding terminal that attaches to melanosomes for cargo transport in the cytosol.

- Kinesin is a motor protein that move along microtubule towards its positive end to the periphery away from the nucleus and is called anterograde transport.
- Dynein is a motor protein that also move along microtubule but towards its negative end next to the nucleus and is called retrograde transport.
- Myosin Va (Myosin Type V in melanocytes) moves along filamentous actin (F-Actin) and usually away from the nucleus and is involved in dispersion of the melanosomes [26].

Although these processes have been elucidated in classic melanocytes such as skin melanocytes, there are no studies to verify their action in the iris melanocytes considering that there very short projections in these melanocytes and there is minimal pigment transfer to the surrounding cells.

Hypothetical theory that one can come up with by these observations is that there is a prominence of Dynein activity in dark iris that accumulates the melanosomes around the nucleus to protect DNA from the harmful UV radiation. Also, there is a prominence of Kinesin and MyosinVa in blue iris that causes the peripheral location and dispersion of melanosomes in their cytoplasm and possible exocytosis and shedding [27].

The stage of maturation is also a major component of the color differences. The melanosomes of dark color eyes are mainly stage IV which the melanosomes are filled with melanin. This is the result of complete task of melanosome biogenesis and maturation without interruption. This process is summarized as follows (Fig. 4.39):

- Stage I: Formation of spherical vacuole by budding off the early endosomes.
- Stage II: Cleavage and formation of anchoring sheets for melanin attachment by MART-1 and PMEL accordingly.
- Stage III: Formation of melanin by TYR, TYRP 1 and TYRP 2 which are packed within Golgi and transported by AP-3 and or AP-1 clathrin coated transport vesicles to melanosomes and attaches to the premelanosome protein (PMEL) induced fibrils.
- Stage IV: The melanin attachment to the PMEL fibrils is being completed and is the result the melanosomes become darkly pigmented and looks like an opaque structure.

PMEL gene is regulated by microphthalmia-associated transcription factor (MITF) in the melanocyte nucleus. After PMEL transfer to melanosomes it will be fragmented to small sections and will produce non-toxic striated amyloid sheets the base for melanin attachment.

In the blue iris this process is incomplete in many stages. The melanosomes are varying from stage I and II and occasional stage III melanosomes, rarely a single incomplete stage IV can be seen in the light color eyes (Fig. 4.27a, b).

The number of fibroblasts on the surface of the iris is very variable and as the result the amount of secreted collagen fibers correlates with the color of the iris. The collagen is produced by fibroblasts (Fig. 4.42).

There are many layers of fibroblasts on the surface of the light color eyes and very few to almost none on the surface of the very dark color eyes. There is a thick fluffy layer of collagen that coats the surface of the blue eye but does not exist on the surface of the dark color irides. The nodules of Wolfflin which is an accumulation of collagen in the surface of blue eyes does not exist in the brown/dark color eyes. The collagen absorption of the red wavelength portion of the full light spectrum causes the reflected rays looks blue as we see in blue nevus example in which the melanin pigment from the nevus that located deep in the dermis of the skin appears blue or the red blood content of blood vessels in the skin looks blue. To emphasize, the appearance of melanin and hemoglobulin that is reflected as blue, when they are located in the deeper layers of the dermis that reflected light has to pass through the collagen and intercellular matrix is due to the same phenomenon.

The blue iris surface layers of collagen can easily be observed by naked eye and/ or by any magnifying devices and on the slit lamp examination. The production of collagen on the surface of the blue eyes will show as whitish blue/white strands,

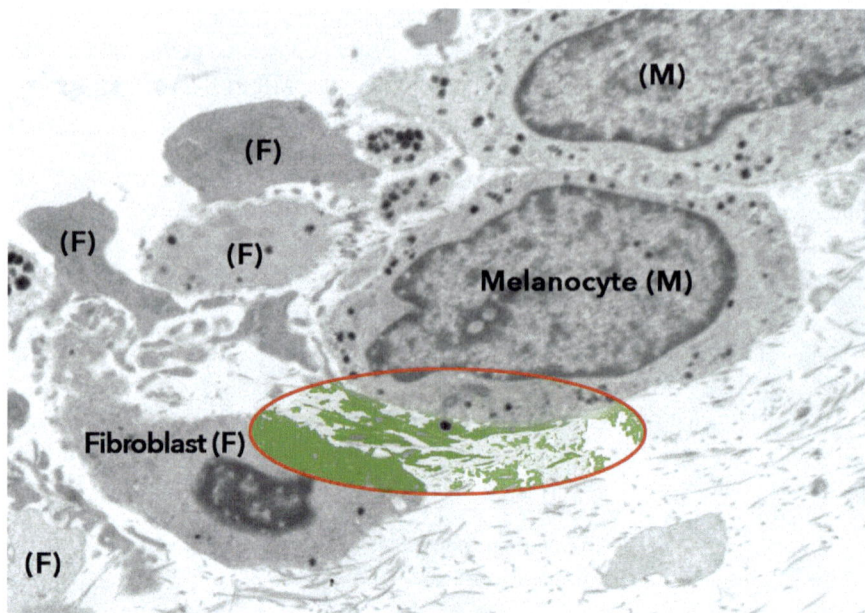

Fig. 4.42 Electron microscopy ×25,000. Blue iris. Collagen coating of melanocytes by fibroblasts are shown in green and circled in red

fluffs and meshwork. The collagen content of the cornea also has an important role on the absorption of the red portion of the reflected wavelengths and as the result the color of the eye. In case of a very dark iris no light reflects back, so the collagen contents of the cornea are irrelevant. In the blue eyes the majority of the light reflects back since it is not absorbed by stroma melanin, as the result the collagen content of iris surface and the participation of the cornea becomes more effective. As we see in the attached pictures when the cornea is removed surgically, the appearance of the iris changes significantly and the color differences become less prominent (Fig. 4.1).

The number and density of pigment Melanin is the same in double layered IPE (Iris Pigment Epithelium) located on the posterior surface of the Iris in all different color eyes.

There are many melanosomes in different stages of maturation that exist in blue eye melanocyte cytoplasm which is not the same as in the dark color eyes. The cytoplasm of the dark eye melanocytes is filled with mature melanosomes.

The lysosomes have the same ancestors as melanosomes as the fate of the off-spring is dictated by the genetic inheritance.

The cytoplasmic vacuoles of the very dark irides are not common in blue eyes. These vacuoles have been reported as the result of aging or increased intraocular pressure [28].

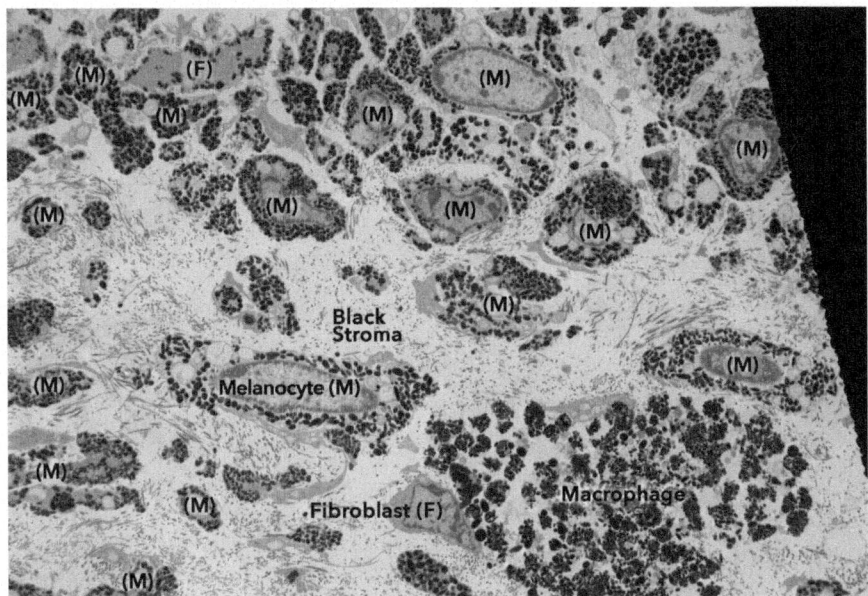

Fig. 4.43 Electron microscopy ×1000. Black iris. Multiple mature melanocytes with stage IV melanosomes occupying the stroma can be seen with a minimal stromal interstitial matrix and collagen

The intra cytoplasmic vacuoles can be due to variety of origins. Usually they are lysosomal origin and can be due to exocytosis or endocytosis or due to autophagy and non-autophagy processes which involves the cell death and survival (Fig. 4.27a).

Lee et al. [29]

Shubin et al. [30]

Number of mitochondria seems more in the blue eyes. As the cytoplasm of the dark melanosome is filled with stage IV melanosomes that obscures the observation of other structures.

Finger like projections are more prominent in blue eyes. No Explanation was found on this observation.

Stromal melanocytes are very rare in blue eyes. There are many stromal melanocytes with high melanin content in the melanosomes in the entire thickness of dark color iris. This makes the dark brown color of the entire thickness of the iris. The anterior surface of the stroma, the stroma and the double layers of post iris pigment epithelium all heavily pigmented in dark color eyes.

This explains unsuccessful attempts to laser ablation of anterior surface of the iris in order to change the color of the eye of very dark irides (Fig. 4.43).

It is important to emphasize that:

1. In dark irides, stroma macrophages, melanocytes and fibroblasts that contain melanin particles, occupying the entire stroma and they are filled with stage IV melanosomes.

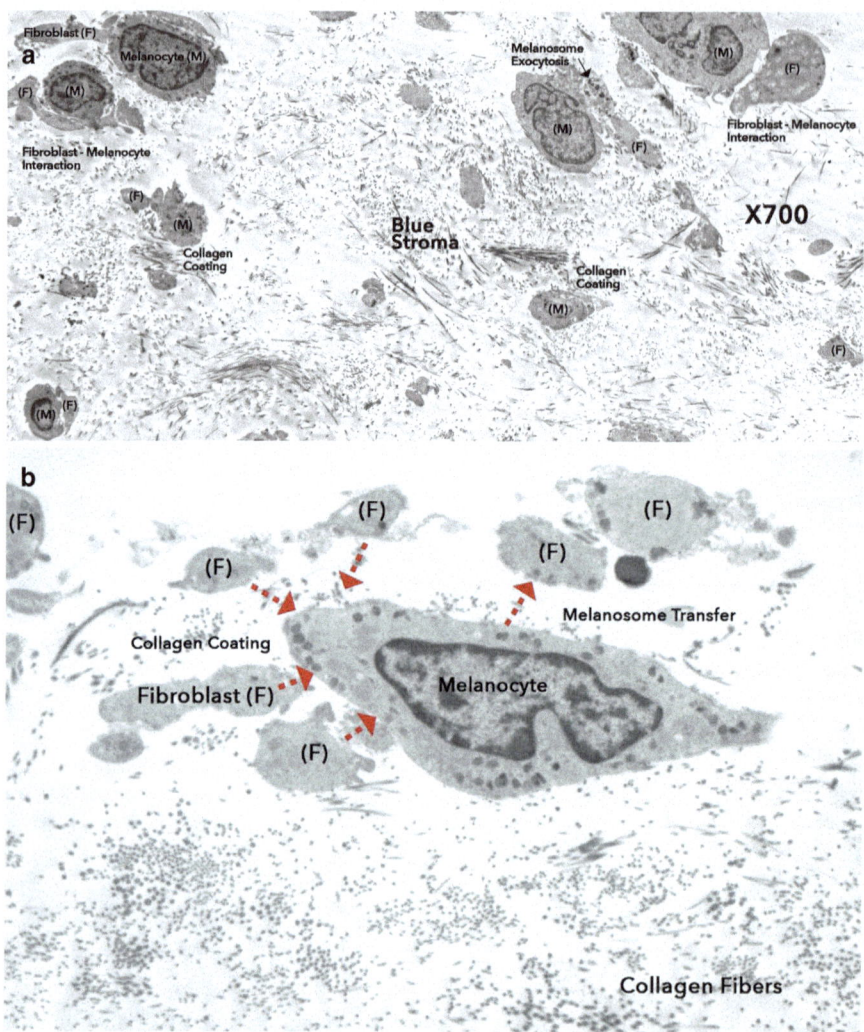

Fig. 4.44 (**a**) Electron microscopy ×700. Blue iris. Few scattered melanocytes with early stages of melanosomes occupying the stroma can be seen with abundant interstitial matrix and collagen in between. (**b**) Electron microscopy ×1200. Blue iris. Fibroblast collagen production and coating of melanocyte. Melanosome shedding by melanocyte and endocytosis by fibroblast are marked by the red arrows

2. In Blue irides, the stroma is not saturated with melanocytes and macrophages and there is a vast number of Fibroblasts which produce extracellular collagen and extracellular matrix in the stroma (Fig. 4.43)

Stromal collagen fibers are minimal in the dark eyes as the number of fibroblasts are less and as the result, production of the collagen is less.

Blue iris stroma is less cellular but contains abundant fibroblasts that produce a lot of collagen fibers and intercellular matrix (Fig. 4.44a, b).

Conclusion

In Conclusion the electron microscopic or ultra-structure of the middle and front portion of the iris is very variable and is responsible for the color variation of the reflected light, in contrast the posterior portion structure of the iris is constant and does not show variation in different iris colors (Fig. 4.45).

Incomplete melanosome maturation and lysosomes at the periphery of the cyto-plasm of the blue iris melanocytes that are in the close proximity and contact with the fibroblast can be observed in the reference images.

Phagocytosis of a cluster of melanosomes by fibroblast can also be seen in the red circle (Fig. 4.46).

The internalization/phagocytosis of melanosomes by skin fibroblasts have been reported.

Kohda et al. [31]

Enhancement of collagen deposition and cross-linking by coupling lysyl oxidase with bone morphogenetic protein-1 and its application in tissue engineering have been described by Rosell-Garcia et al. [32].

In the following recent article, the importance of autophagy is elucidated in the skin, fibroblasts and melanocytes. There are no references or studies on autophagy in the iris, fibroblasts and melanocytes. We hope that there will be more studies on these topics regarding the iris [33].

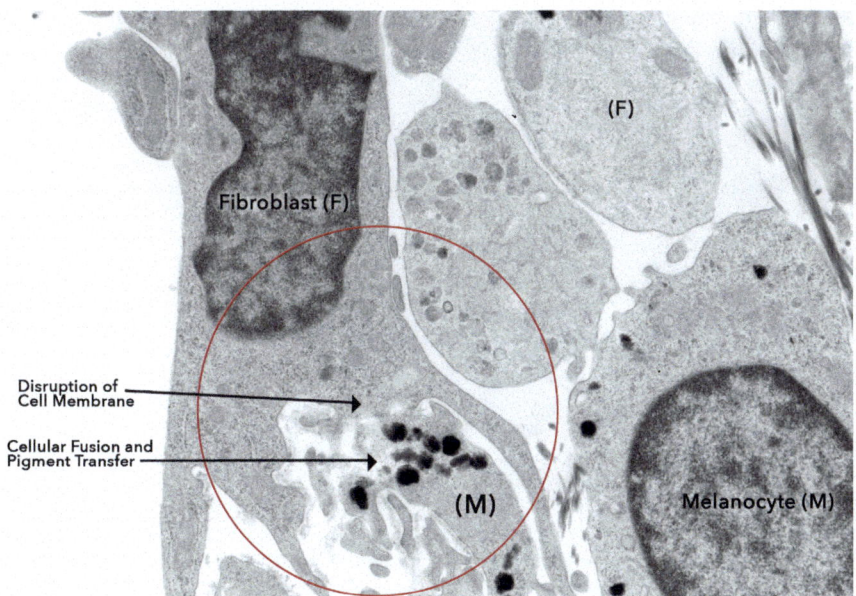

Fig. 4.45 Electron microscopy ×6000. Blue iris. Membrane fusion between melanocyte and fibro-blast for melanosome transfer, circled in red

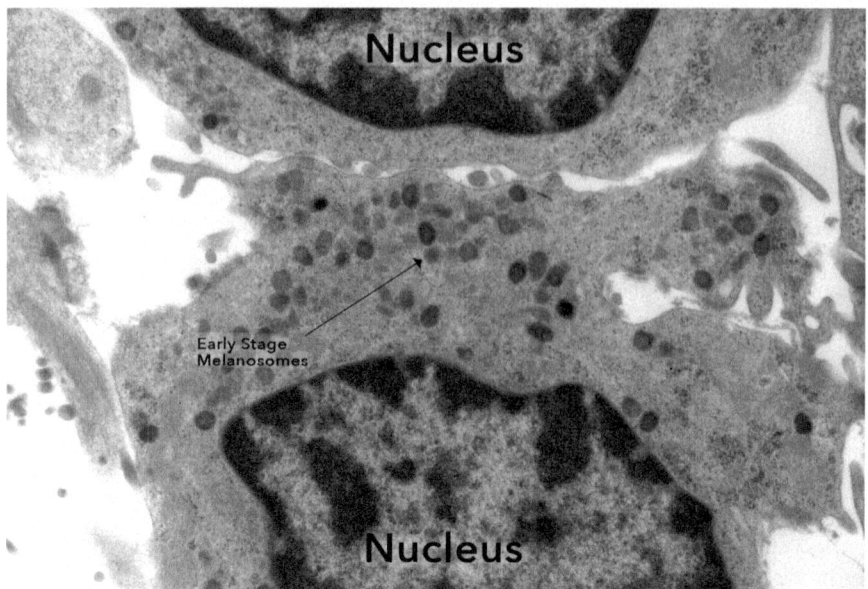

Fig. 4.46 Electron microscopy ×10,000. Blue iris. Melanosomes adjacent to each other with scattered immature stages I, II, and III melanosomes

Bibliography

1. Imesch PD, Bindley CD, Khademian Z, Ladd B, Gangnon R, Albert DM, Wallow IH. Melanocytes and iris color: electron microscopic findings. Arch Ophthalmol. 1996;114(4):443–7. [Online]. Available at: https://www.ncbi.nlm.nih.gov/pubmed/8602783.
2. Wilkerson CL, Syed NA, Fisher MR, Robinson NL, Albert DM. Melanocytes and iris color: light microscopic findings. Arch Ophthalmol. 1996;114(4):437–42. https://doi.org/10.1001/archopht.1996.01100130433014. [Online]. Available at: https://jamanetwork.com/journals/jamaophthalmology/article-abstract/641593.
3. McCartney AC, Riordan-Eva P, Howes RC, Spalton DJ. Horner's syndrome: an electron microscopic study of a human iris. Br J Ophthalmol. 1992;76(12):746–9. [Online]. Available at: https://doi.org/10.1136/bjo.76.12.746.
4. Stuart-Fox D, Moussalli A, Whiting MJ. Predator-specific camouflage in chameleons. Biol Lett. 2008;4(4):326–9.
5. Akkaynak D, Siemann LA, Barbosa A, Mäthger LM. Changeable camouflage: how well can flounder resemble the colour and spatial scale of substrates in their natural habitats? R Soc Open Sci. 2017;4(3):160824.
6. Kural C, Serpinskaya AS, Chou YH, Goldman RD, Gelfand VI, Selvin PR. Tracking melanosomes inside a cell to study molecular motors and their interaction. Proc Nat Acad Sci. 2007;104(13):5378–82. [Online]. Available at: https://www.pnas.org/content/104/13/5378.
7. Reilein AR, Serpinskaya AS, Karcher RL, Dujardin DL, Vallee RB, Gelfand VI. Differential regulation of dynein-driven melanosome movement. Biochem Biophy Res Commun. 2003;309(3):652–8. [Online]. Available at: https://www.ncbi.nlm.nih.gov/pubmed/12963040.
8. Wang Y, Viennet C, Robin S, Berthon JY, He L, Humbert P. Precise role of dermal fibroblasts on melanocyte pigmentation. J Dermatol Sci. 2017;88(2):159–66. [Online]. Available at: https://doi.org/10.1016/j.jdermsci.2017.06.018. Epub 2017 Jul 1.

9. Hedley SJ, Layton C, Heaton M, Chakrabarty KH, Dawson RA, Gawkrodger DJ, Neil SM. Fibroblasts play a regulatory role in the control of pigmentation in reconstructed human skin from skin types I and II. Pigment Cell Res. 2002;15(1):49–56. [Online]. Available at: https://onlinelibrary.wiley.com/doi/full/10.1034/j.1600-0749.2002.00067.x

10. Wu X, Hammer JA. Melanosome transfer: it is best to give and receive. Curr Opin Cell Biol. 2014;29:1–7. [Online]. Available at: https://doi.org/10.1016/j.ceb.2014.02.003.

11. Xu Z, Chen L, Jiang M, Wang Q, Zhang C, Xiang LF. CCN1/Cyr61 stimulates melanogenesis through Integrin α6β1, p38 MAPK, and ERK1/2 signaling pathways in human epidermal melanocytes. J Invest Dermatol. 2018;138(8):1825–33. [Online]. Available at: https://doi.org/10.1016/j.jid.2018.02.029. Epub 2018 Mar 3.

12. Üstün Y, Reibetanz M, Brachvogel B, Nischt R, Eckes B, Zigrino P, Krieg T. Dual role of laminin-511 in regulating melanocyte migration and differentiation. Matrix Biol. 2019;80:59–71. [Online]. Available at: https://doi.org/10.1016/j.matbio.2018.09.006.

13. Noor O, Elston D, Flamm A, Hall LD, Cha J. A recurrent melanocytic nevus phenomenon in the setting of Hailey–Hailey disease. J Cutan Pathol. 2015;42(8):574–7. [Online]. Available at: https://doi.org/10.1111/cup.12511.

14. Kim NH, Choi SH, Lee TR, Lee CH, Lee AY. Cadherin 11 involved in basement membrane damage and dermal changes in melasma. Acta Derm Venereol. 2016;96(5):635–41. [Online]. Available at: https://doi.org/10.2340/00015555-2315.

15. Singh P, Carraher C, Schwarzbauer JE. Assembly of fibronectin extracellular matrix. Annu Rev Cell Dev Biol. 2010;26:397–419. [Online]. Available at: https://doi.org/10.1146/annurev-cellbio-100109-104020.

16. Baranska A, Shawket A, Jouve M, Baratin M, Malosse C, Voluzan O, Vu Manh TP, Fiore F, Bajénoff M, Benaroch P, Dalod M, Malissen M, Henri S, Malissen B. Unveiling skin macrophage dynamics explains both tattoo persistence and strenuous removal. J Exp Med. 2018;215(4):1115–33. [Online]. Available at: https://doi.org/10.1084/jem.20171608.

17. Guerra L, Odorisio T, Zambruno G, Castiglia D. Stromal microenvironment in type VII collagen-deficient skin: the ground for squamous cell carcinoma development. Matrix Biol. 2017;63:1–10. [Online]. Available at: https://doi.org/10.1016/j.matbio.2017.01.002.

18. Sugita A, Ishibashi R, Shiotani N, Yoshioka H. Morphological features of iris fibroblasts in dilator muscle region. Jpn J Ophthalmol. 1988;32(2):151–8. [Online]. Available at: https://www.ncbi.nlm.nih.gov/pubmed/3184548.

19. Fuchs E. Normal pigmentierte und albinotische iris. Graefes Arch Clin Exp Ophthalmol. 1913;84/85:521. [Online]. Available at: https://link.springer.com/article/10.1007%2FBF02080373?LI=true.

20. Dieterich CE. The fine structure of melanocytes in the human iris. Graefes Arch Clin Exp Ophthalmol. 1972;183(4):317–33. [Online]. Available at: https://link.springer.com/article/10.1007%2FBF00496159.

21. Eagle Jr RC. Iris pigmentation and pigmented lesions: an ultra-structural study. Trans Am Ophthalmol Soc. 1988;86:581–687. . [Online]. Available at: https://www.ncbi.nlm.nih.gov/pmc/articles/PMC1298824/.

22. Prota G, Hu DN, Vincensi MR, McCormick SA, Napolitano A. Characterization of melanins in human irides and cultured uveal melanocytes from eyes of different colors. Exp Eye Res. 1998;67(3):293–9. [Online]. Available at: https://doi.org/10.1006/exer.1998.0518.

23. Imesch PD, Wallow IH, Albert DM. The color of the human eye: a review of morphologic correlates and of some conditions that affect iridial pigmentation. Surv Ophthalmol. 1997;41:S117–23. [Online]. Available at: https://doi.org/10.1016/S0039-6257(97)80018-5.

24. Meertens L, Bertaux C, Dragic T. Hepatitis C virus entry requires a critical postinternalization step and delivery to early endosomes via clathrin-coated vesicles. J Virol. 2006;80(23):11571–8. [Online]. Available at: https://doi.org/10.1128/JVI.01717-06.

25. Liggins MC, Flesher JL, Jahid S, Vasudeva P, Eby V, Takasuga S, Sasaki J, Sasaki T, Boissy RE, Ganesan AK. PIKfyve regulates melanosome biogenesis. PLoS Genet. 2018;14(3):e1007290. PLOS Genetics. [Online]. Available at: https://doi.org/10.1371/journal.pgen.1007290.

26. Byers HR, Yaar M, Eller MS, Jalbert NL, Gilchrest BA. Role of cytoplasmic dynein in mela-nosome transport in human melanocytes. J Invest Dermatol. 2000;114(5):990–7. [Online]. Available at: https://doi.org/10.1046/j.1523-1747.2000.00957.x.
27. Robinson CL, Evans RD, Sivarasa K, Ramalho JS, Briggs DA, Hume AN. The adaptor pro-tein melanophilin regulates dynamic myosin-Va: cargo interaction and dendrite develop-ment in melanocytes. Mol Biol Cell. 2019;30(6):742–52. [Online]. Available at: https://doi.org/10.1091/mbc.E18-04-0237.
28. Zinn KM, Mockel-Pohl S, Villanueva V, Furman M. The fine structure of iris melano-somes in man. Am J Ophthalmol. 1973;76(5):721–9. [Online]. Available at: https://doi.org/10.1016/0002-9394(73)90568-0.
29. Lee WJ, Chien MH, Chow JM, Chang JL, Wen YC, Lin YW, Cheng CW, Lai GM, Hsiao M, Lee LM. Nonautophagic cytoplasmic vacuolation death induction in human PC-3M prostate cancer by curcumin through reactive oxygen species-mediated endoplasmic reticulum stress. Sci Rep. 2015;5:10420. [Online]. Available at: https://doi.org/10.1038/srep10420.
30. Shubin AV, Demidyuk IV, Komissarov AA, Rafieva LM, Kostrov SV. Cytoplasmic vacuoliza-tion in cell death and survival. Oncotarget. 2016;7(34):55863. [Online]. Available at: https://doi.org/10.18632/oncotarget.10150.
31. Kohda H, Ishikawa M, Ishii H, Ando H, Ichihashi M, Nishikata T. Studies on the melanosome-phagocytic activity of Human Dermal Fibroblast (HDF). J Dermatol Sci. 2016;84(1):e178. [Online]. Available at: https://doi.org/10.1016/j.jdermsci.2016.08.524.
32. Rosell-Garcia, F. Rodriguez-Pascual. Enhancement of collagen deposition and cross-linking by coupling lysyl oxidase with bone morphogenetic protein-1 and its application in tissue engineering. Scientific Reports. 2018;8(1).
33. Wang Y, Wen X, Hao D, Zhou M, Li X, He G, Jiang X. Insights into autophagy machinery in cells related to skin diseases and strategies for therapeutic modulation. Biomed Pharmacother. 2019;113:108775. [Online]. Available at: https://doi.org/10.1016/j.biopha.2019.108775.

Chapter 5
Molecular Biology of Iris

Abstract The iris main cellular residents are fibroblasts and melanocytes similar to the skin, with the exception or lack of Keratinocytes in the iris. There are constant molecular cross talking and interactions between these cells via paracrine, and autocrine messaging. In order to understand these interactions, the comparison of iris and skin seems crucial and relevant.

The activity of melanocytes very much depends on their neighboring cells and their receptors. In the skin melanocytes are mainly interact with skin cells "keratinocytes" and the role of fibroblasts are important but limited. In the Iris due to the lack of keratinocytes, the main interaction of melanocytes is with fibroblasts. The Iris melanocyte receptors are also different from skin melanocytes. The main and most prominent receptor in skin melanocytes are the family of MC1R which gets activated by ACTH and alpha MSH, which is non-functioning or do not exist in Iris melanocytes. The variants of MC1R have been discussed in the literature in skin melanocytes but not in iris melanocytes.

The signaling pathways will elucidate in molecular level, what happens in iris tissue due to different physiological or pathological phenomenon.

Another major difference is that the skin melanocytes have active and functioning prostaglandin FP receptors, yet the iris melanocytes lack FP receptors and their interaction with Prostaglandins are depend on FP receptors from adjacent fibroblasts.

Examples are the lack of changes in the color of the iris by sun exposure, or the iris color changes due to use of prostaglandin analogue for treatment of glaucoma. Other examples of iris color changes in humans are the color changes associated with viral infections such as Ebola, or iris color change due to the lack of sympathetic innervation of the iris as have been described in Horner's syndrome, which will be discussed in this chapter.

Finally, the role of basement membrane and fibroblasts on melanocytes hemostasis and biogenesis are discussed as an important paracrine factor.

Discussion

Molecular Biology is the future of medical science. As we are entering this new era of science, more information becomes available every day and many unsolved questions are being answered.

Due to complexity of the molecular pathways and their interactions, only simplified versions and essentials relevant to the iris will be discussed here. The comparison of iris to the skin is necessary and is only to facilitate better understanding of this organ.

Due to the fact that the majority of the bulk of iris is made of fibroblasts, melanocytes, and Iris Pigment Epithelium (IPE). Reviewing of the molecular biology of these cellular structures are very crucial to understand iris molecular biology and thus its structure and appearance.

Molecular Development of Iris

The development of the iris is a complex process. The anatomic developmental process has been discussed earlier in chapter on embryology.

In this chapter we review the molecular biology of the iris development. The main pathways for this process are Retinoic Acid (RA), Pitx2 and Wnt regulatory pathways [39]:

Anterior chamber formation starts with the migration of the Neural Crest (NC) mesenchyme and expression of Foxc1, Foxc2, Lmx1b and Pitx2.

First step is the involvement of RA/PITX2/Wnt which is associated with the migration of the neural crest mesenchyme between the newly formed lens vesicle and the Surface ectoderm.

After organization and condensation of the mesenchyme the gene expression of Foxc1, Foxc2, Lmx1b, and Pitx2 are required to develop the anterior segment.

Retinoic acid, the Metabolite of Vitamin A is an essential autocrine and paracrine signaling molecule that binds to the nuclear receptors that activates necessary transcription factors.

Nuclear receptors for RA are from different protein molecular structures:

- Retinoic Acid Receptors (RAR) alpha, Beta, y. These proteins bind to both all-trans and 9-cis-RA
- Retinoid X Receptors (RXR) Alpha Beta, y. which bind only to 9-cis-RA.

Cellular Receptors and Signaling Pathways

In order to focus on molecular biology of the Iris we have to identify the specific cells and their receptors and their cellular communications and their signaling transduction pathways.

The following subjects will be discussed to better understand the iris structural variation and its color dissimilarity:

- Fibroblasts
- Melanocytes
- Macrophages
- Surface receptors
- Melanogenesis process
- Essential relevant molecular signaling pathways such as (MITF and PI3K/ Akt, Etc.)
- Viral effect and endocytosis
- PGA's effect
- Inflammatory cascade
- Malignant transformation

As we mentioned earlier the comparison of Iris structure with the skin will help to clarify and facilitate the understand of the basics. What is unique about the structure of the iris and as a result its reflected color, can be greatly elucidated by molecular biology.

Literature references to melanocytes studies have been mainly focused on skin melanocytes and little attention have been paid on iridial melanocytes. Iridial melanocytes which are part of Uveal melanocytes, behave very differently from the other melanocytes in many aspects. There are also physiologcal and structural differences between the iridial melanocytes of different eye colors.

To understand many of these unanswered questions regarding the structural differences of iris melanocytes and the variety of eye colors we have to pay attention to the following questions:

- Why the eye color does not change (tan) similar to the skin by sun exposure?
- Why the color of the iris changes with certain glaucoma drops (Prostaglandin analogues).
- Why the color of the eye changed in some patients with Ebola infection.
- Why the color of the eye changes in Horner's syndrome.
- Why it is so difficult to change the color of the eye by medications or small molecules.

The color of the skin is directly and mainly depending on the amount of melanin pigment in the specific organelles called melanosomes that are located in the cytoplasm of the pigment cells called melanocytes and also depends the amount of pigment that has been transferred by melanocytes to their adjacent skin cells, Keratinocytes (Fig. 5.1a–c).

The color of the iris is a much more complex phenomenon and not only depends on the amount of Melanin pigment in the melanocytes of the anterior surface of the Iris but also depends on many other cofactors in which we will discuss in detail in this chapter.

The skin and the iris have both melanocytes with the same embryonic origin. They both are originating from Neural Crest (NC) and then migrate via mesoderm to their very different final destinations. The new settlements which for the skin melanocytes are on the basement membrane in the basal layer of the epidermis

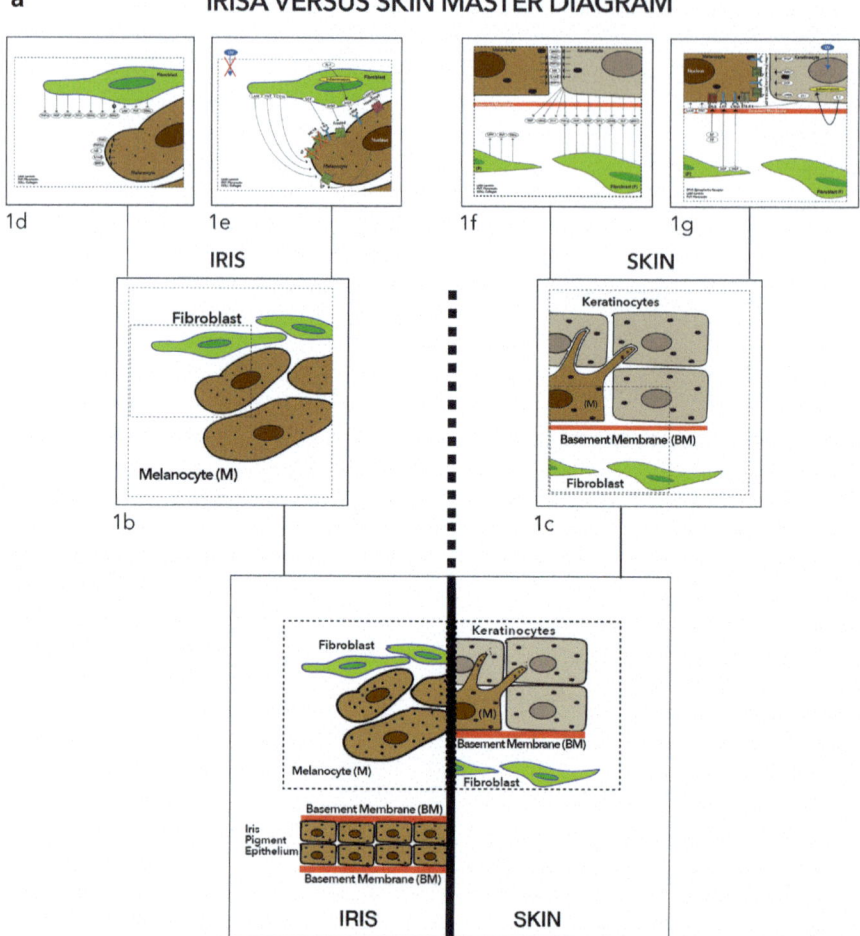

Fig. 5.1 (**a**) Illustrated comparison of iris versus skin protein synthesis and receptors magnified in stages. (**b**) Cellular residence of both the iris and skin are shown for comparison. Emphasis is placed on the location of the basement membrane and its relationship to the neighboring cellular structures. (**c**) Magnified portion of the iris structure image. The emphasis is on the proximity of the different cellular structures (Melanocytes [M] and fibroblasts). (**d**) Magnified portion of the skin structure. The emphasis is on the proximity of the different cellular structures (Melanocytes [M], keratinocytes, and fibroblasts). (**e**) Summary of molecular synthesis by individual cells in the iris. Molecular synthesis of fiberblasts and melanocytes are only by direct contact. The role of the basement membrane is played by the fibroblast in the iris. (**f**) Schematic figure of iris melanocyte receptors and the effect of fibroblasts on melanocytes. (**g**) Summary of molecular synthesis by individual cells in the skin. Molecular synthesis of fiberblasts and melanocytes can infiltrate through the basement membrane, whereas the interaction between the keratinocytes and melanocytes are by direct contact. (**h**) Schematic figure of skin melanocyte receptors and the effect of keratinocytes and fibroblasts on melanocytes

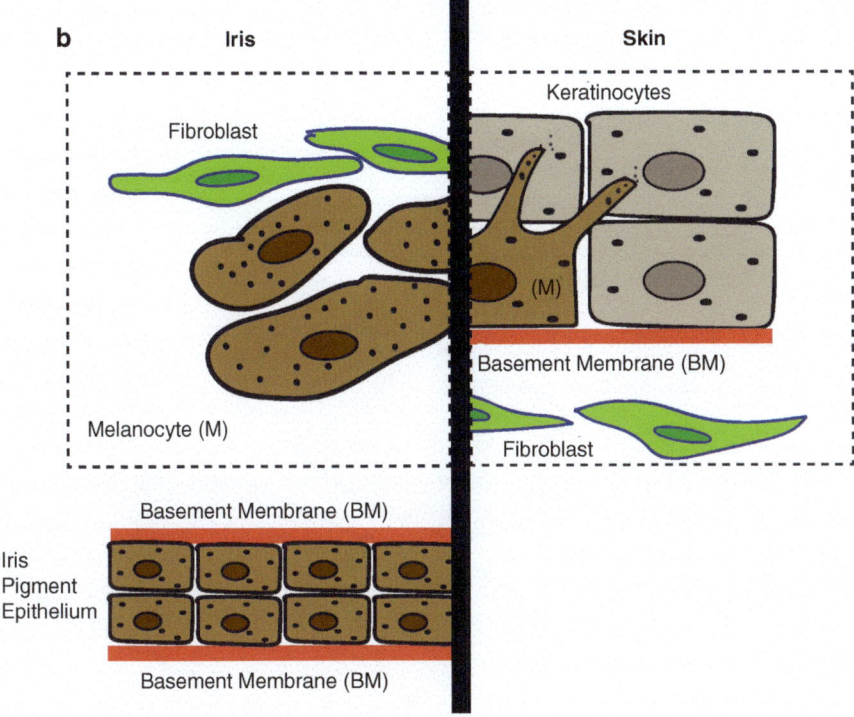

Fig. 5.1 (continued)

c   **Iris fibroblast-melanocyte interaction**

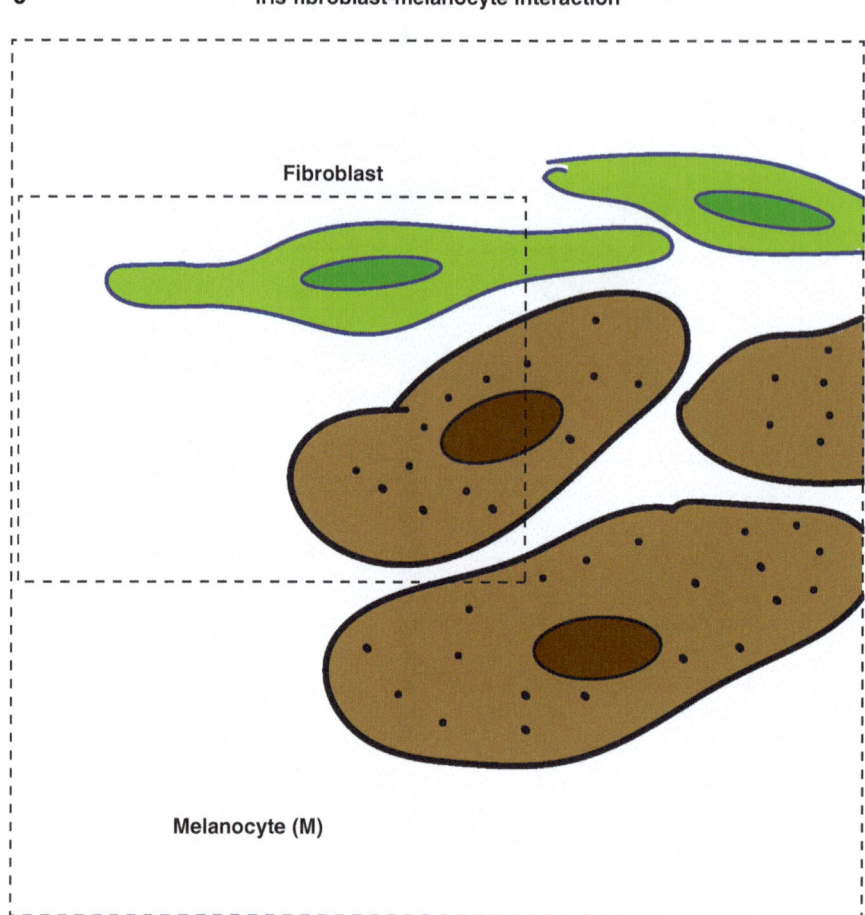

Fig. 5.1 (continued)

d   **Skin fibroblast-melanocyte interaction**

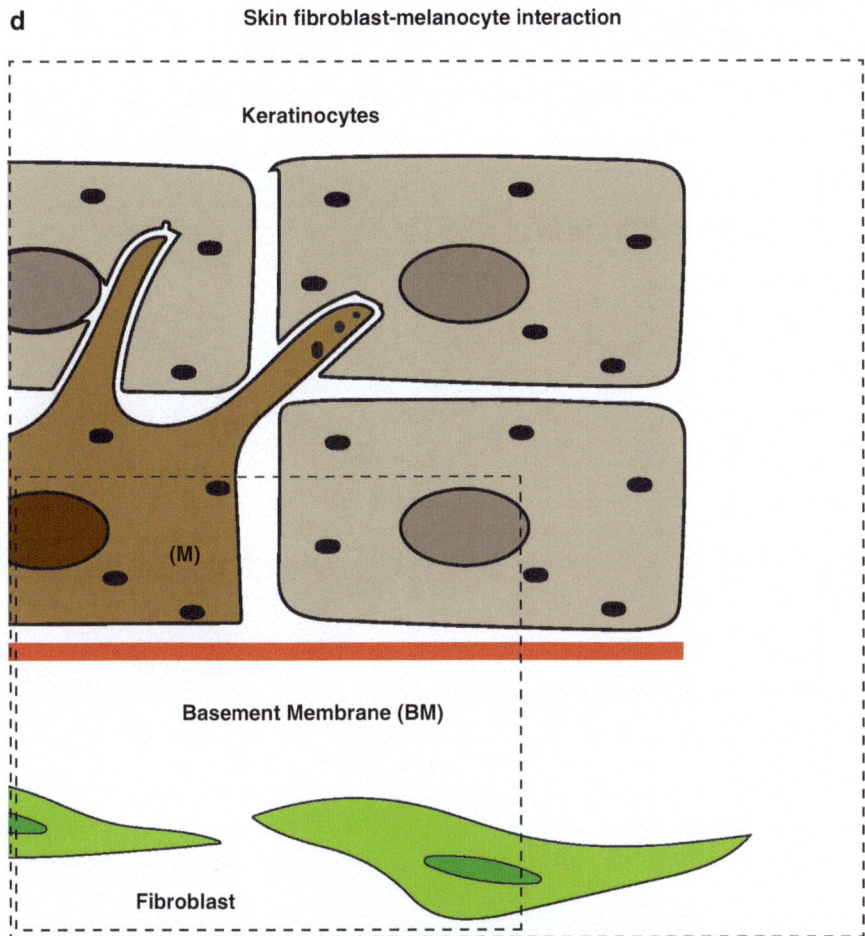

Fig. 5.1 (continued)

e   **Mollecular synthesis by iris melanocytes & fibroblasts**

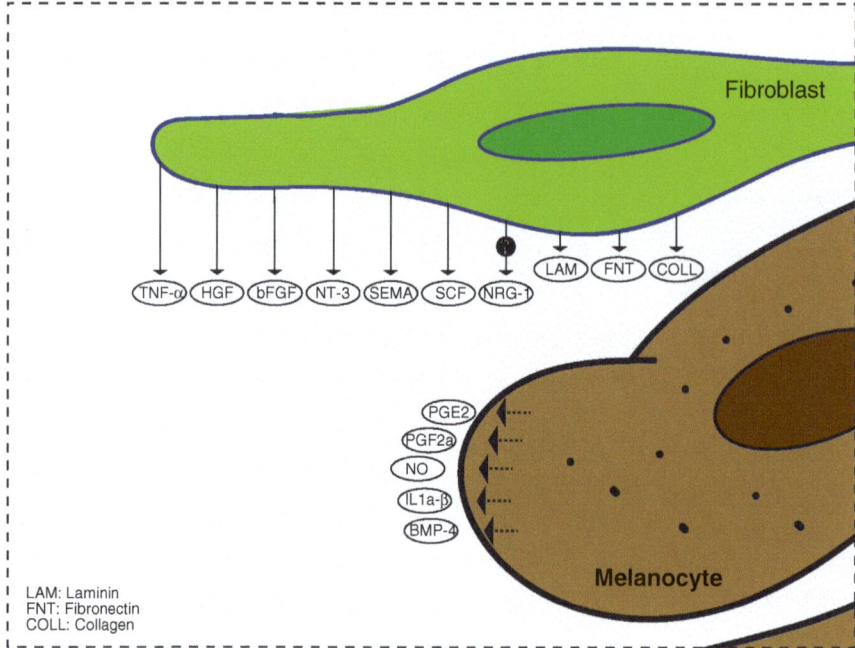

f   **Iris melanocyte receptors**

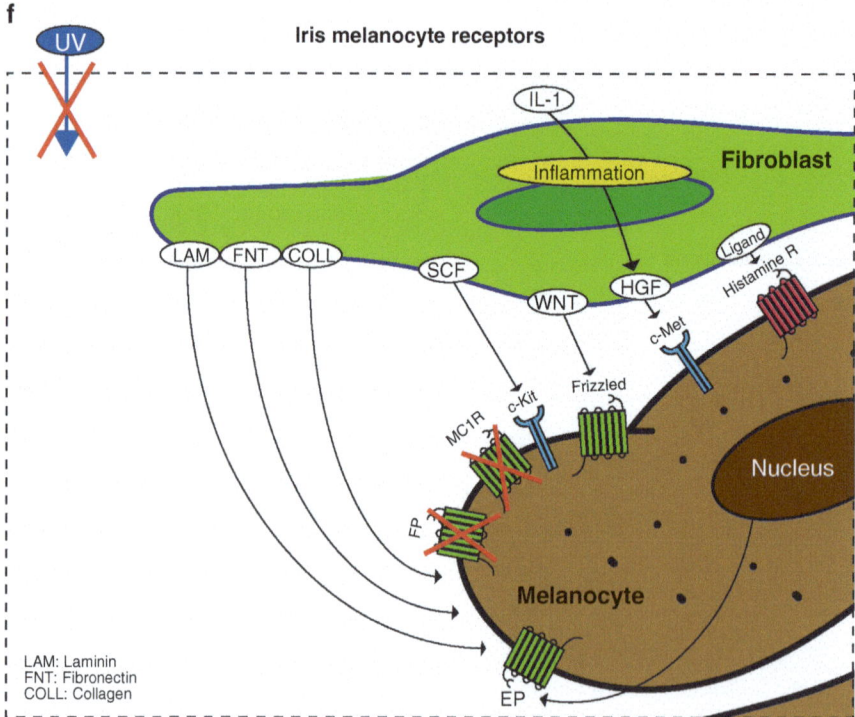

Fig. 5.1 (continued)

g   **Mollecular synthesis bykeratinocytes,
                              melanocytes & fibroblasts**

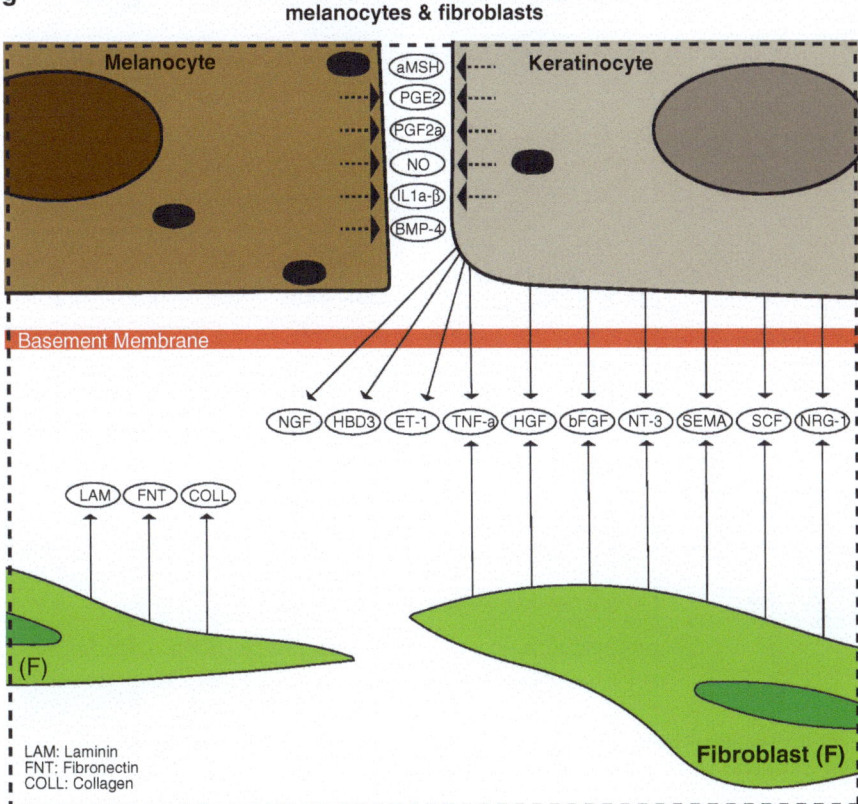

Fig. 5.1 (continued)

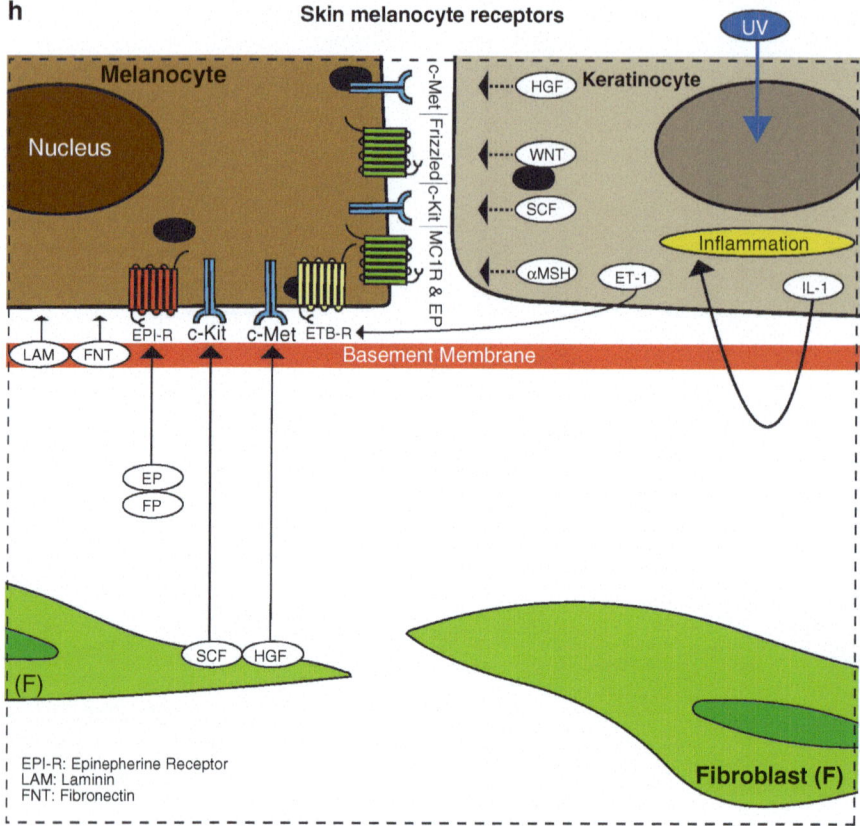

Fig. 5.1 (continued)

and for the iris melanocytes are in the iris stroma specially in the anterior layer of iris stroma.

Molecular biology explains the answer to the above questions by reviewing the molecular structures and interactions that resulting in different behavior and function between the skin and Iris melanocytes. Many parts of the process of the molecular biology of embryology of the iris from "Neural Crest Development" and their migration [26] to their final destination and finally their interaction to their microenvironment and cell to cell communications with their specific receptors have been discovered in recent years [24].

The fundamental differences in melanocytes are being discussed in the iris of different colors in this chapter and also in other chapters of this book.

The scope of molecular biology has become so vast and complex that cannot be discussed in full detail in this chapter. Here the summary and the relevance of this complex system to the iris is being discussed that can be helpful to more general audiences rather than molecular biologists. This includes other fields of science and technology and visual sience profesionals and practitioners such as ophthalmologists and medical students.

Iris Fibroblasts

Iris fibroblasts like all connective tissue cells originates from primitive mesenchyme. It's the most common type of cell in human connective tissue. It produces the collagen and extracellular matrix (EM) that is the structural framework of the iris. The ability of these cells in tissue structure formation and wound healing make them a very important cells in the body in general [2].

Fibroblasts are spindle shape cells with the oval nucleus in the center with elongated processes that attach to other cells, as shown in (Fig. 4.33).

Fibroblast function can be summarized and not yet completed as new information is being discovered as time goes by: (Fig. 5.1d–f)

- Formation of collagen I and III fibers Vimelin, Tropocollagen (Matrix)
- Production of extracellular matrix (glycoproteins & polyssacarides) the ground substances surrounding the collagen fibers.
- Production of Laminin and Fibronectin similar to basement membrane (BM) which controls and interacts with melanocytes.
- Constant paracrine and direct contact interaction with melanocytes.
- Interactive function in tissue repair in wound healing process (limited in Iris).
- Ability to endocytose and phagocytose similar to macrophages.
- Paracrine communication with surrounding cells including melanocytes via Hepatic growth factor (HGF) Stem cell factor (SCF) basic fibroblast growth factor (bFGF), Neurotrophine 3(NT3), Semaphorin 7a, Neuregulin-1 (NRG-1) (Fig. 5.1d–f)
- Multiple surface receptors (Fig. 5.1–g)
- Facilitate angiogenesis
- Stablish 3-dimensional space for other cells to move in.
- Fibroblasts are easy to culture in the laboratory make them valuable for research.
- Fibroblasts transfection is a commonly used method in research in molecular and cell biology.
- Similar to leukocytes, Fibroblasts are able to directly mobilize by expression of Formyl Peptide Receptors (FPR) that can cause calcium mobilization, actin polymerization, and adhesion [53].

Fibroblast growth factors (FGFs) are a family of many different ligands that bind with variable affinity to different FGF receptors [55].

Iris Melanocytes

In General melanocytes are protective pigmented cells that migrate from neural crest to their final destination in different organs. They have a common characteristic and yet at the final different destinations they adopt their new specifications according their neighboring tissues.

The common characteristics are:

- Synthesis of melanin

- Storage of melanin in special organelles called melanosome.
- Synthesis of autocrine and paracrine signaling products (Fig. 5.1d, f).
- Multiple specific receptors (Fig. 5.2a, b).
- Low proliferation potential
- Long life span almost immortal
- Resistant to apoptosis by expression of protein Bc12
- Potential to become malignant (Melanoma)

The specific characteristics are mainly due to their paracrine networking with surrounding cells.

These communications cause very different functional and behavioral response to their environment.

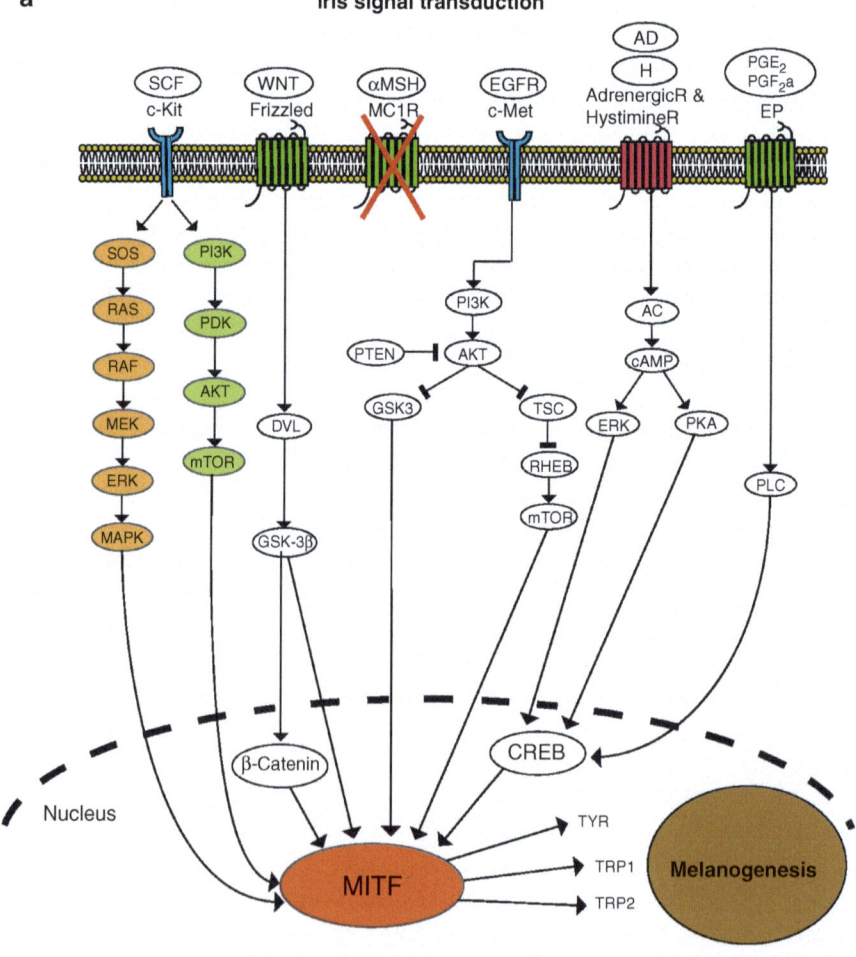

Fig. 5.2 (**a**) Schematic figure of various pathways of signal transduction in iris melanocytes with the destination to MITF and induction of melanogenesis. (**b**) Schematic figure of various pathways of signal transduction in the skin melanocytes with the destination to MITF and induction of melanogenesis

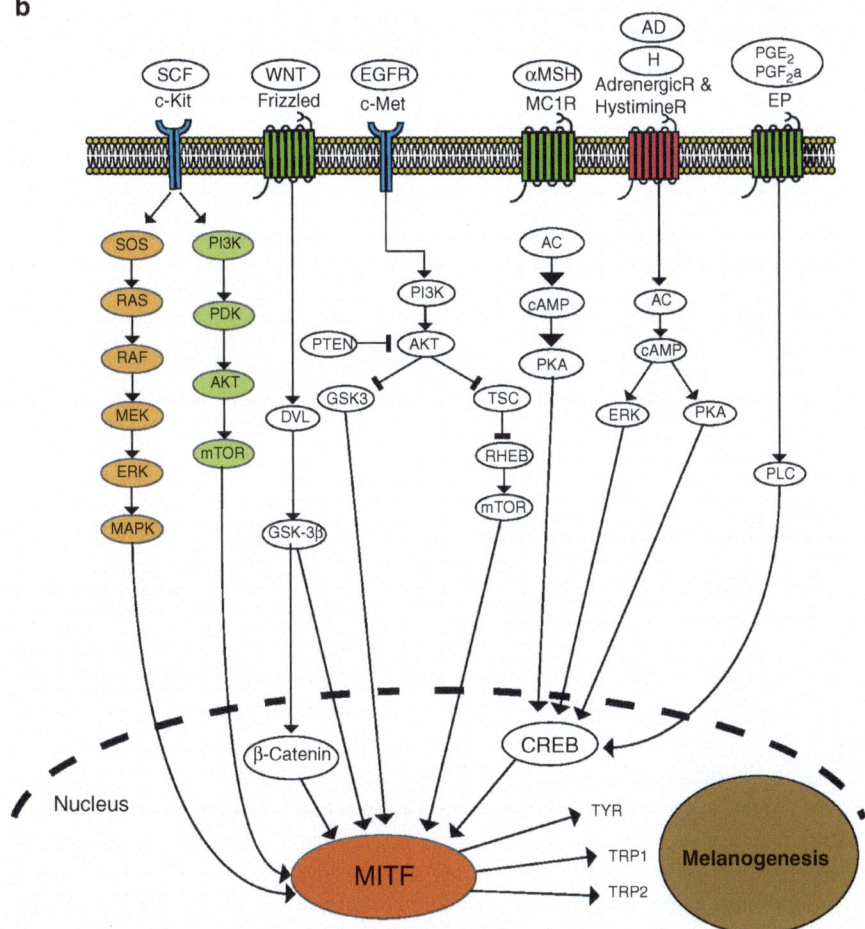

Fig. 5.2 (continued)

For example, iris melanocytes do not respond to the alfa-MSH and ACTH which are the main Hormonal stimulator of melanin formation in the skin melanocytes. Also, the lack of iris melanocytes response to UV light is correlated to lack of or non-functioning MC1R which is very abundant receptor in skin melanocytes. Lack of response MC1 Receptors in Uveal melanocytes was describe but there is no explanation for its nonfunctioning phenomena in the iris [28].

Iris melanocytes are from 2 different embryonic origins and have different functions. The melanocytes in the stroma originates from neural crest and migrate via mesoderm into the anterior iris border and stroma. The iris pigment epithelium that is a double layer of pigment epithelium that transported via neural ectoderm and is located on the posterior surface of the iris.

The stromal melanocytes are very variable in number and pigment content in different individuals with different eye colors but the iris pigment epithelium in contrast is packed with melanin containing melanosomes and does not change in different individuals with different eye colors.

Melanocytes carry the pigment melanin in their specific intra-cytoplasmic organelles called melanosomes. The process of pigment melanin synthesis and transport to the melanosomes will be discussed here. This complex phenomenon involves many steps and stages.

The most important evolutionary survival function of melanin is to protect the DNA from UV damage.

Melanocytes are generally classified into cutaneous and non- cutaneous type.

Cutaneous melanocytes:

• Epidermal melanocytes
• Dermal melanocytes

Non-Cutaneous melanocytes:

• Eye
• Inner Ear
• Heart
• Brain (Fig. 5.3)

There are many differences in the structures of melanocytes, specially between the cutaneous and iris melanocytes.

As we mentioned before what is unique about the iris melanocytes is that they are not very active as compare to skin melanocytes. Iris melanocytes are just maintaining their hemostasis and get influenced by surrounding fibroblasts by production of basement membrane like proteins and coating the melanocytes with collagen. As the result iris melanocytes are controlled by fibroblasts by their paracrine influence and by production of collagen, laminin and Fibronectin and by endocytosis of melanosomes and/or melanocytes. Adrenergic and cholinergic neurotransmitters, and macrophages also have direct effect on iris melanocytes.

External influences like the lack of neural stimulation, use of prostaglandin analogues (PGA's), viral infection and inflammation also affects the pigmentation of the iris which will be discussed in this chapter.

Starting with categorical differences, we include all differences between the skin versus iris melanosomes (Cutaneous vs non-cutaneous melanocytes).

In general, in molecular biology there are few important notations that deserve attention.

• Non-cutaneous melanocytes are not responsive to MC1R and are highly dependent on Endothelin3 (ET3) and Hepatocyte Growth Factor (HGF) signaling pathways and less dependent (although not totally independent) on Stem cell growth factor (SCF, c-KIT) signaling.
• Cutaneous melanocytes highly responsive to MC1R and are also dependent to KIT signaling and also responsive to ET3 and HGF [29].
• As we mentioned Iris melanocytes lack functional MC1R receptors in contrast to the skin melanocytes that has many functional MC1R receptors. Again, there is no description of the reason for the nonfunctioning phenomena [20].
• Lack of FP receptors in iris melanocytes [60], in contrast with skin melanocytes which respond to prostaglandin ligands.

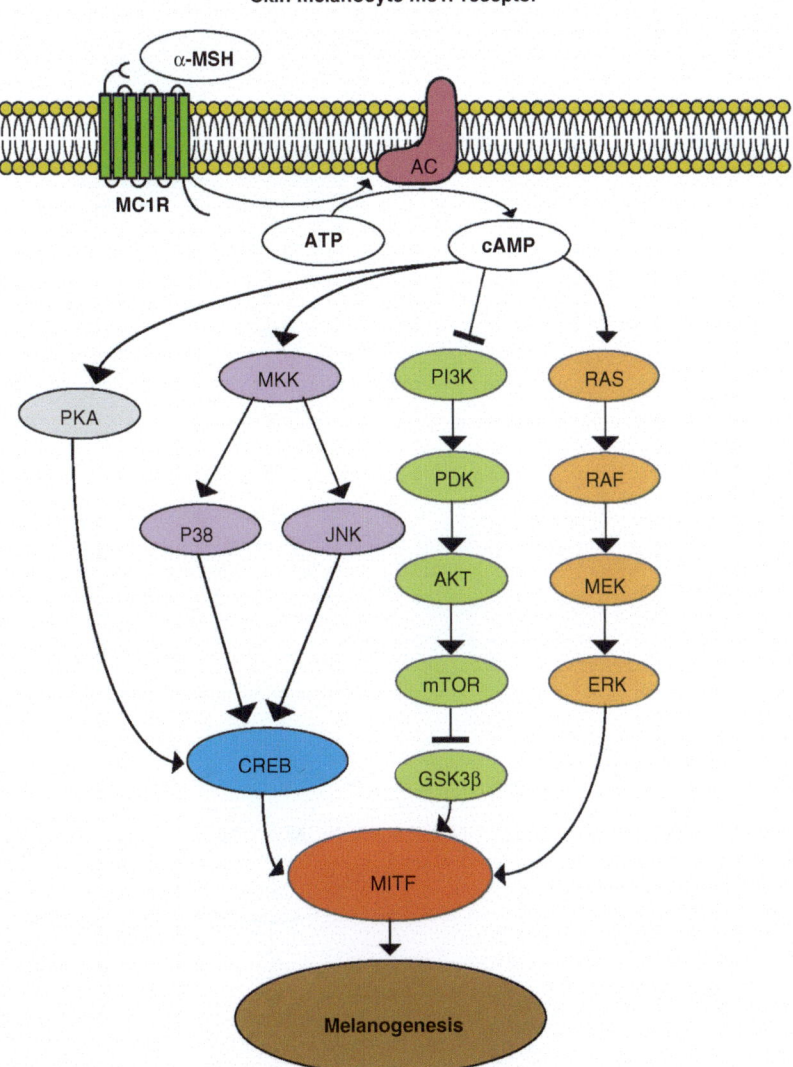

Fig. 5.3 Schematic figure of melanocortin 1 receptor transduction pathways with the destination to MITF with resultant melanogenesis

The importance of alpha-MSH- MC1R pathway is that by producing cAMP it triggers many different signal transduction pathways to produce melanin synthesis as shown in Fig. 5.3

- Cholinergic and adrenergic synapses exist between terminal nerve endings and iris melanocytes in the iris stroma. Interruption of theses communications can cause depigmentation of the iris as seen in Horner's syndrome (Fig. 5.4) [34].
- Neuronal contact with melanocytes of the iris would get activated by hormonal effect of epinephrine released from the synaptic vesicles on the melanocytes surface receptors [59].

Fig. 5.4 Neuro-
transmitter pathway.
Attachment of
adrenaline to the
G-protein coupled
neuroreceptor
activating adenylyl
cyclase to release
cAMP with the
destination to MITF

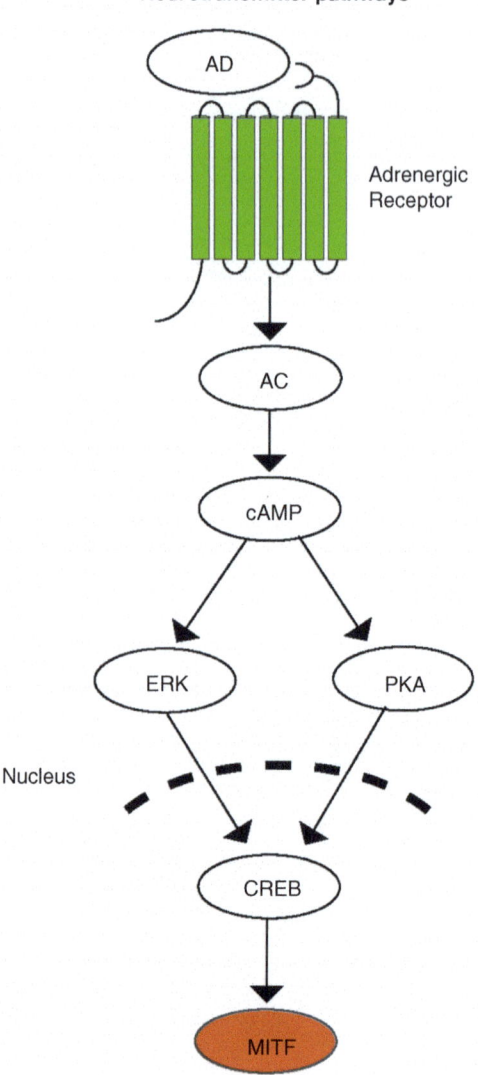

Neuroendocrine Functions of the Melanocyte

Skin melanocytes produce classical stress neurotransmitters, neuropeptides and
hormones, and this production is stimulated by ultraviolet radiation, biological factors and other agents that act within the skin neuroendocrine system. Specifically,
melanocytes produce corticotropin releasing factor (CRF) and related CRF receptors types 1 and 2 (CRF1 and CRF2). Signal transduction through the CRF receptors can proceed with different second messengers including cAMP, PI3k and Ca^{+2}
to regulate melanogenesis.

Skin melanocytes express proopiomelanocortin (POMC) that is processed to adrenocorticotropic hormone (ACTH), α-MSH and β-endorphin express MC1-R, MC2-R, MC-4, and opioid receptors.

Iris melanocytes response to neurotransmitters have been studied in animals with ability to change the color of their eyes due to stress, mating or for camouflage. In humans the slow process of depigmentation of the iris can occur as the result of sympathetic denervation of the iris such as in Horner's syndrome.

The neurotransmitter receptors in melanocytes are from the family of G protein-Coupled receptors (GPCRs). They composed of seven transmembrane receptors and are one of the largest receptor classes for drug targeting. The secondary messengers include: cAMP, PI3k and Ca^{+2} to regulate melanogenesis (Fig. 5.5).

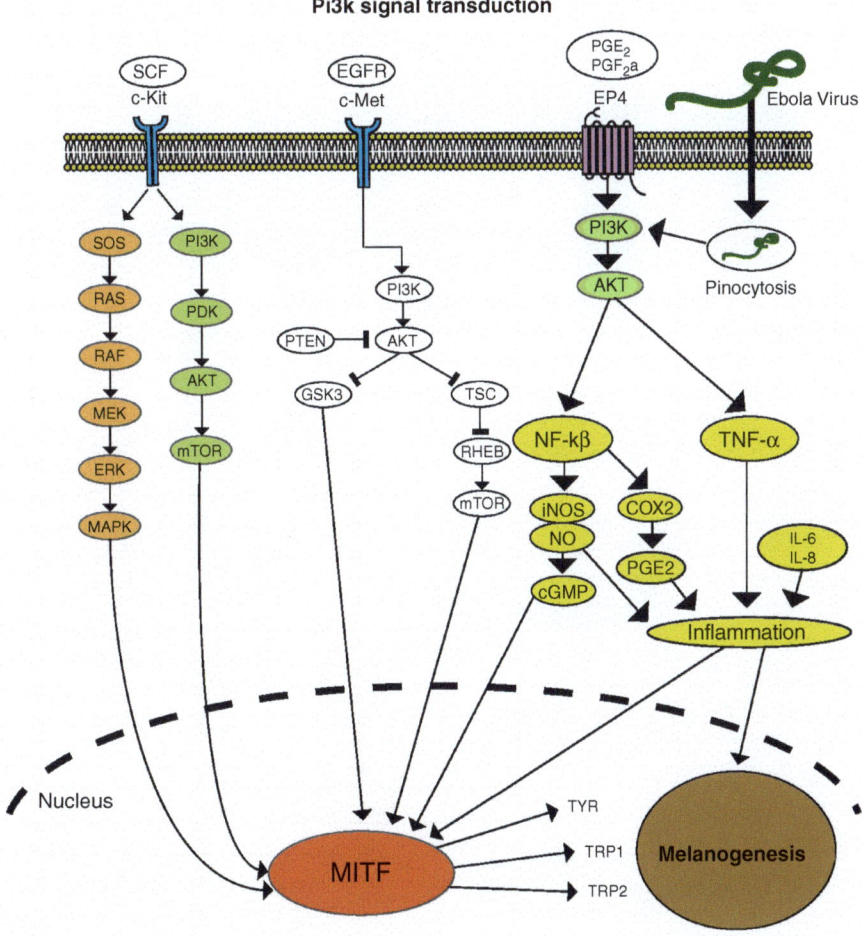

Fig. 5.5 Schematic figure of various pathways of signal transduction of PI3K pathways with the destination to MITF and induction of melanogenesis

There are many studies on the effect of prostaglandin analogs (PGA's) on melanocytes.

In one study [60], the role of fibroblasts discussed as the iris melanosomes responds to PGA's via the fibroblast receptors. These responses were through iris fibroblast FP prostaglandin receptors, Histamine receptors and IL receptors.

In general FP prostaglandin receptors and histamine receptors coupled to phospholipase C to generate cAMP to initiate melanogenesis. Iris melanocytes lack functionally active FP receptors (Fig. 5.6).

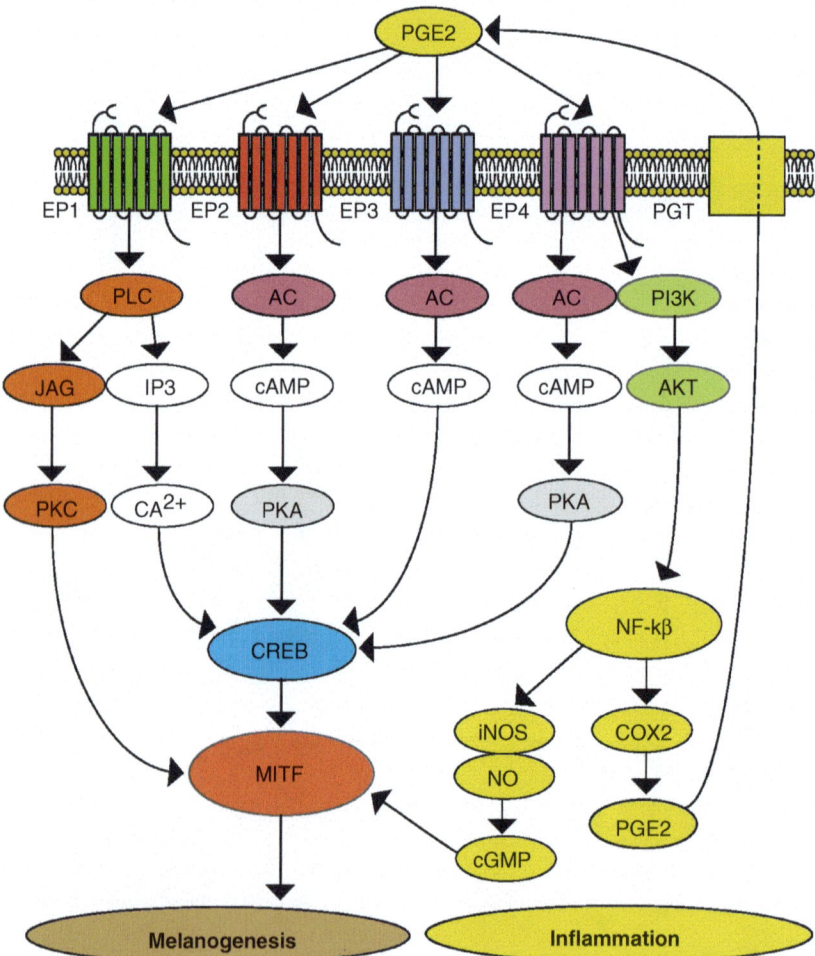

Fig. 5.6 Schematic figure of iris prostaglanden receptors with the destination to MITF with resultant melanogenesis and inflammatory signal transduction loop

There is a very important guideline for studying and research on iris melano-cytes as there is a need for co-culture of iris melanocytes with fibroblasts in order to evaluate the iris pigmentary change studies. This is due to limited receptor func-tion on iris melanocytes and the influence of fibroblasts.

Both iris melanocytes and fibroblasts in one study responded equally to endothe-lin 1 receptor (ET1) activation (Fig. 5.7) [56, 57].

The iris melanocytes do not respond to UV light due to lack of response to MC1R and there for to ACTH and will not change by exposure to the UV light. Also, the role of fibroblasts in this process has been discussed earlier.

It should be noted that the Iris freckle melanocytes behave more like a nevus melanocyte, which can change and increase in size by sun exposure.

A recent study proposed the association between iris freckle formation due to exposure to UV light as a biomarker for dermatological sun damage.

They have concluded that iris freckles can increase in number size and pig-mentation by sun exposure [52].

- Iris Melanocytes Paracrine receptors are responding to adjacent Fibroblasts in Connective tissue [56, 57].
- Skin Melanocytes Paracrine receptors are responding to adjacent Keratinocytes (Skin cells) with different receptors [23].

These different receptors have been summarized in (Fig. 5.1e, g) and will be discussed.

Macrophages

Macrophages have an important role in tissue hemostasis which includes:

- Clearance of apoptotic cells
- Phagocytosis of foreign material
- Growth factor secretion
- Pro-inflammatory cytokines production

Phagocyte Response initiates as an initial response to infection or insult such as injury or an acute inflammatory processes. The process is initiate by resident mac-rophages and dendritic cells that are previously present in affected tissues.

The initial inflammation cascade starts by secreting signaling proteins (cytokines and chemokines).

These cells are able to recognize the molecules that are linked to groups of the pathogens that releases from injured cells:

- Pathogen-associated molecular patterns (PAMPs)
- Damage-associated molecular patterns (DAMPs)

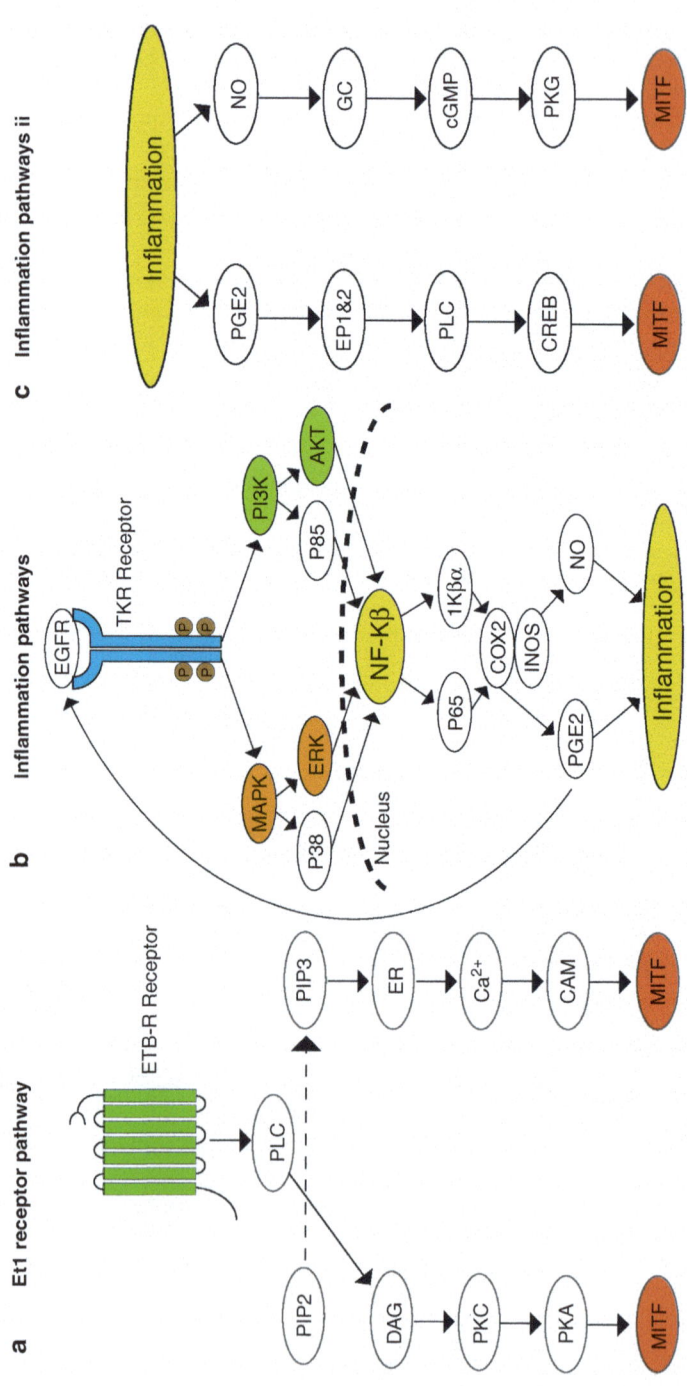

Fig. 5.7 (**a**) Schematic figure of ET1 receptor pathway with different destinations to MITF. There are different pathways leading from the ETB-Rt receptor, which is a variety of the G-protein coupled receptor. (**b**) Inflammatory pathways with activation of intranuclear NF-κβ and formation of endogenous PGE2 and NO, which can reactivate the receptor, as shown in the illustration above. (**c**) Downstream inflammatory pathway with activation of PGE2 and NO, with the destination to MITF, as shown in the illustration above

The surface receptors for these cells are:

- Pattern recognition receptors (PRRs), for example, phagocytic C-type lectin receptors.
- Scavenger receptors
- nucleotide-binding oligomerization domain-like receptors (NLRs)
- Transmembrane signaling Toll-like receptors (TLRs)
- Binding PRRs to PAMPs triggers immediate cellular and molecular response.

Macrophages release different toxic products that help phagocyte microorganisms.

- Antimicrobial peptides,
- Reactive nitrogen species (NO)
- Reactive oxygen species (ROS), such as superoxide anion
- Hydrogen peroxide (H_2O_2).

Macrophages also can activate other immune system cells and recruit them in an immune response and proteolytic activation of pro-inflammatory cytokines IL-1β and IL-18.

Macrophage Activation:

Macrophages have the ability to express variety of functional phenotypes in response to environmental signals. They can accordingly express receptor expression, effector function, cytokine and chemokine products.

- M1 Proinflammatory (Classic activation) by T helper cell 1(Th1) responses and IFNγ production: IFNγ, lipopolysaccharide, TNF, GM-CSF, or Toll-like receptor ligands
- M2 Anti-inflammatory (alternative activated): IL4, IL10, IL13, IL21, IL33, or TGF-β.

Resident and infiltrated macrophages play an important role in uveitis as effectors of innate immunity and inductors of acquired immunity [31].

Prostaglandin Receptors and Prostaglandin Analogues (PGA)

In recent years, there have been many synthetic derivatives of natural prostaglandin PGF2a that have become available in the market for the treatment of glaucoma. PGA's have powerful effect on lowering the intra ocular pressure in order to protect the nerve fiber layer of the retina and optic nerve [68].

Prostanoid receptors FP and EP (EP1, EP2, EP3, EP4) subtypes have different signal transduction pathways.

- FP and EP1 stimulate intracellular Ca+ and have constrictor properties.
- EP2 and EP4 activates Adenylate Cyclase (AC) and have relaxant properties.
- EP3 inhibits Adenylate Cyclase and have Constrictor properties.

The specific location and expression of FP and EP prostanoid receptors have been discussed [51] and location of these receptors have been identified in the ocular tissue (Fig. 5.6).

PGF2a is a ligand for FP receptor and its effect have many responses in the surrounding microenvironment which includes:

- Contraction of smooth muscles such as ciliary or trabecular meshwork.
- Remodeling of the extracellular matrix.
- Cytoskeletal alterations.
- Melanogenesis in the skin melanocytes by production of PGF2a which binds to FP receptor as an autocrine activation.
- Melanogenesis in the iris melanocytes is fibroblast dependent [60] probably by autocrine prostaglandin production by Cox2 and decreasing production of collagen, fibronectin and Laminin by fibroblasts.

In one study the effect of Latanoprost which is a (Prostaglandin analogue), a synthetic derivative of prostaglandin F2a (PGF2a) on nerve fibers was evaluated. The study revealed increased levels of Akt and mTOR expression through an FP receptor-mediated by modulation of the PI3K-Akt-mTOR signaling pathway (Fig. 5.5) [77].

In another study Latanoprost acid (PGF2a) effect was evaluated on the production of endogenous Prostaglandins in iridial melanocytes leading to increased pigmentation. This effect on melanogenesis was mediated by cyclo-oxygenase 2 (Cox2) and associated autocrine and paracrine signaling pathways [6].

latanoprost and travoprost are selective agonists for the prostaglandin F(2alpha) receptor [61].

There is a feedback loop in Cox-2 production of intracrine PGE2 uptake by the prostaglandin transporter (PGT) via hypoxia-inducible factor-1(HIF-1a) by increased epidermal growth factor transactivation. This amplification leads to activation of PI3K/AKT transduction pathway [32].

Signal Transduction Pathways in Melanocytes

The process of melanogenesis in melanocytes starts with the attachment of a ligand to the cell surface receptors. There are different receptors or receptor function in iris melanocytes as compare to skin melanocytes and due to close contact with fibroblasts, iris melanocytes can be influenced by using fibroblasts receptors in vivo. Again, this is a very important factor to be considered when studying melanogenesis in vitro to get accurate results.

The melanocytes most important surface receptors are:

- MC1R (Ligand = Adrenocorticotropin Hormone, ACTH & alpha-Melanocyte-stimulating Hormone, alpha-MSH)

  Structure: G-Protein-coupled receptor

Note: (non-functioning in iris melanocytes) (Fig. 5.3).

• Frizzled (Ligand = Wingless+Int-1, Wnt)

  Structure: G-Protein-coupled receptor (Fig. 5.8).

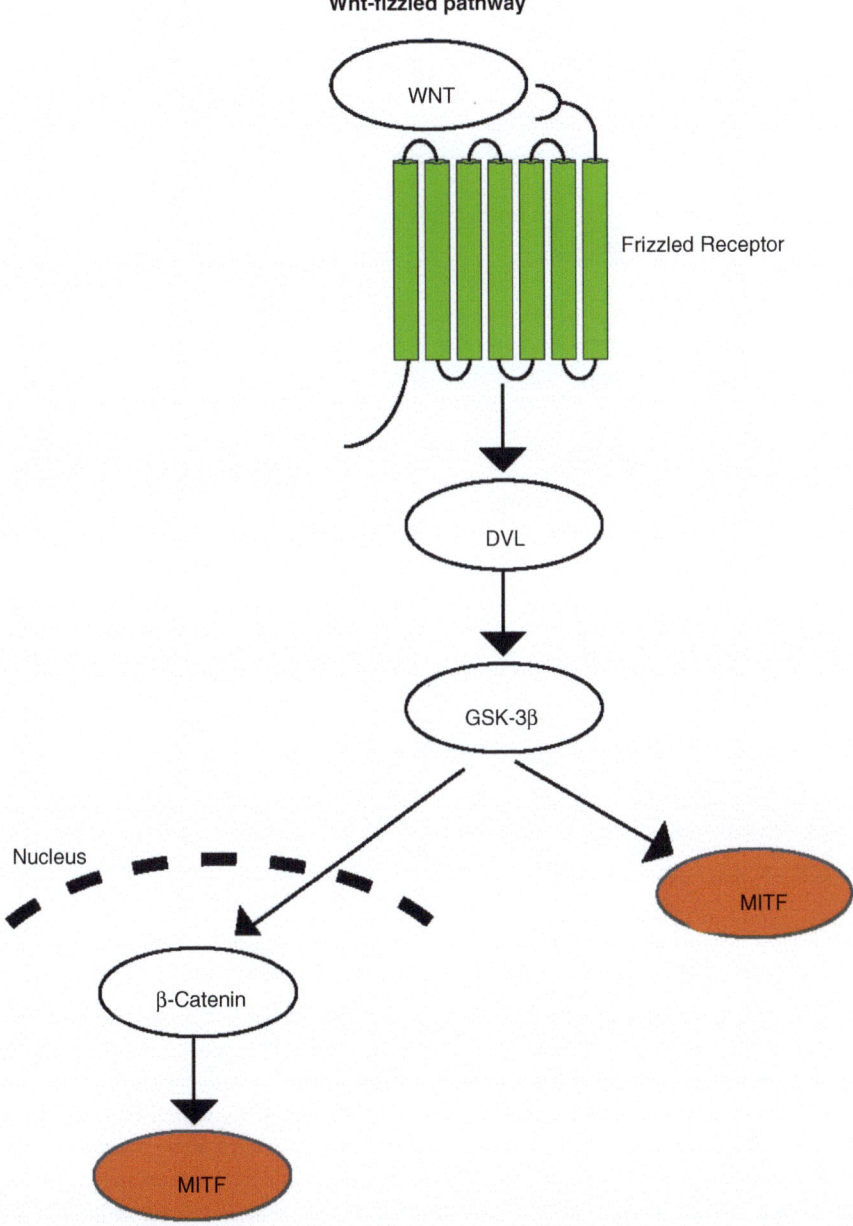

Fig. 5.8 WNT Frizzled pathway with different pathways leading from the Frizzled receptor, which is a G-coupled protein receptor

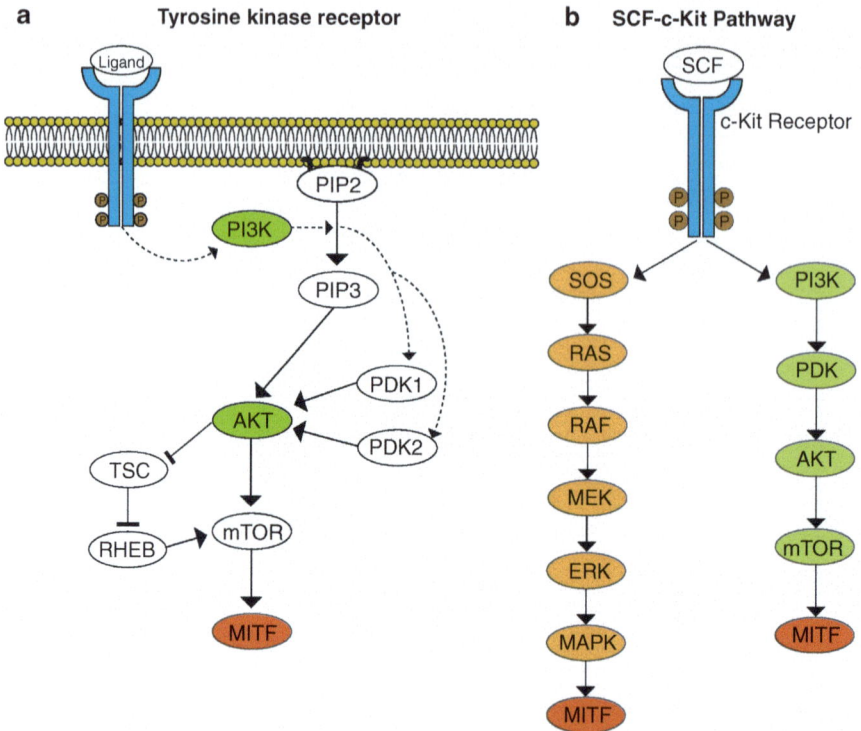

Fig. 5.9 (**a**) Transduction pathways affecting mTOR via TSC inhibition by AKT, as shown in the illustration above. (**b**) Schematic figure of SCF – cKit pathway with the destination to MITF. There are different pathways leading from the c-Kit receptor, which is a variety of tyrosine kinase receptor

- c-Kit (Ligand = Stem Cell Growth Factor, SCF)

  Structure: Tyrosine Kinase Receptor (TKR).
  Phosphoinositide dependent protein kinase1(PDK1) (Fig. 5.9a, b)

- ETB-R (Ligand = Endothelin-1, ET-1)

  Structure: G-Protein-coupled receptor.

- Folate receptors (FRα, FRβ and FRγ) (Ligand = Folic Acid)

  Structure: cysteine-rich cell-surface glycoproteins that bind folate Melanoma cells.
     The PI3K/TSC/mTORC1/AKT/GSK3β/β-catenin/MITF play a central role in regulating melanogenesis in iris melanocytes (Fig. 5.5).

  There are multiple steps in the process of melanogenesis which behave like a domino effect that starts with a ligand attachment to the receptor to initiate the activation and phosphorylation of many downstream secondary messengers from the cytoplasm to the nucleus to produce necessary enzymes for the production of melanin.

This process of signal transduction in a normal pigment cell causes melanocyte to produce melanin pigment to store in melanosomes in order to shield and protect the DNA. In normal melanocyte there is a physiological activation of PI3k and Akt and as a result inactivation of TSC complex (TSC1-RSC2). This will cause activation of mTORC1 and retain activity of AKT which phosphorylate GSK3b which reduces the b-Catenin phosphorylation. Nuclear entry of b-catenin activates TCF/LEF1 which increase the expression of MITF which leads to pigment formation (melanogenesis) with subsequent production of tyrosinase and other genes required for melanogenesis (Fig. 5.2a, b).

MITF expression is dependent on other transcription factors such as:

- (PAX3) Paired box 3
- (CREB) cAMP-response element-binding protein
- B-catenin
- (TCF/LEF1) T cell transcription factor/lymphoid enhancer-binding1

Microphthalmia-associated transcription factor MITF controls the transcription of other genes by binding to E-boxes [CAC(G/A)TG] or M-boxes [TCAC(G/A)TG] in their promoter regions:

- *(TYR) tyrosinase*
- (PMEL) premelanosome protein,
- (DCT) dopachrome tautomerase
- (MLANA) MelanA [*MLANA*])

Mutations in *MITF* cause the autosomal dominant disorder Waardenburg syndrome type 2A (WS2A), in which aberrant pigmentation of the iris, skin and hair and is associated with deafness.

WNT/β-catenin signaling is required for the developmental pathway that leads to melanocyte derivation from the neural crest (Fig. 5.8) [9].

mTOR

The mechanistic target of rapamycin (mTOR) is an evolutionary-conserved serine-threonine protein kinase.

mTOR complex is composed of two distinct complexes, mTORC1 and mTORC2 but both have growth factor sensing.

mTOR complex have many regulatory functions:

- Melanogenesis
- Cell growth
- Proliferation
- Survival
- Balance between cell growth and cell death
- Modulator of autophagy

These functions are in response to:

- Nutritional status
- Stress signals
- Growth factors

Growth factors bind to their receptors triggers a cascade of events that activates PI3K which activates protein kinase (AKT), which is an essential regulator of mTOR. Also the effect of extra cellular signal-regulated kinase (ERK) and ribosomal S6 kinase with ultimately affect the Tuberous sclerosis complex (TSC1 and TSC2). TSC complex is an essential regulator of mTOR1. Reduced expression of TSC complex causes reduced melanogenesis through mTORC1 activation which results in hyperactivation of glycogen synthase kinase 3b (GSK3b) followed by phosphorylation and loss of b-cathenin from the nucleus which reduces the expression of MITF.

mTORC1/GSK3β signaling may support a less differentiated phenotype in melanocytes with reduced MITF-regulated pigment biosynthetic pathway activity, while mTORC2/AKT signaling may promote increased differentiation and pigment biosynthesis.

There is dual regulatory mechanism mTOR signaling which the (mTORC1) reducing pigment synthesis and the (mTORC2) promoting it.

$$TSC > mTORC1 > AKT > GSK3b > beta - catenin$$
$$> MITF > Tyr > Melanin\ Synthesis$$

Rheb is ubiquitously expressed in on mTORC1. Rheb directly binds to the amino-terminal part of the mTORC1 catalytic domain for activation (Fig. 5.9a).

Recent studies have revealed that mTORC1 activation is responsible for degeneration of retinal pigment epithelium [21].

Loss of TSC1 or TSC2 leads to activated GSK3β signaling and decreased MITF expression, which causes pigmentation loss via mTORC1 activation.

TSC 1/2 complex has shown to translocate to the lysosomal membranes in close proximity of mTORC1 for its inactivation in response to stress such as amino-acid starvation or growth factor removal, while growth factor promotes its dissociation from the lysosomal membranes [21].

Functions of mTORC1

- Regulation of melanogenesis via tuberous sclerosis complex (TSC) [9].
- Detection of nutrient abundance: mTORC1 by activated RAG anchors to lysosomal membrane in order to regulate, sense and detect the amino acids specifically Leucine and glutamine.

- Detection of energy level ATP: Multiple mechanisms involved including relaying information by another major kinase, the AMP-activated protein kinase (AMPK) which phosphorylate TSC2 to inhibit mTORC1.
- Detection of Hypoxia: Hypoxia induced transcription factor (HIF) binds to hypoxia-response elements (HREs) to activate the expression of hypoxia-response genes.
- Detection of other external stresses includes radiation, high salt concentration, DNA topoisomerase inhibitors and histone deacetylase inhibitors.
- Regulation of autophagy: As we mentioned the AMPK gets activated during energy starvation which the ratio on AMP to ATP is increased in the cell. AMP binds to autophagy activated kinase (ULK1) by direct phosphorylation and promote autophagy initiation and autophagosome maturation.

Metformin activates AMPK indirectly by inhibiting the mitochondrial respiratory chain complex I, thus increasing the cellular AMP/ATP ratio and inhibition of mTOR [43].

Phosphatidylinositol 3 Kinase (PI3K) Pathway

The PI3K pathway has a vital role in many diverse cellular activities. It is part of the network that integrate environmental and extracellular stimuli and translating them into intracellular signals (Fig. 5.5).

The PI3k/AKT/mTOR signaling pathway regulates many cellular processes such as glucose homeostasis, protein synthesis, cell growth, increased cell cycle, migration, motility, cellular proliferation, survival and vesicular trafficking and melanogenesis.

The activity of PI3k is regulated by growth factor receptors. The large family of growth factors such as fibroblast growth factors (FGFs) binds and activates isoforms of receptor tyrosine kinase (RTKs).

The binding of a ligand (usually a growth factor) to the receptor for example receptor tyrosine kinase (RTK) causes conformation of receptor by dimerization and autophosphorylation which activates PI3K. There are different ways that the PI3K can be activated at this point (Fig. 5.5).

- By direct attachment to the phosphorylated monomer of RTK
- Bind to IRS1 that is attached to the phosphorylated monomer of RTK
- Binding to membrane bound gtp-RAS [17].

The activation of PI3K phosphorylate phosphatidylinositol-(4,5) bisphosphate (PIP2) located on the lipid cell membrane to phosphatidylinositol (3,4,5)-trisphosphate (PIP3).

PIP3 is an important second messenger of PI3K. This process facilitates the activation of AKT which is a Serine and Threonine kinase.

PIP3 recruits PDK1 to directly phosphorylate and activate AKT or indirectly by activation and phosphorylation of mTORC2 [74].

A main negative regulator of PI3K is the tumor suppressor PTEN, which antagonizes the PI3K activity by its intrinsic lipid phosphatase activity, converting PIP3 back into PIP2 [73].

PI3k has a central role on development and progression of many forms of cancer.

Mutation activation of epidermal growth factor receptor (EGFR) as an activator of PI3k is a major contributor to carcinogenesis in non-small cell lung cancer.

Mutation of PI3k gene have been associated with many human cancer types such as breast endometrial and colorectal neoplasms.

PI3K role in viral infections and melanogenesis:

Activation of PI3k by membrane bound receptor tyrosine kinase (RTKs) serve as entry point for endocytosis of Many viruses including Zaire strain of Ebola Virus (ZEBOV) and other strains of Ebola viruses [15]. It was suggested that early activation of the PI3K-Akt pathway by ZEBOV may also have implications in pathogenesis of Ebola hemorrhagic fever [49].

The report of an eye color change in an individual with Ebola infection is supporting this theory as the virus can be detected in the aqueous humor for up to 9 weeks after the clearance of viremia [70].

As the targeted viral infected macrophages produce many pro-inflammatory cytokines and chemokines including TNF-alpha, IL-6 and IL-8, severe inflammatory response will be produced. The inflammatory process will then proceed as an inflammatory pathway to melanogenesis (Fig. 5.10).

The Ebola virus envelop glycoproteins also may play a vital role in proinflammatory cytokines response induced by the virus even in the absence of virus replication.

There is also evidence that the PI3K-Akt pathway contributes significantly toward regulation of each of these cytokines.

PI3K-Akt pathway activation does also lead to increased vascular permeability and vascular deregulation and hemorrhage which is the characteristic of these infections [3, 10].

PI3K also participate in cellular entry and endocytosis of bovine ephemeral fever virus (BEFV) through clathrin-mediated and dynamin 2-dependent endocytosis pathways.

The virus also triggers Cox-2-catalysed prostaglandin E2 (PGE2) synthesis and induces expressions of G-protein-coupled E-prostanoid (EP) receptors 2 and 4, leading to amplify signal cascades of Src-JNK-AP1 and PI3K-Akt-NF-κB, which elevates both clathrin and dynamin 2 expressions.

Macropinocytosis has been described as a source for Ebola virus entry to the host cell [64].

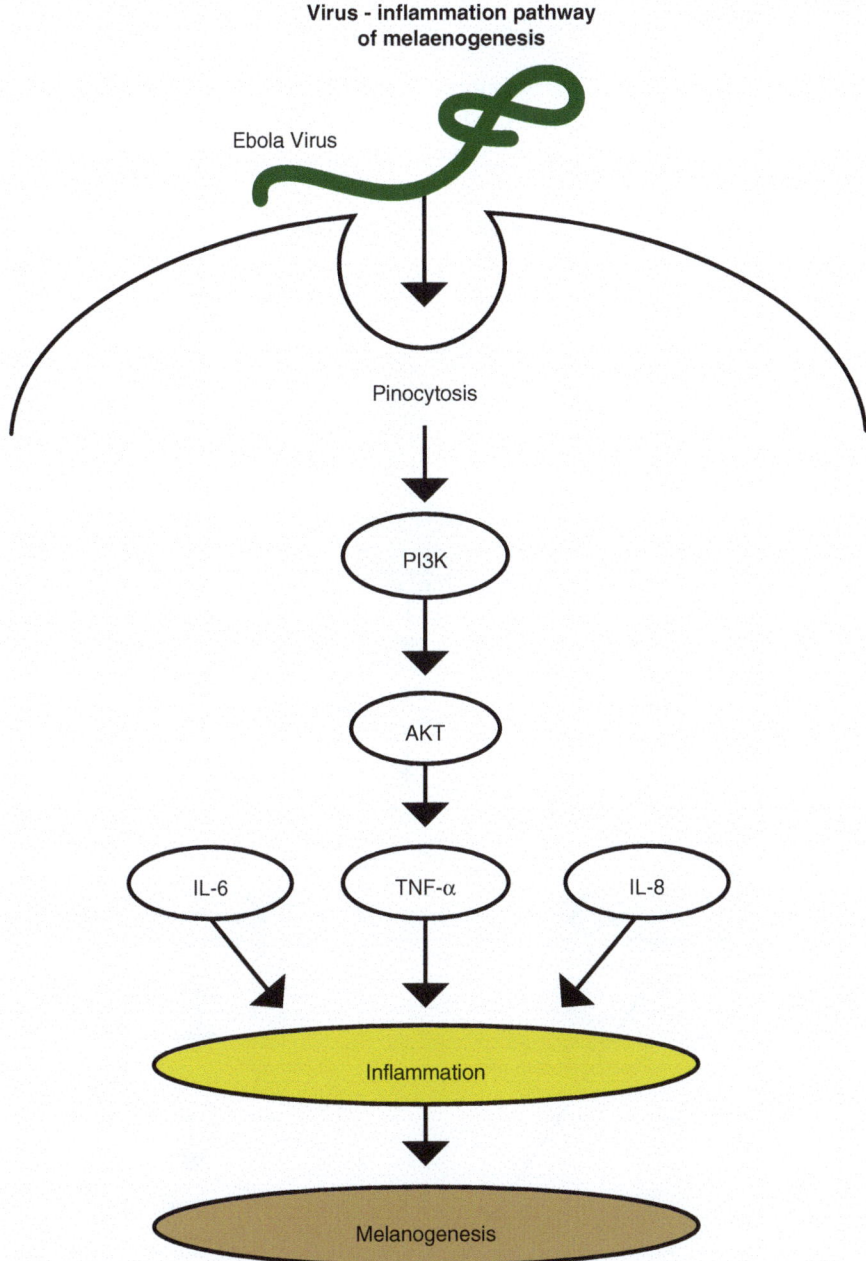

Fig. 5.10 Melanogenesis induced by ebola virus through activation of intracellular inflammatory pathways, as shown in the illustration above

Akt Signaling

Akt or protein kinase B (PKB) compose of 3 different isoforms with similar protein structures. Inactive Akt normally exist in the cytosol in an inactive form. When activated by PI3K it will translocate to the plasma membrane (Fig. 5.11).

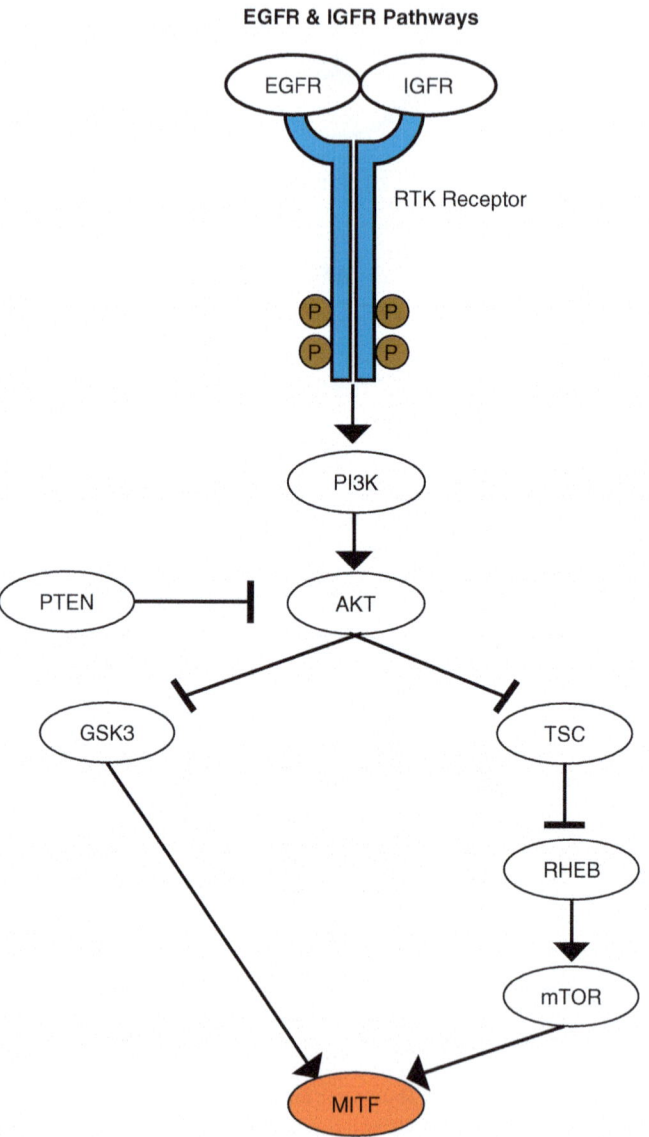

Fig. 5.11 Schematic figure EGFR and IGFR pathways with the destination to MITF. There are different pathways leading from the RTK receptor, which is a variety of tyrosine kinase receptor, with multiple activators and inhibitors, as seen above

AKT is a Serine and Threonine kinase which is regulated by growth factor signals. By attachment of a growth factor to the cell membrane receptor tyrosine kinase (RTK) and activation of AKT multiple activation and inhibition cascades will initiate which involves in apoptosis, DNA repair, cell cycle, glucose metabolism, cell growth, motility, invasion, angiogenesis and melanogenesis.

The main target of Akt is mammalian target of rapamycin (mTOR), which has a central role in PI3K-Akt pathway and cancer. Regularly, mTOR as we mentioned earlier plays a crucial part in the regulation of cell growth and proliferation by monitoring nutrient availability, cellular energy, oxygen levels, and mitogenic signals.

- AKT inhibition by TSC complex
- AKT signaling negatively regulates GSK3
- mTORC1 activation counter-regulate PI3K/AKT signaling and reduce AKT
- AKT inhibit TSC complex which inhibits Rheb and as a result activates mTORC1 [14].

Melanogenesis

The process of melanogenesis is extremely complex and involve in many different ligands, receptors, secondary messengers, signaling pathways and nuclear transcription factors. From formation of early endosomes to the process of melanosome maturation and development and the chemical process of melanin synthesis in the melanosomes is a complex task that require many signaling pathways and enzymes (Fig. 5.12). The early stage is well described in the literature [22].

Cyclooxygenase-2 (COX-2)

Cox 2 is an enzyme induced in response to multiple mitogenic and inflammatory stimuli, including UV light. UV-induced COX-2 expression induces production of prostaglandin E2 (PGE2) in keratinocytes, which mediates inflammation and cell proliferation. COX-2 Increases the expressions of tyrosinase, TRP-1, TRP-2, gp100 and MITF, which also increase tyrosinase enzyme activity (Fig. 5.6) [16, 41, 50, 71].

Mitogen-Activated Protein Kinase(MAP Kinase)

The MAP kinase family, including ERK, JNK and p38. MAPKs are also involved in mammalian melanogenesis.

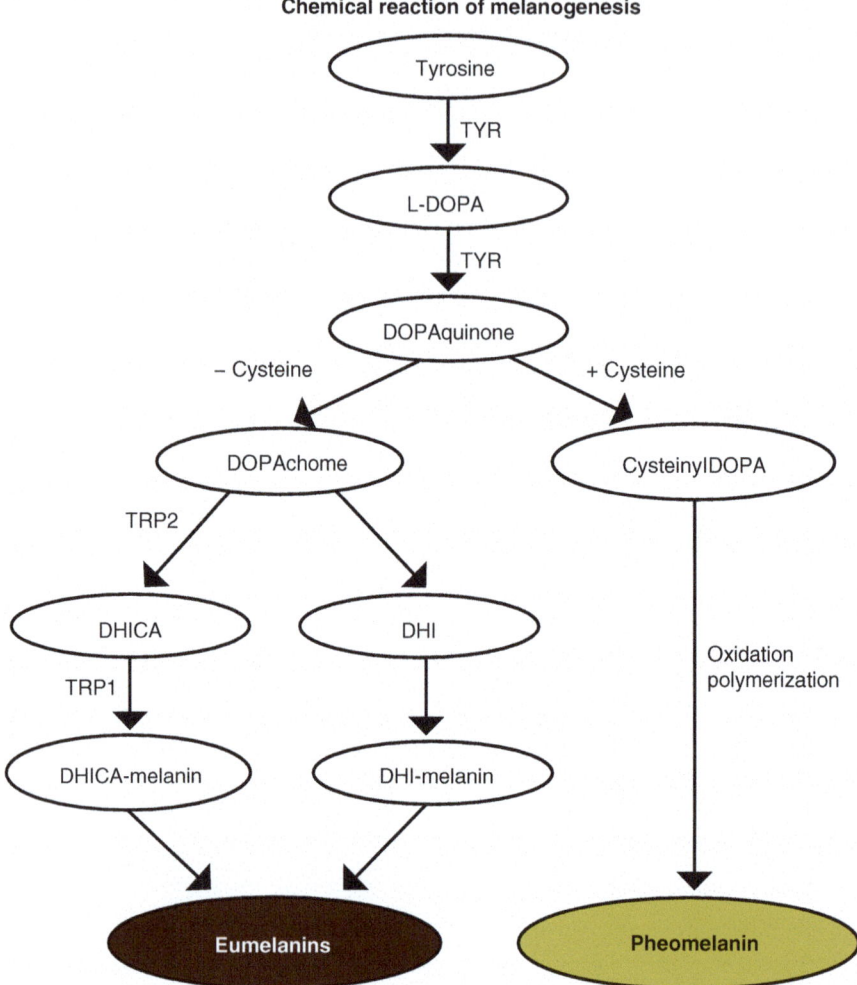

Fig. 5.12 Schematic of the chemical sequences of the synthesis of both eumelanin and pheomelanin production

cAMP Response Element-Binding Protein (CREB)

α-melanocyte-stimulating hormone (α-MSH), through activation of its receptor, melanocortin-1 receptor (MC1R), is a stimulator of melanogenesis by inducing MITF expression. α-MSH-mediated signaling, such as ERK and cAMP response element-binding protein (CREB), causes MITF overexpression and melanogenesis. The receptor MC1R is nonfunctional or absent in iris melanocytes (Fig. 5.13) [75].

Fig. 5.13 α-MSH pathway
leading from the MC1R
receptor, which is a
G-coupled protein receptor
with the
destination to MITF

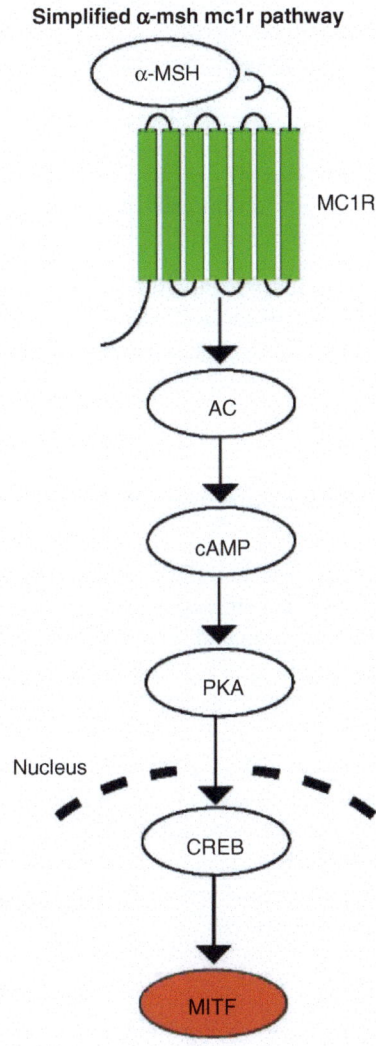

WNT Pathway

In humans, Wnt proteins compose a family of 19 glycoproteins that act through a variety of receptors to stimulate distinct intracellular cascades involved with melanogenesis.

These pathways are typically involved in embryonic development, cell growth, migration, and differentiation of melanocytes.

The Wnt signaling is also required throughout life for the homeostatic balance of self-renewing melanocytes.

Wnt pathways may be subdivided into following categories:

- The canonical Wnt pathway, which includes the intracellular transcriptional co-activator β-catenin as a central component, through the binding to Frizzled receptors (FRZD1-7) [40].
- Non-canonical Wnt pathway.
- Non-canonical WNT/Calcium pathway

Wnt specific receptor FRZDs are composed of seven transmembrane domain (TM). These cell surface receptors belong to the large family of GPCRs (Fig. 5.8).

Mutations in the genes has been reported to cause familial exudative vitreoretinopathy [54].

Microphthalmia-Associated Transcription Factor (MITF)

MITF is a basic helix-loop-helix leucine zipper transcription factor involved in lineage-specific pathway regulation of many types of cells including melanocytes.

The transcription factor MITF, have been reported to be involved in many genes in pigment cells, and is an essential regulator for melanocyte development.

MITF has multiple role in proliferation and survival, and the expression of enzymes and structural proteins necessary for the production of melanin [69].

MITF is a transcriptional factor that activates several genes which encode melanosome-localized proteins involved both in melanin synthesis and in melanosome biogenesis and transport. Mutations in these genes are associated with human oculocutaneous and ocular forms of albinism.

MITF also coordinates cell-cycle progression, cell migration, metabolism, and lysosome biogenesis.

The structure of MITF includes three critically important regions.

- The helix-loop-helix motif
- The leucine-zipper motif
- The above two motifs are critical for protein interactions. These motifs allow molecules of MITF to interact with each other or with other proteins with a similar structure, creating a two-protein unit (dimer) that functions as a transcription factor.
- The basic motif, binds to specific areas of DNA, allowing the dimer to control gene activity [36].

Many signaling pathways affect MITF.

BRAF/MAPK and GSK3 signaling converge to control MITF nuclear export MAPK, PI3K, and WNT signaling pathways affect MITF and involve in the development of cancer [18, 27].

p21-activated kinase 4 (PAK4) is a key regulator of cAMP-response element–binding protein (CREB) that acts upstream of microphthalmia-associated transcription factor (MITF). Melanocytes express both PAK2 and PAK4 isoforms. Inhibition of PAK4 over several days markedly decreased the levels of CREB, MITF, and tyrosinase in melanocytes. PAK4 promotes α-MSH/UVB-induced melanogenesis via the CREB and Wnt/β-catenin signaling pathways in the skin but not in Iris [76].

Prostaglandin E2 activation (PGE2/EP) receptor signaling amplify Src-JNK-AP1 and PI3K-Akt-NF-κB pathways in an autocrine or paracrine fashion to enhance melanogenesis (Fig. 5.6).

Inflammation and Melanogenesis

Inflammation Cascade: Inhibition of inflammation by stimulating the p38-cyclooxygenase-2 (COX-2)–prostaglandin E2 (PGE2) pathway in keratinocytes activates nuclear factor erythroid 2-related factor-2 (Nrf2) and inhibits the production of reactive oxygen species (ROS) [72].

Both the p38 signaling pathway and PGE2 play crucial roles in melanogenesis. The transcription factor Nrf2 protects against oxidative stress and represses melanogenesis by modulating PI3K/Akt signaling (Fig. 5.6) [11].

Activation of AKT by PI3K in turn activates NFkB a fast-acting transcription factor. NFκB regulates production of inflammatory mediators and induces transcription of pro-inflammatory genes. NFκB also contributes to the regulation of cell proliferation and survival.

NFκB-mediated secretion of cytokines (such as TNFα, IL-1β, IL-6), expression of COX-2 and production of PGE2 in UVB-exposed skin.

In addition, p53 and NFκB signaling have many mutually antagonistic functions; specifically p53 can inhibit NFκB signaling (Fig. 5.7a) [7, 42].

Nuclear Factor κ-Light-Chain-Enhancer of Activated B Cell (NFκB) Pathway

The nuclear factor κ-light-chain-enhancer of activated B cell (NF-κB) pathway is a positive modulator of inflammation and immune response. NF-κB signaling is required during early development and its molecules are involved in many physiological activities and conditions.

NF-κB activation is triggered by a diverse range of stimuli;

* Cytokines
* Tumor necrosis factor α (TNF-α)
* Interleukin 1 (IL-1)
* Growth factors
* Bacterial lipopolysaccharide (LPS)
* ROS
* UV
* Ionizing radiation

The result is the transcription of a variety of target genes, including interleukins, chemokines, proteases, and apoptosis-related genes, leading to stress response, immunity, cell proliferation, and apoptosis.

By being involved in the induction of proliferation genes, inhibition of apoptosis, and regulation of immune and inflammatory responses.

NF-κB comprises a family of transcription factors that act as homo- or heterodimers and, upon activation, translocate into the nucleus where they interact with specific location in DNA structures that modulate target gene expression [5].

In the absence of stimulus, NF-κB dimers are typically sequestered and inactivated in the cytoplasm by inhibitors of NF-κB inhibitor of NF-κB (IκB family).

The prototypical dimer in the canonical NF-κB (or classical) pathway is mainly activated by:

* TNF-α, IL-1 and Toll-like receptors (TNF-α receptor (TNFR),
* IL-1 receptor (IL-1R)
* TLR

Down the line is the activation of p38 MAPK and MAP3K MEKK3, which promote cascades for further polyubiquitination and proteasome-dependent degradation.

The non-canonical pathway, which is activated by lymphotoxin-β (LTβ), B-cell activating factor (BAFF), assemble in distinct conformations in the canonical and non-canonical NF-κB pathway.

The cascade that regulate selective immune responses, such as lymphoid organogenesis and B-cell maturation and survival [14].

Transforming Growth Factor-β (TGF-β) Pathway

TGF-β signaling has important roles in embryogenesis and tissue homeostasis and melanogenesis.

TGF-β1 is known to have hypopigmentation effects and can independently regulate the expression of enzymes such as tyrosinase and related proteins (eg, TYRP1 and DCT) [7].

Transforming growth factor beta1 also mediates hypopigmentation of B16 mouse melanoma cells by inhibition of melanin formation and melanosome maturation [33].

The other effects of TGF-β includes:

- Regulating cell proliferation,
- Migration,
- Cell differentiation,
- Synthesis of extracellular matrix.
- Cell adhesion
- Cell fate determination
- Apoptosis.

More than 30 TGF-β members have been described in humans, and they can be divided into different families as TGF-βs, bone morphogenetic proteins (BMPs), and Nodal. The mature ligands are prone to form homo or heterodimers and interact with two types of serine/threonine kinase receptors to initiate the signaling.

Its similarity of signal transduction to ECF (Epidermal growth factor) has been elaborated in the literature [38].

In humans, distinct type I and type II TGF-β receptors have been identified which they signal to different transcriptional targets.

Smads are intracellular mediator proteins that participate on the TGF-β signaling, and are involved in transducing the signals from the receptors to the nucleus (Fig. 5.14).

Upon ligand binding, type II receptor phosphorylates the type I receptor, exposing its Smad-binding site and enabling R-Smad activation by phosphorylation. The receptor activation, driven by distinct TGF-β ligands, induces different transcription factor responses.

Activated TGF-β receptors can further stimulate other pathways in a Smad-independent manner, PI3K and Akt can also be activated by TGF-β receptors and, in particular, Akt is able to regulate Smad3 activity either by sequestering it on the cytosol or by preventing its phosphorylation and degradation. Both Smad and non-Smad pathway activation seems important for epithelial to mesenchymal transition (EMT), which is associated with tumor metastasis and fibrosis.

Notch Pathway

The Notch pathway has an important role in cell fate determination, proliferation, differentiation, and survival. The Notch signaling cascade modulates a broad range of cellular processes, including cell cycle arrest regulation, apoptosis/survival, differentiation, and stem cell maintenance, as well as the cross talk with hypoxia response.

The Notch protein family is composed by cell surface receptors that transduce signals by interacting with the transmembrane ligands Delta-like (DLL) and Jagged

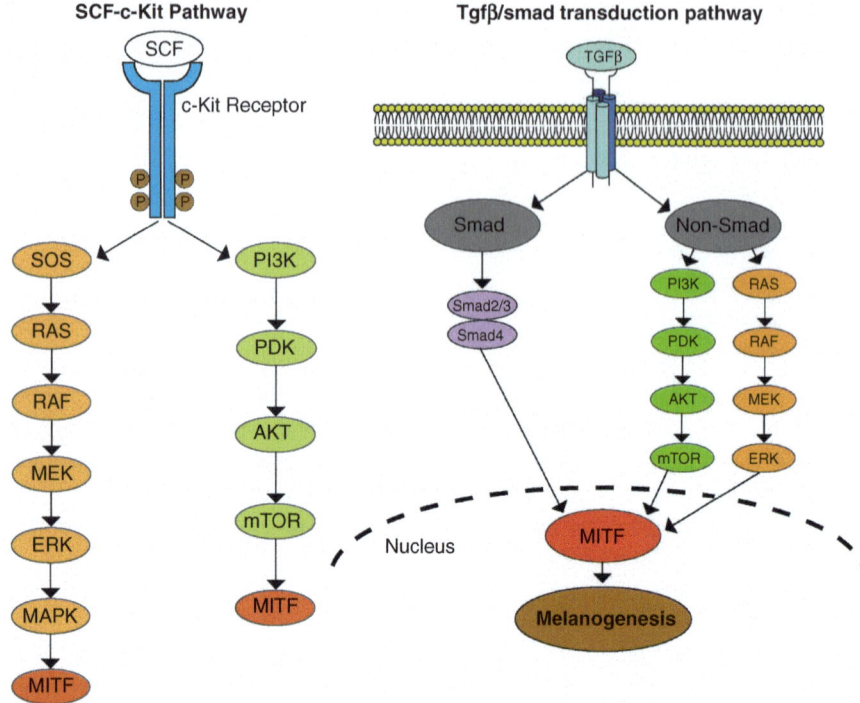

Fig. 5.14 Schematic figure of TGFβ pathway with Smad and non-Smad transduction pathways, and destination to MITF with resultant melanogenesis

(JAG) on neighboring cells. The Notch receptors are composed by two major domains:

- Extracellular domain (Notch extracellular domain (NECD).
- Intracellular domain (Notch intracellular domain (NICD).

The Notch receptor is translocated to the trans-Golgi network as a full-length protein which is cleaved to form membrane-attached heterodimeric receptor. The signaling cascade initiates after binding of the ligands JAG1 and 2 or DSL 1, 3, and 4 to the Notch receptor between neighboring cells. The binding initiates two successive proteolytic cleavages that culminate in the release of the NICD, which is translocated into the nucleus, where it interacts with the transcription factors.

The triggering mechanism of the canonical Notch signaling involves proteolytic cleavages at three sites of the Notch protein: S1, S2, and S3. This cleavage generates two subunits (NECD and NICD) interconnected by the TM. These processed subunits are then transported to the plasma membrane, where they associate as non-covalently bound heterodimers to form the functional Notch receptor.

Notch signaling may also interact with other pathways:

- PI3K,
- mTORC2,
- Wnt,
- NF-κβ,
- HIF-1α,
- Integrin
- Notch canonical signaling is required for many normal cellular functions such as homeostasis and regulation of melanocytes.
- Notch non-canonical signals Participate in many pathological conditions such as cancer or auto-immune disorders.

Melanogenesis

Melanogenesis is a complex process of synthesis and storage of melanin in the specific cytoplasmic organelles of pigment cells (melanocytes) which is called melanosomes. Melanin synthesis regulated by microphthalmia-associated transcription factor (MITF), a key transcription factor controlling the expression of melanogenesis-related enzymes including tyrosinase, tyrosinase-related proteins 1 (TRP-1) and TRP-2 (Fig. 5.12).

Tyrosinase plays an essential role in melanogenesis. Its catalytic effect takes part in the two rate-limiting steps in melanogenesis:

- The hydroxylation of tyrosine to 3,4-dihydroxyphenylalanine (DOPA).
- The oxidation of DOPA to DOPA quinone (Fig. 5.14).
- The melanin production is predominantly dependent on tyrosinase expression and activity and the transcriptional activity of MITF.
- Post-translational regulation is by extracellular signal-regulated kinase (ERK) and phosphatidylinositol 3-kinase (PI3K)/Akt signaling pathways [25].
- Many different transcription factors participate in the transactivation of the genes in melanocytes:
- The paired box-containing transcription factor PAX3,
- Sex determining region Y (SRY) family member SOX10,
- The Wnt/β-catenin pathway effector LEF-1.
- The cAMP pathway effector cAMP response element binding (CREB).
- Many other promoters and indirect activators of the MITF has been reported previously [69].

It is also known that melanogenesis is regulated by the balance between a variety of signal transduction pathways:

- The cyclic adenosine monophosphate/protein kinase A (cAMP/PKA)
- p38 mitogen-activated protein kinase (p38 MAPK)
- Extracellular signal-regulated kinase (ERK)
- Phosphoinositide 3-kinase/Akt (PI3K/Akt) pathways
- Nuclear factor erythroid 2 (Nrf2), The phosphorylation statuses of several signaling molecules after Nrf2 via CREB, p38 MAPK and ERK mTOR and S6 kinase substrate. Nrf2 decreases melanogenesis by activating the PI3K/Akt /mTOR pathway [58].

Signal Transduction and Cancer

The mutation in signaling pathways have been associated with many cancers. The two major pathways frequently mutated in human cancer such as colorectal, are the Ras-MAPK- and the PI3K/AKT-signaling pathways.

These pathways are also is used by Epstein-Barr virus protein LMP2A to activate Ras-MAPK-AKT to stablish a latent infection in host B cells and later development of variety of malignancies [44].

These alterations can occur in both upstream and downstream components of the pathways. Most commonly, constitutive activation of the Ras-MAPK pathway occurs via mutations.

As already mentioned, COX-2-derived PGE2 is able to signal via the PI3K/AKT- and Ras-MAPK/ERK-signaling pathways to enhance cell survival.

There is a possibility that the COX-2/PGE2 pathway represents an alternative mechanism by which tumors acquire growth factor autonomy.

Aberrant activation of the COX-2/PGE2 pathway might phenocopy-activating mutations in the PI3K/AKT and/or Ras-MAPK pathways, which could play an important role in melanogenesis and promoting tumor progression.

Deregulation of the COX-2/PGE2 pathway activate Ras resulting in a positive feedback loop that increase COX-2 expression and further stimulation of melanogenesis.

During hypoxia, the transcription factor hypoxia-inducible factor-1 (HIF-1) directly up-regulates COX-2 expression and increases PGE2 production.

Activation of the Ras-MAPK pathway, act in a positive feedback loop to maintain an active pro-survival COX-2/PGE2 pathway during hostile microenvironmental conditions [19].

Sox10

The Sox (Sry-related box) family of genes is involved in the development processes of testis, oligodendrocytes, the central nervous system, and chondrocytes.

Sox10 plays an important role in neural crest cell and melanocyte development, and mutations in Sox10 result in Waardenburg–Shah syndrome. Afflicted individuals exhibit pigmentary alterations and nervous system defects.

- Sox10 directly regulates expression of MITF and other genes essential in melanin synthesis.
- Sox10 in synergy with PAX3 bind directly to the MITF promoter to regulate MITF expression.
- Sox10 is a useful tissue biomarker in melanocytic neoplasms.
- Similar to MITF, Sox10 protein is expressed in the nucleus, and the utility of Sox10 in evaluation of melanocytic lesions parallels that of MITF.
- Sox10 is also expressed in Schwann cells, myoepithelial cells, granular cells, adnexal structures, and salivary glands.
- The expression of Sox10 has been limited to tumors of melanocytic, Schwann cell, or myoepithelial differentiation, Sox10 has become useful in differential diagnosis of melanoma.
- Sox10 expression is absent in fibroblasts and macrophages and thus can aid in evaluating excision specimens for residual tumor.

Molecular Biology of Malignant Melanoma of Iris

Iris melanoma is a malignant transformation of the uveal melanocytes. The eye creates an immunosuppressive environment in order to protect eyesight. UM cells use similar processes to escape immune surveillance. Regarding innate immunity the production of macrophage inhibiting factor (MIF) and TGF-β, added to MHC class I upregulation, inhibits the action of natural killer (NK) cells.

- Uveal Melanoma cells produce cytokines such as IL-6 and IL-10 that favor macrophage differentiation to the M2 subtype, which promote tumor growth instead of an effective immune response.
- Uveal Melanoma cells also impair the adaptive immune response through production of indoleamine 2,3-dioxygenase (IDO), overexpression of programmed death ligand-1 (PD-L1), alteration of FasL expression, and resistance to perforin.

The clinical and metastatic behavior of Uveal Melanoma differs from cutaneous melanoma because of its initially purely hematogenous dissemination and its tendency to metastasize to the liver.

GNA11 (GNAQ/11) have been identified in 80% of primary UMs. GNAQ/11 activate signaling pathways, including the mitogen-activated protein kinase (MAPK) pathway, similar to the way that BRAF mutation does in cutaneous melanoma.

The immune-privileged nature of the eye promotes and exploits by uveal melanoma (UM).

The uvea, constituted by the iris, the ciliary body and the choroid, has two main functions; nutrition and gas exchange. The Uvea consist of vascular tissue, immune cells and melanocytes. Melanocytes are the cells that UM develops from.

The eye is considered an immune-privileged organ. It has a unique ability to defend itself against uncontrolled inflammation that could damage its highly specialized cells. This immune privilege influences the immune response against UM cells and provides escape mechanisms for UM. Different factors play a role in the immune-privilege of the eye.

- Immunosuppressive proteins such as transforming growth factor β (TGF-β),
- Vasoactive intestinal peptide (VIP),
- α-melanocyte-stimulating hormone (α-MSH)
- Complement regulatory proteins (CRP's)
- The blood-eye barrier restricts inflammatory cell access to the eye excpt in the iris
- Eye cells reduce major histocompatibility complex (MHC) class Ia expression provides escape cytotoxic mediated lyses.
- Ocular cells express PD-L1 which inhibits T cell response.
- Anterior chamber-associated immune deviation (ACAID) active immune cells interact with the immune system to induce unusual suppression of the systemic immune response when an antigen is detected in the anterior chamber.

The eye, the thymus, the spleen, and the sympathetic nervous system are also involved in ACAID.

Minimal to moderate inflammation against antigens presented into the eye is an evolutionary adaptation to prevent the loss of eyesight.

The innate immune system is the nonspecific part of the immune system that responds to pathogens in a generic way without conferring long-lasting or protective immunity on the host. Two cell types of the innate immune system might play an important role in UM;

- The natural killer (NK) cells.
- The macrophages.

NK cells protect us against viral infections and neoplasms. Their main function is to recognize and kill any cell failing to express major histocompatibilty (MHC) class I molecules.

The endothelial cells that line the anterior chamber of the eye as well as UM cells seem to express little or no MHC class I molecules.

Several other mechanisms have been described in order to explain how UM cells avoid NK destruction by the effect of the following cytokines:

- Macrophage migration inhibitory factor (MIF)
- Inhibitory molecules FasL, or TRAIL on tumor cell membranes in response to different pro-inflammatory cytokines such TNF-β and IFN-α.

Macrophages have different functions depending on the subtype.

The M1 subtype has an immunostimulatory role acting as antigen-presenting cells (APCs).

The M2 subtype favors angiogenesis and works as myeloid-derived suppressor cells (MDSC). Inflammatory infiltrates in the tumor microenvironment are critical for the development of malignancies, and UM cells might take advantage of this inflammatory environment through the recruitment of macrophages in the tumor that drive the pro-angiogenic and immunosuppressive function.

Tumor-Associated Macrophages (TAM)s-driven angiogenesis is vital to tumor growth in UM.

This might be mediated by cytokines produced not only by the tumor cells but also by normal cells such as IL-6, IL-10, TGF-β, MIF, GM-CSF, and VEGF.

Most of those cytokines are immunosuppressive and are known to polarize macrophages to the M2 subtype.

Activated T-cells, both T-helper and T-cytotoxic, are present in UM, and they can be inhibited by tumor cells using a variety of processes.

- The production of indoleamine 2,3-dioxygenase (IDO), which is an enzyme that leads to tryptophan depletion, impairing lymphocyte proliferation (66).
- Metabolites produced by this IDO act as immune suppressors at other cellular levels such as NK-cells and macrophages.
- Expression of an altered Fas Ligand, resistance to perforin action via INF-γ secretion

The most relevant mechanism to inhibit T-cell action by melanoma cells is the overexpression of PD-L1 when exposed to IFN-γ.

INF-γ in the tumor local microenvironment promotes up-regulation of the PD-L1 expression by UM, promoting immune escape by impairing T-cell function.

In summary T-cell function is affected and compromised by many factors such as:

- PD-L1 expression is dynamic and tied to INF-γ expression, and IL-2 production from
- PD-L1 contributes to suppression of T-cells by decreasing IL-2 production.
- UM cells do not constitutively express PD-L1 while they are in the immunoprivileged ocular microenvironment, but when they metastasize, these cells come in contact with normal microenvironment.
- IFN-γ produced PD-L1 is up-regulated which is leading to T-cell apoptosis and a decrease in the production of cytokines.
- INF-γ cytokines has an inhibitory effect on T-cells. Increase in the MHC class I, suppresses their MHC class I-restricted destruction by CD8+ lymphocytes [65].

Affected T cells no longer function as hypersensitivity-mediating T cells, but as regulatory T cells (Treg's). Pigmented epithelial cells of the iris can also induce regulatory activity in T cells through contact. IPE cells promote conversion of T cells into Tregs solely through a contact-dependent mechanism. T cells exposed to IPE cells acquire full regulatory capacity [37, 62].

As we mentioned earlier, Malignant Melanoma is a malignant transformation of melanocytes. Uveal melanoma is the most common primary intraocular malignancy in adults with specific characterizations:

- The incidence of Uveal melanoma in the western world is about 7 in one million.
- The incidence of Iris melanoma is about 4–10% of Uveal melanomas.
- There is no difference in incidence of iris melanoma between men and women.
- There is a higher incidence of iris melanoma in Caucasian population with the light color iris.

Iris Melanoma can be presented in variety of sizes and shapes.

The treatment is based on individual size, location and characteristics of the tumors.

The treatment is depending on many individual factors and includes:

- Excision
- Enucleation
- proton beam radiation
- Radioactive implants

Unfortunately, none of the above have a predicted result.

Diffuse iris melanoma can also occur that has a greater risk of metastasis.

There are many factors that affects the increased risk of metastasis and survival which are as follows:

- Association with High intraocular pressure
- Angle involvement
- Tumor thickness
- Extraocular extension
- Increased age

There are many mutations that involves signaling pathways and transductions that are involved in tumor genesis and malignant transformation of melanocytes.

Here only the essential pathways and transcription factors that have a major role in melanoma formation will be summarized.

MAPK and Melanoma

- MAPK signaling is the most external signaling pathway which is activated by cell surface membrane receptors MC1R, c-Kit, c-Met, IGFR and WNT.

The most common cause of deregulation of MAPK towards malignant transformation are mutations in upstream N-Ras and /or BRAF genes.

N-Ras downstream is activation of Raf or MEK which activates JNK and ERK which activates nuclear targets for transcription.

• BRAF mutations in melanocytes involves in a thymine to adenine DNA base point mutation that replaces the amino acid valine with glutamic acid at the 600 position (BRAF V600E). This mutation causes the aberrant activation of the MAPK signaling pathway to promote melanoma.
• Activation of Ras-Raf-MAPK-Erk also involves with the production of immuno-suppressive cytokines such as IL-6, IL10, and VEGF by melanoma cells [63].

There are many interactions between the different signal transductions pathways that are beyond the scope of this book and can be reviewed in detail on the "Melanoma development" textbook by Anja Bosserhoff.

MITF and Melanoma

MITF (microphthalmia-associated transcription factor) functions in the development and differentiation of a variety of cell types, including melanocytes.

• MITF is involved in induction of Melanoma.
• From many isoforms of MITF, the M isoform is specifically expressed in melanocytes.
• Melanin synthesis is regulated by MITF via transcription of melanogenesis genes (tyrosinase, tyrosinase-related protein 1&2.)
• MITF expression can be used as the differential diagnosis of melanoma from other forms of tumors such as dermatofibrosarcoma, leiomyosarcoma, neurofibroma, and schwannoma.

MITF and Sox10 in Melanoma

• Sox10 directly regulates expression of MITF and other genes essential in melanin synthesis and malignancy transformation.
• Sox10 has become useful in differential diagnosis of melanoma due to the fact that the expression of Sox10 has been limited to tumors of melanocytic, Schwannian, or myoepithelial differentiation.
• Sox10 has also been reported to be a reliable marker in evaluating sentinel lymph nodes for metastatic melanoma.

PTEN-PI3K-AKT Pathway

PI3K (Phosphoinositol-3-Kinase) pathway is one of the most frequently deregulated pathways in melanoma cells [3]. PI3k is activated by IGFR and c-Met receptors.

PI3K activates PIP2 into secondary lipid signaling molecule PIP3 which activates AKT which is affected in melanoma cells. PTEN is a negative regulator of AKT. PTEN is commonly mutated in Melanoma cells.

It also has been suggested that Melanoma activates PI3K pathway by inactivation of PTEN [47].

NF-kB Regulation

As we mentioned earlier NFκB regulates production of inflammatory mediators and induces transcription of proinflammatory genes.

NF-kB signaling has an important role in melanogenesis and melanoma growth and survival. It is activated by variety of cytokines and chemokines via AKT-signaling and MAPK-signaling and NIK (NFKB Interacting Kinase) [48].

In the absence of stimuli NF-kB is localized in cytoplasm in a protein bind format and in an inactive state. When activated with above signaling pathways it dissociates from binding proteins and translocate in the nucleus to activate transcription genes.

HGF/c-MET Signaling Pathway in Melanoma

HGF/c-MET pathways contributes to several processes that are crucial for melanoma development. Stimulation of these pathways is responsible for proliferation, survival, motility, and invasion of the melanoma cells including distant metastasis [13].

SMAD/SKI

SMAD 2/3 are activated by binding of Transforming Growth Factor (TGF) family to their receptors. When phosphorylated they will bind to SMAD 4 and will function as transcription factor in the nucleus [35].

SKI is mostly localized in the cytoplasm in high levels. SKI inhibits SMAD driven transcription of P21 in melanoma.

SKI is a potent stimulator of WNT/beta-Catenin signaling pathway which in turn activated MITF.

SKI participates in regulation of melanoma progression by activating beta-catenin signaling and repressing the TGF-beta pathway.

HIF1a (Hypoxia–Inducible Factor 1alfa)

HIF1 is the main transcription regulator of cellular response to hypoxia consists of HIF 1 alpha and HIF 1 Beta which are also the target of MITF [8].

HIF1a is regulated by the PI3K/AKT and MAPK/ERK and influenced by PTEN [78].

P53

P53 is one of the most important Tumor suppressors in human [30]. The function are as follows responses:

- Control of DNA damage
- Cell cycle progression
- Apoptosis

P53 activates the melanogenesis response via transcriptional activation of the POMC promoter in Keratinocytes which encodes alpha-MSH [12].

Melanoma Biomarkers

Several melanocytic tissue biomarkers are available that can facilitate the histo-pathologic and mutational status of this disease [67].

These biomarkers are helpful to assess melanocytic differentiation, vascular invasion, mitotic capacity, and mutation status.

MiTF and Sox10 are both useful biomarkers in identification of melanocytic differentiation and carcinoma.

Anti-BRAFV600E identifies melanomas with BRAFV600E mutation and is a useful surrogate marker to evaluate BRAF mutation status in melanoma patients [66].

Two-pore channel 2 (TPC2) Another protein component of melanogenesis process that regulates human pigmentation is TPC2 which is located in melanosomes, where melanin is synthesized. TPC2 regulates the pH and size of melanosomes, thus controlling the amount of melanin produced [4].

Autophagy and Melanogenesis

The role of autophagy in melanogenesis have been reported recently. This pathway is via Microtubule-associated protein light chain 3 (LC3) by regulation of MITF expression in melanocytes [75].

Autophagy plays an important role in melanogenesis by regulating melanosome degradation and biogenesis in melanocytes (Fig. 5.15).

LC3 contributes to melanogenesis by increasing ERK-dependent MITF expression, the signaling network that links autophagy to melanogenesis.

Microphthalmia-associated transcription factor (MITF) is critical for melanogenic enzyme transcription. MITF enhances the expression of tyrosinase, tyrosine-related protein 1 (TRP-1) and TPR-2 and the melanogenic gene PMEL17 which inducing formation of functional fibrils in melanosomes.

Autophagy is essential for tissue homeostasis, adaption to starvation, and removal of dysfunctional organelles or pathogens. Autophagy regulators may have prominent roles in the initial stages of melanosome formation, a lysosome-related organelle in which melanin is synthesized [46]. Co-localization of LC3 in melanosomes with amyloid protein PMEL17 highlights the importance of the autophagy pathway in regulation of melanosome biogenesis.

Autophagy is activated to maintain cellular homeostasis under various stress conditions. Autophagy activation takes place in melanogenic regions which can be precisely determined by preventing autophagosome–lysosome fusion and subsequent autophagosomal degradation. The autophagy activator rapamycin increased LC3-II expression in association with decreased expression of p62, a known substrate for autophagic degradation. Rapamycin-induced autophagy also enhanced melanin synthesis in melanocytes [45].

Autophagy activation correlates with melanogenesis in melanocytic nevi.

- Autophagy activation occurs during melanosome biogenesis.
- LC3 may be an intracellular mediator of melanogenesis.
- LC3 mediates diverse cellular functions in various cells as a signaling molecule distinct from other autophagic factors by associating with microtubules and localizing to nuclei.
- The mechanisms guiding autophagic regulator proteins during melanogenic signaling may vary with respect to cell type or environmental stimuli.

MITF is linked to melanogenic potential via an MITF-mediated increase of tyrosinase activity. Depletion of the serine/threonine kinase mTOR leads to increased MITF transcription, whereas depletion of autophagy protein WIPI1 increases TORC1 activity, which leads to repression of TORC2, activation of GSK3β, increased β-catenin degradation, and decreased MITF transcription.

MITF is a critical mediator of LC3-II-dependent melanogenesis during rapamycin-induced autophagy. LC3-II enhanced α-MSH-dependent melanogenesis by increasing MITF expression via its ability to activate ERK.

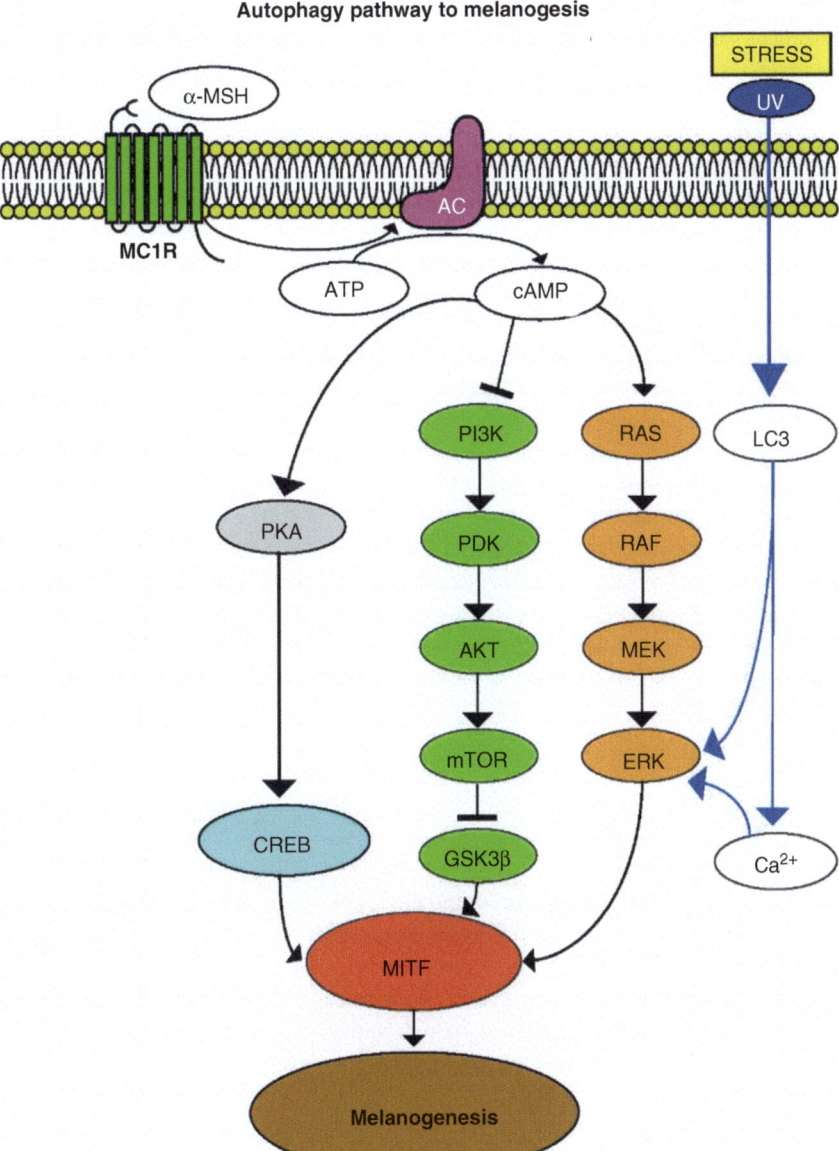

Fig. 5.15 Schematic figure of autophagy transduction pathways with the destination to MITF with resultant melanogenesis

LC3-II likely promotes ERK phosphorylation, thus initiating a pathway that transduces an upstream signal for α-MSH-induced MITF expression during melanogenesis.

Possible mechanistic explanation of autophagy-induced melanogenesis is that mobilization Ca2+ via α-MSH activation leads to induction of ERK activity and autophagy intracellular Ca2+ signaling machinery.

Ca2+ activates CREB, a well-characterized target of MITF, via the Rap1-ERK pathway during normal neuronal function.

α-MSH induces cAMP production via activation of adenyl cyclase and phosphorylation of CREB, which directly stimulates MITF transcription and ultimately contributes to melanogenesis.

Therefore, multiple relationships between intracellular Ca2+ signaling and autophagy and with subsequent CREB/MITF activation via ERK activity may influence melanogenesis.

Activation of stress-mediated autophagy triggers lipidation of LC3 to form LC3-II in melanocytes, which induced phosphorylation of ERK, likely through an increased intracellular Ca2+ release.

Once in the presence of melanogenic stimuli, such as α-MSH, LC3-II-dependent ERK activation increases phosphorylation of CREB and subsequent MITF expression, leading to induction of melanogenic gene expression (e.g. TYR, PMEL17). Thus, LC3-II, elevated during autophagy activation, appears to participate in and/or modulate a mechanism that links autophagic and melanogenic pathways under certain stress conditions.

Conclusion

The study of molecular interaction in the microenvironment of iris between its cellular contents is essential to understand its function and structural variations and color.

The role of fibroblasts in control and coordination the melanocytes of the iris has not been elaborated and emphasized enough in the past. In the previous chapter the structural aspect of these interactions has been shown in electron microscopy images.

Here the molecular interactions between the cellular structures of the iris have been discussed and described.

There are many molecular signaling pathways involved in iris that was discussed in this chapter. Fibroblasts have the main effect on melanosomes by coating the iris melanocytes with collagen, Laminin and Fibronectin. These effects are complimented by endocytosis of released melanosomes by the fibroblasts. (Refer to Figures in Chap. 4).

Fibroblasts function mimics basement membrane by controlling and moderating the function and the activity of the melanocytes. As the number of melanocytes are very limited and scars in dark irides the melanocytes have no limitation on melanin production and continue to proliferate and produce more pigment. In contrast in blue iris there are numerous fibroblasts that engulf and coat the melanocytes and prevent them from proliferation and pigment production. Fibroblasts also engulf and phagocytose (exocytosis/endocytosis) melanosomes at the melanocyte projections.

The surface receptors and signaling pathways are very different in iris melanocytes compare to the skin melanocytes. Understanding these pathways elucidates and explains many of the unanswered question regarding the physiologic and pathological changes that occur in the iris.

By understanding the molecular signaling pathways and the specification of their receptors in iris, we are able to answer the questions that was brought up at the beginning of the chapter;

Why the eye color does not change (tan) similar to the skin by sun exposure? The lack of functional MC1R receptor in iris melanocytes and the lack of paracrine signaling and participation of keratinocytes are responsible for this phenomenon. As we know the keratinocytes on exposure to UV light produce multiple paracrine factors such as alpha MSH which is the ligand for MC1R that starts the process of melanogenesis via multiple transduction pathways. Figure [1].

Why the color of the iris changes with certain glaucoma drops (Prostaglandin analogues)?

Prostaglandin analogues behave like prostaglandins and activate the EP receptors of the iris melanocytes and start the process of melanogenesis via multiple transduction pathways. Figure.

The iris melanocytes lack FP receptors and receive paracrine signaling from FP receptors of adjacent fibroblasts.

- Why the color of the eye changed in some patients with Ebola infection.

- Ebola virus activates the PI3K signal transduction and inflammatory transduction pathways that activates the process of melanogenesis. Figure.
- Why the color of the eye changes in Horner's syndrome.
- Iris melanocytes are directly connected to the autonomic neural network via synapsis which is necessary for the iris melanocyte cellular hemostasis. The lack of neural stimulation in a long period of time results in decrease melanogenesis as seen in Horner's syndrome.
- Why it is so difficult to change the color of the eye by medications or small molecules.

- The complexity of anatomical, histological and cellular molecular biology of iris structure and its melanocytes makes it very difficult to alter the pigmentation, however with a correct and specific strategy this task could be achievable.

Bibliography

1. Abdel-Malek ZA. Fueling melanocytes with ATP from keratinocytes accelerates melanin synthesis. J Invest Dermatol. 2019;139(7):1424–6. https://doi.org/10.1016/j.jid.2019.03.1137.
2. Akl MR, Nagpal P, Ayoub NM, Tai B, Prabhu SA, Capac CM, Gliksman M, Goy A, Suh KS. Molecular and clinical significance of fibroblast growth factor 2 (FGF2/bFGF) in malignancies of solid and hematological cancers for personalized therapies. Oncotarget. 2016;7(28):44735.. Available at: https://www.researchgate.net/publication/299396648
3. Saeed MF, Kolokoltsov AA, Freiberg AN, Holbrook MR, Davey RA. Phosphoinositide-3 kinase-Akt pathway controls cellular entry of Ebola virus. PLoS Pathog. 2008;4(8). https://doi.org/10.1371/journal.ppat.1000141.
4. Ambrosio AL, Boyle JA, Aradi AE, Christian KA, Di Pietro SM. TPC2 controls pigmentation by regulating melanosome pH and size. Proc Natl Acad Sci USA. 2016;113(20):5622–7. https://doi.org/10.1073/pnas.1600108113.
5. Bak MJ, Hong SG, Lee JW, Jeong WS. Red ginseng marc oil inhibits iNOS and COX-2 via NFκB and p38 pathways in LPS-stimulated RAW 264.7 macrophages. Molecules. 2012;17(12):13769–86. https://doi.org/10.3390/molecules171213769.
6. Bergh K, Wentzel P, Stjernschantz J. Production of prostaglandin E2 by Iridial melanocytes exposed to latanoprost acid, a prostaglandin F2 α analogue. J Ocular Pharmacol Ther. 2002;18(5):391–400. https://doi.org/10.1089/10807680260362678.
7. Bhardwaj S, Bhatia A, Kumaran MS, Parsad D. Role of IL-17A receptor blocking in melanocyte survival: a strategic intervention against vitiligo. Exp Dermatol. 2019;28(6):682–9. https://doi.org/10.1111/exd.13773.
8. Buscà R, Berra E, Gaggioli C, Khaled M, Bille K, Marchetti B, Thyss R, Fitsialos G, Larribère L, Bertolotto C, Virolle T, Barbry P, Pouysségur J, Ponzio G, Ballotti R. Hypoxia-inducible factor 1α is a new target of microphthalmia-associated transcription factor (MITF) in melanoma cells. Journal of Cell Biology. 2005;170(1):49–59.
9. Cao J, Tyburczy ME, Moss J, Darling TN, Widlund HR, Kwiatkowski DJ. Tuberous sclerosis complex inactivation disrupts melanogenesis via mTORC1 activation. J Clin Invest. 2017;127(1):349–64. https://doi.org/10.1172/JCI84262.
10. Cheng CY, Huang WR, Chi PI, Chiu HC, Liu HJ. Cell entry of bovine ephemeral fever virus requires activation of S rc-JNK-AP 1 and PI 3 K-A kt-NF-κ B pathways as well as C ox-2-mediated PGE 2/EP receptor signalling to enhance clathrin-mediated virus endocytosis. Cell Microbiol. 2015;17(7):967–87. https://doi.org/10.1111/cmi.12414.
11. Chung BY, Kim SY, Jung JM, Won CH, Choi JH, Lee MW, Chang SE. The antimycotic agent clotrimazole inhibits melanogenesis by accelerating ERK and PI 3K-/Akt-mediated tyrosinase degradation. Exp Dermatol. 2015;24(5):386–8. https://doi.org/10.1111/exd.12669.
12. Cui R, Widlund HR, Feige E, Lin JY, Wilensky DL, Igras VE, D'Orazio J, Fung CY, Schanbacher CF, Granter SR, Fisher DE. Central Role of p53 in the Suntan Response and Pathologic Hyperpigmentation. Cell. 2007;128(5):853–64.
13. Czyz M. HGF/c-MET signaling in melanocytes and melanoma. Int J Mol Sci. 2018;19(12):3844. https://doi.org/10.3390/ijms19123844.
14. Dantonio PM, Klein MO, Freire MR, Araujo CN, Chiacetti AC, Correa RG. Exploring major signaling cascades in melanomagenesis: a rationale route for targetted skin cancer therapy. Biosci Rep 2018;38(5). https://doi.org/10.1042/BSR20180511.
15. Diehl N, Schaal H. Make yourself at home: viral hijacking of the PI3K/Akt signaling pathway. Viruses. 2013;5(12):3192–212. Available at: www.mdpi.com/journal/viruses.
16. Eo SH, Kim SJ. Resveratrol-mediated inhibition of cyclooxygenase-2 in melanocytes suppresses melanogenesis through extracellular signal-regulated kinase 1/2 and phosphoinositide 3-kinase/Akt signalling. Eur J Pharmacol. 2019;860:172586. https://doi.org/10.1016/j.ejphar.2019.172586.

17. Eswarakumar VP, Lax I, Schlessinger J. Cellular signaling by fibroblast growth factor receptors. Cytokine Growth Factor Rev. 2005;16(2):139–49. https://doi.org/10.1016/j.cytogfr.2005.01.001.

18. Goding C, Ngeow KC, Friedrichsen HJ, Li L, Zeng Z, Andrews S, Berridge G, Picaud S, Fischer R, Lisle R, Knapp S. BRAF/MAPK and GSK3 signalling converge to control MITF nuclear export. Proc Natl Acad Sci U S A. 2018:115(37). https://doi.org/10.1073/pnas.1810498115.

19. Greenhough A, Smartt HJ, Moore AE, Roberts HR, Williams AC, Paraskeva C, Kaidi A. The COX-2/PGE 2 pathway: key roles in the hallmarks of cancer and adaptation to the tumour microenvironment. Carcinogenesis. 2009;30(3):377–86. https://doi.org/10.1093/carcin/bgp014.

20. Hu DN, McCormick SA, Seedor JA, Ritterband DC, Shah MK. Isolation, purification and cultivation of conjunctival melanocytes. Exp Eye Res. 2007;84(4):655–62. https://doi.org/10.1034/j.1600-0749.13.s8.15.x.

21. Huang J, Gu S, Chen M, Zhang SJ, Jiang Z, Chen X, Jiang C, Liu G, Radu RA, Sun X, Vollrath D. Abnormal mTORC1 signaling leads to retinal pigment epithelium degeneration. Theranostics. 2019;9(4):1170. https://doi.org/10.7150/thno.26281.

22. Huizing M, Helip-Wooley A, Westbroek W, Gunay-Aygun M, Gahl WA. Disorders of lysosome-related organelle biogenesis: clinical and molecular genetics. Annu Rev Genomics Hum Genet. 2008;9:359–86. https://doi.org/10.1146/annurev.genom.9.081307.164303.

23. Imokawa G. Melanocyte Activation Mechanisms and Rational Therapeutic Treatments of Solar Lentigos. International Journal of Molecular Sciences. 2019;20(15):3666.

24. Ke CY, Mathias CJ, Green MA. The folate receptor as a molecular target for tumor-selective radionuclide delivery. Nucl Med Biol. 2003;30(8):811–7. https://doi.org/10.5021/ad.2013.25.1.36.

25. Lee MS, Yoon HD, Kim JI, Choi JS, Byun DS, Kim HR. Dioxinodehydroeckol inhibits melanin synthesis through PI3K/Akt signalling pathway in α-melanocyte-stimulating hormone-treated B16F10 cells. Exp Dermatol. 2012;21(6):471–3. https://doi.org/10.1111/j.1600-0625.2012.01508.x.

26. Lee JS, Kim DH, Choi DK, Kim CD, Ahn GB, Yoon TY, Lee JH, Lee JY. Comparison of gene expression profiles between keratinocytes, melanocytes and fibroblasts. Ann Dermatol. 2013;25(1):36–45.

27. Lee HJ, Lee WJ, Chang SE, Lee GY. Hesperidin, a popular antioxidant inhibits melanogenesis via Erk1/2 mediated MITF degradation. Int J Mol Sci. 2015;16(8):18384–95. https://doi.org/10.3390/ijms160818384.

28. Li L, Hu DN, Zhao H, McCormick SA, Nordlund JJ, Boissy RE. Uveal melanocytes do not respond to or express receptors for α-melanocyte-stimulating hormone. Invest Ophthalmol Visual Sci. 2006;47(10):4507–12. Available at: https://iovs.arvojournals.org/article.aspx?articleid=2124882.

29. Li P, Schille C, Schweizer E, Rupp F, Heiss A, Legner C, Klotz UE, Geis-Gerstorfer J, Scheideler L, et al. Mechanical characteristics, in vitro degradation, cytotoxicity, and antibacterial evaluation of Zn-4.0 Ag alloy as a biodegradable material. Int J Mol Sci. 2018;19:755. https://doi.org/10.3390/ijms19051475.

30. Liu J, Zhang C, Hu W, Feng Z, Verma CS. Tumor suppressor p53 and metabolism. Journal of Molecular Cell Biology. 2019;11(4):284–92.

31. Luke JJ, Triozzi PL, McKenna KC, Van Meir EG, Gershenwald JE, Bastian BC, Gutkind JS, Bowcock AM, Streicher HZ, Patel PM, Sato T. Biology of advanced uveal melanoma and next steps for clinical therapeutics. Pigment Cell Melanoma Res. 2015;28(2):135–47. https://doi.org/10.1111/pcmr.12304.

32. Madrigal-Martínez A, Constâncio V, Lucio-Cazaña FJ, Fernández-Martínez AB. PROSTAGLANDIN E2 stimulates cancer-related phenotypes in prostate cancer PC3 cells through cyclooxygenase-2. J Cell Physiol. 2019;234(5):7548–59. https://doi.org/10.1002/jcp.27515.

33. Martínez-Esparza M, Ferrer C, Castells MT, García-Borrón JC, Zuasti A. Transforming growth factor β1 mediates hypopigmentation of B16 mouse melanoma cells by inhibition of melanin formation and melanosome maturation. Int J Biochem Cell Biol. 2001;33(10):971–83. Available at: https://www.ncbi.nlm.nih.gov/pubmed/11470231?dopt=Abstract.

34. Mukuno K, Witmer R. Innervation of melanocytes in human iris. Albrecht von Graefes Archiv für klinische und Exp Ophthalmol. 1977;203(1):1–8. Available at: https://link.springer.com/article/10.1007/BF00410042.

35. Nakao A. TGF-beta receptor-mediated signalling through Smad2, Smad3 and Smad4. The EMBO Journal. 1997;16(17):5353–62.

36. NIH. MITF gene. 2019. [Online] Available at: https://ghr.nlm.nih.gov/gene/MITF.

37. Oliva M, Rullan AJ, Piulats JM. Uveal melanoma as a target for immune-therapy. Ann Transl Med. 2016;4(9) https://doi.org/10.21037/atm.2016.05.04.

38. Organ SL, Tsao MS. An overview of the c-MET signaling pathway. Ther Adv Med Oncol. 2011;3(1_suppl):S7–19. https://doi.org/10.1177/1758834011422556.

39. Osei-Sarfo K, Gudas LJ. Retinoic Acid Suppresses the Canonical Wnt Signaling Pathway in Embryonic Stem Cells and Activates the Noncanonical Wnt Signaling Pathway. STEM CELLS. 2014: 32(8):2061–71.

40. Sturm RA. Molecular genetics of human pigmentation diversity. Hum Mol Genet. 2009 Apr 15;18(R1):R9–17. https://doi.org/10.1002/stem.1706.

41. Paglia D, Dubielzig RR, Kado-Fong HK, Maggs DJ. Expression of cyclooxygenase-2 in canine uveal melanocytic neoplasms. Am J Vet Res. 2009;70(10):1284–90. https://doi.org/10.2460/ajvr.70.10.1284.

42. Pal HC, Athar M, Elmets CA, Afaq F. Fisetin inhibits UVB-induced cutaneous inflammation and activation of PI3K/AKT/NFκB signaling pathways in SKH-1 hairless mice. Photochem Photobiol. 2015;91(1):225–34. https://doi.org/10.1111/php.12337.

43. Paquette M, El-Houjeiri L, Pause A. mTOR pathways in cancer and autophagy. Cancers. 2018;10(1):18. https://doi.org/10.3390/cancers10010018.

44. Portis T, Longnecker R. Epstein–Barr virus (EBV) LMP2A mediates B-lymphocyte survival through constitutive activation of the Ras/PI3K/Akt pathway. Oncogene. 2004;23(53):8619–28. Available at: https://www.nature.com/articles/1207905

45. Qomaladewi NP, Kim MY, Cho JY. Rottlerin reduces cAMP/CREB-mediated melanogenesis via regulation of autophagy. Int J Mol Sci. 2019;20(9):2081. https://doi.org/10.3390/ijms20092081.

46. Raposo G, Marks MS. The Dark Side of Lysosome-Related Organelles: Specialization of the Endocytic Pathway for Melanosome Biogenesis. Traffic. 2002;3(4):237–48.

47. Reifenberger J, Wolter M, Boström J, Büschges R, Megahed M, Ruzicka T, Schulte KW, Reifenberger G. Allelic losses on chromosome arm 10q and mutation of the PTEN (MMAC1) tumour suppressor gene in primary and metastatic malignant melanomas. Virchows Archiv. 2000;436(5):487–93.

48. Richmond A. NF-κB, chemokine gene transcription and tumour growth. Nature Reviews Immunology. 2002;2(9):664–74.

49. Saeed MF, Kolokoltsov AA, Freiberg AN, Holbrook MR, Davey RA. Phosphoinositide-3 kinase-Akt pathway controls cellular entry of Ebola virus. PLoS Pathog. 2008;4(8). https://doi.org/10.1371/journal.ppat.1000141.

50. Sandulache VC, Parekh A, Li-Korotky H, Dohar JE, Hebda PA. Prostaglandin E2 inhibition of keloid fibroblast migration, contraction, and transforming growth factor (TGF)-β1–induced collagen synthesis. Wound Repair Regeneration. 2007;15(1):122–33. https://doi.org/10.1111/j.1524-475X.2006.00193.x.

51. Schlötzer-Schrehardt U, Zenkel M, Nüsing M. Expression and localization of FP and EP prostanoid receptor subtypes in human ocular tissues. Invest Ophthalmol Visual Sci. 2002;43(5):1475–87. Available at: https://iovs.arvojournals.org/article.aspx?articleid=2123539.

52. Schwab C, Mayer C, Zalaudek I, Riedl R, Richtig M, Wackernagel W, Hofmann-Wellenhof R, Richtig G, Langmann G, Tarmann L, Wedrich A. Iris freckles a potential biomarker for chronic

sun damage. Invest Ophthalmol Visual Sci. 2017;58(6):BIO174–9. https://doi.org/10.1167/iovs.17-21751.

53. VanCompernolle SE, Clark KL, Rummel KA, Todd SC. Expression and function of formyl peptide receptors on human fibroblast cells. J Immunol. 2003;171(4):2050–6. Available at: http://www.jimmunol.org/content/171/4/2050

54. Seemab S, Pervaiz N, Zehra R, Anwar S, Bao Y, Abbasi AA. Molecular evolutionary and structural analysis of familial exudative vitreoretinopathy associated FZD4 gene. BMC Evol Biol. 2019;19(1):72. Available at: https://bmcevolbiol.biomedcentral.com/articles/10.1186/s12862-019-1400-9.

55. Shao L, Wang J, Karatas OF, Feng S, Zhang Y, Creighton CJ, Ittmann M. Fibroblast growth factor receptor signaling plays a key role in transformation induced by the TMPRSS2/ERG fusion gene and decreased PTEN. Oncotarget. 2018;9(18):14456. https://doi.org/10.18632/oncotarget.24470.

56. Sharif NA, Crider JY. Intracellular signaling in human iridial fibroblasts and iridial melanocytes in response to prostaglandins, endothelin, isoproterenol, and other pharmacological agents. Curr Eye Res. 2011;36(4):310–20. https://doi.org/10.1111/j.1600-0625.2009.00892.x.

57. Sharif NA, Crider JY. Intracellular signaling in human iridial fibroblasts and iridial melanocytes in response to prostaglandins, endothelin, isoproterenol, and other pharmacological agents. Curr Eye Res. 2011;36(4):310–20. Available at: https://www.ncbi.nlm.nih.gov/pubmed

58. Shin JM, Kim MY, Sohn KC, Jung SY, Lee HE, Lim JW, Kim S, Lee YH, Im M, Seo YJ, Kim CD. Nrf2 negatively regulates melanogenesis by modulating PI3K/Akt signaling. PLoS One. 2014;9(4) https://doi.org/10.1371/journal.pone.0096035.

59. Slominski A. Neuroendocrine activity of the melanocyte. Exp Dermatol. 2009;18(9):760–3. https://doi.org/10.1111/j.1600-0625.2009.00892.x.

60. Smith-Thomas L, Moustafa M, Spada CS, Shi L, Dawson RA, Wagner M, Balafa C, Kedzie KM, Reagan JW, Krauss AP, Woodward DF. Latanoprost-induced pigmentation in human iridial melanocytes is fibroblast dependent. Exp Eye Res. 2004;78(5):973–85. https://doi.org/10.1016/j.exer.2003.12.003.

61. Stjernschantz JW, Albert DM, Hu DN, Drago F, Wistrand PJ. Mechanism and clinical significance of prostaglandin-induced iris pigmentation. Surv Ophthalmol. 2002;47:S162–75. https://doi.org/10.1016/s0039-6257(02)00292-8.

62. Sugita S, Keino H, Futagami Y, Takase H, Mochizuki M, Stein-Streilein J, Streilein JW. B7+ iris pigment epithelial cells convert T cells into CTLA-4+, B7-expressing CD8+ regulatory T cells. Invest Ophthalmol Visual Sci. 2006;47(12):5376–84. https://doi.org/10.1167/iovs.05-1354.

63. Sumimoto H, Imabayashi F, Iwata T, Kawakami Y. The BRAF–MAPK signaling pathway is essential for cancer-immune evasion in human melanoma cells. Journal of Experimental Medicine. 2006;203(7):1651–6.

64. Swanson JA, King JS. The breadth of macropinocytosis research. 2018. Available at: https://doi.org/10.1098/rstb.2018.0146.

65. Taylor AW. Ocular immune privilege and transplantation. Front Immunol. 2016;7:37. https://doi.org/10.3389/fimmu.2016.00037.

66. Tetzlaff MT, Pattanaprichakul P, Wargo J, Fox PS, Patel KP, Estrella JS, Broaddus RR, Williams MD, Davies MA, Routbort MJ, Lazar AJ, Woodman SE, Hwu W-J, Gershenwald JE, Prieto VG, Torres-Cabala CA, Curry J. Utility of BRAF V600E Immunohistochemistry Expression Pattern as a Surrogate of BRAF Mutation Status in 154 Patients with Advanced Melanoma. Human Pathology. 2015;46(8):1101–10.

67. Tetzlaff MT, Torres-Cabala CA, Pattanaprichakul P, Rapini RP, Prieto VG, Curry JL. Emerging clinical applications of selected biomarkers in melanoma. Clin Cosmetic Invest Dermat. 2015;8:35. https://doi.org/10.2147/CCID.S49578.

68. Tripathy K, Geetha R. Latanoprost. In StatPearls [Internet] 2019. StatPearls Publishing. Available at: https://www.ncbi.nlm.nih.gov/books/NBK540978/.

69. Vachtenheim J, Borovanský J. "Transcription physiology" of pigment formation in melanocytes: central role of MITF. Exp Dermatol. 2010;19(7):617–27. https://doi.org/10.1111/j.1600-0625.2009.01053.x.
70. Varkey JB, Shantha JG, Crozier I, Kraft CS, Lyon GM, Mehta AK, Kumar G, Smith JR, Kainulainen MH, Whitmer S, Ströher U. Persistence of Ebola virus in ocular fluid during convalescence. N Engl J Med. 2015;372(25):2423–7. https://doi.org/10.1056/NEJMoa1500306.
71. Wentzel P, Bergh K, Wallin Ö, Niemelä P, Stjernschantz J. Transcription of prostanoid receptor genes and cyclooxygenase enzyme genes in cultivated human iridial melanocytes from eyes of different colours. Pigm Cell Res. 2003;16(1):43–9. Available at: https://www.ncbi.nlm.nih.gov/pubmed/12519124.
72. Yao C, Hirata T, Soontrapa K, Ma X, Takemori H, Narumiya S. Prostaglandin E 2 promotes Th1 differentiation via synergistic amplification of IL-12 signalling by cAMP and PI3-kinase. Nat Commun. 2013;4(1):1–5. Available at: https://www.nature.com/articles/ncomms2684.
73. Yao X, Jing X, Ye Y, Guo J, Sun K, Guo F. Fibroblast growth factor 18 exerts anti-osteoarthritic effects through PI3K-AKT signaling and mitochondrial fusion and fission. Pharmacol Res. 2019;139:314–24. https://doi.org/10.1016/j.phrs.2018.09.026.
74. Yao X, Zhang J, Jing X, Ye Y, Guo J, Sun K, Guo F. Fibroblast growth factor 18 exerts anti-osteoarthritic effects through PI3K-AKT signaling and mitochondrial fusion and fission. Pharmacological Research. 2019;139:314–24.
75. Yun WJ, Kim EY, Park JE, Jo SY, Bang SH, Chang EJ, Chang SE. Microtubule-associated protein light chain 3 is involved in melanogenesis via regulation of MITF expression in melanocytes. Sci Rep. 2016;6(1):1–1. https://doi.org/10.1038/srep19914.
76. Yun CY, You ST, Kim JH, Chung JH, Han SB, Shin EY, Kim EG. p21-activated kinase 4 critically regulates melanogenesis via activation of the CREB/MITF and β-catenin/MITF pathways. J Invest Dermatol. 2015;135(5):1385–94. https://doi.org/10.1038/jid.2014.548.
77. Zheng J, Feng X, Hou L, Cui Y, Zhu L, Ma J, Xia Z, Zhou W, Chen H. Latanoprost promotes neurite outgrowth in differentiated RGC-5 cells via the PI3K-Akt-mTOR signaling pathway. Cell Mol Neurobiol. 2011;31(4):597–604. https://doi.org/10.1007/s10571-011-9653-x.
78. Zhang Z, Yao L, Yang J, Wang Z, Du G. PI3K/Akt and HIF-1 signaling pathway in hypoxia-ischemia (Review). Molecular Medicine Reports. 2018.

Chapter 6
Iris Immunology and Wound Healing

Abstract The immunology and wound healing of the iris has not been described well in the past and deserve more attention. The iris has specific characteristics when discussing its immune response and its healing process in physiologic and pathologic conditions.

Iris is a part of anterior segment of the eye that is protected from inflammation by the existence of its immune privilege that is being discussed.

The wound healing of the iris is also very restricted due to many factors form lack of bleeding due to characteristic elastic cuffing of its blood vessels to the lack of inflammatory processes that are required for the healing and scar formation. The lack of collagen VII in the iris tissue is also contribute to the process of non-healing of iris tissue.

Immunology of Iris

Iris located in the anterior chamber of the eye and is floating in the Aqueous Humor that has specific immunological privilege. Due to the fact that there are no epithelium/endothelium on the anterior surface of the iris its tissue is in constant exposure to the anterior chamber environment.

The anterior chamber of the eye, like the brain, uterus, and testis, is one of the body's immune privilege sites. This presents evolutionary adaptation designed to protect itself from damaging effect of immunologic inflammation.

This immunological privilege is very essential for the eye in order to protect its sensitive and delicate structures to damage from inflammatory responses. Cornea also benefit from immunological privilege and that makes corneal and corneal endothelial cell transplants very successful [10].

The intraocular immune privilege is not always sufficient to protect its contents. Inflammation can occur in the eye if the immune privilege is overwhelmed by internal or external insults which is called Iritis and/or uveitis due to diseases and injuries.

© Springer Nature Switzerland AG 2020

K. T. Moazed, *The Iris*, https://doi.org/10.1007/978-3-030-45756-3_6

Many other different etiologies can induce severe inflammation in the eye. Viral infections such as herpes simplex or Herpes Zoster, Bacterial infections, autoimmune diseases, malignancies, Etc [3].

Uveitis is the inflammation and irritation of the Uveal tissue, this pigmented layer of the eye composed of choroid, ciliary body and the iris. Iritis is when the inflammation is more localized in the iris.

Uveitis may also affect adjacent ocular structures, such as the retina, vitreous, and optic nerve. Uvea is a very vascular tissue and contain melanocytes, fibroblasts, macrophages, mast cells, and plasma cells.

Multiple factors involved in this immune privilege state of the anterior chamber. These factors are a combination of anatomic, structural, physiological and immuno-regulatory processes that are unique in the eye.

Active tolerance to foreign antigens can occur through the following mechanisms:

- Induction of apoptosis,
- Promotion of anti-inflammatory cytokines.
- Mediation and activation of antigen-specific regulatory immunity.
- The sealed blood-ocular barriers (the blood-aqueous barrier and the blood-retinal barrier) limit the passage of inflammatory cells and molecules from blood into the eye except in the ciliary body and Iris.
- Lack of intraocular traditional lymphatics
- Lack of lymphatic intraocular immune modulators.
- Lack of Major histocompatibility complex (MHC)
- Anterior chamber (AC) cell membrane molecules (FasL, PD-L1, TRAIL) induce apoptosis and suppress activation of immune cells entering the AC.
- Circadian rhythm induced inflammation.
- Induction of T regulatory cells (Tregs).

Retinal blood vessels have non-fenestrated endothelium that are interconnected by tight junctions and covered by foot branches of astrocytes which limits the entrance of inflammatory cells and molecules into the eye.

Nonpigmented ciliary epithelium of the ciliary body and Iris vessels have fenestrated endothelium. This barrier is permeable to cellular migration of inflammatory cells and leukocytes into the anterior chamber which can occur in Uveitis and Iritis.

Retinal blood vessels are not fenestrated and prevent infiltration of inflammatory cells in the retina [5].

Anterior chamber-associated immune deviation (ACAID) is a crucial mechanism for maintaining the eye's immune privilege [6] (Fig. 6.1).

ACAID is a response to intraocular antigens which induces antigen-specific CD8+ T regulatory cells (Tregs).

- Treg cells suppress the induction and expression of T-helper cell type 1 (Th1) and Th2 immune expression systems.
- Treg cells prevent autoimmune diseases by induction of noncomplement-fixing antibodies.

Systemic, antigen-specific, active immunologic tolerance is mediated by specific class I major histocompatibility complex- (MHC I-) and restriction of Tregs which affect the macrophages, and B-cells, form an integral part of the immune system.

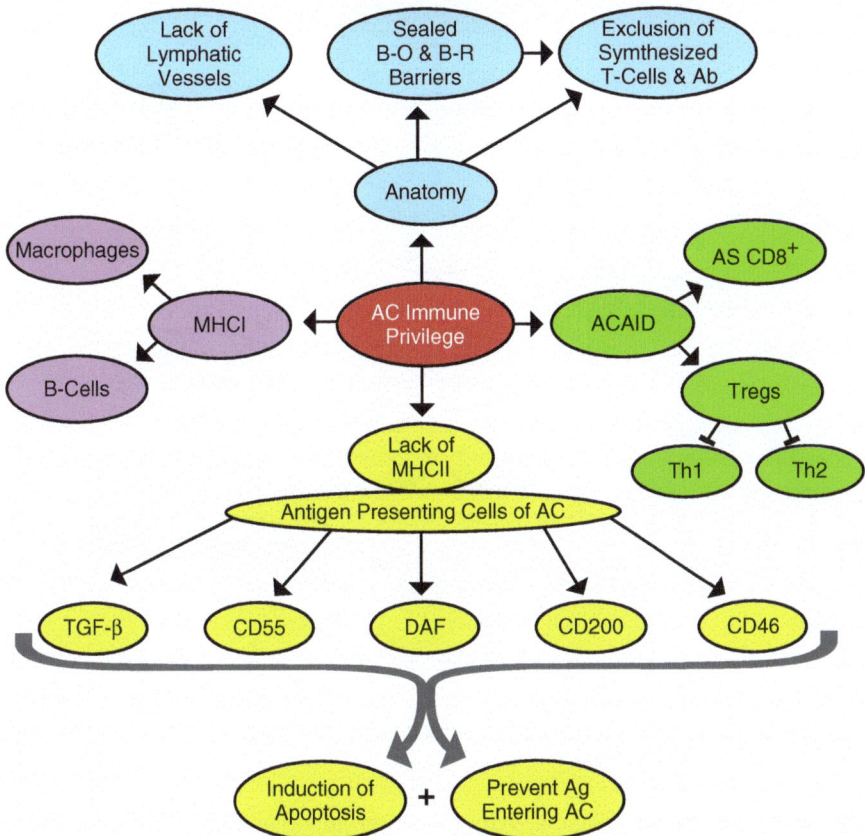

Fig. 6.1 Schematic figure of various pathways of the anterior chamber immune privilege interactions as well as the cause of anatomic and cellular influences

Other mechanisms that support the eye's immune privilege include absence of MHC class II plus professional antigen-presenting cells:

- The presence of immune modulators, such as TGF-β
- Complement decay accelerating factor (CD55 or DAF)
- Cluster of differentiation 200 (CD200) and 46 (CD46)
- Macrophage migratory inhibition factor (MIF).
- Lack of intraocular traditional lymphatic system.

T cell involvement is a crucial factor involved in anterior chamber immune responses which includes:

- Sensitized T-Cells and antibodies are mostly excluded from blood-ocular barriers.
- Induction of Treg cells by TGF-Beta, Interlukin 10 and chemokine C.
- Treg cells production of IFN-gama and inhibition of T-cell proliferation.
- Induction of Treg cells suppress the induction and expression of T-helper 1 and 2 [9].

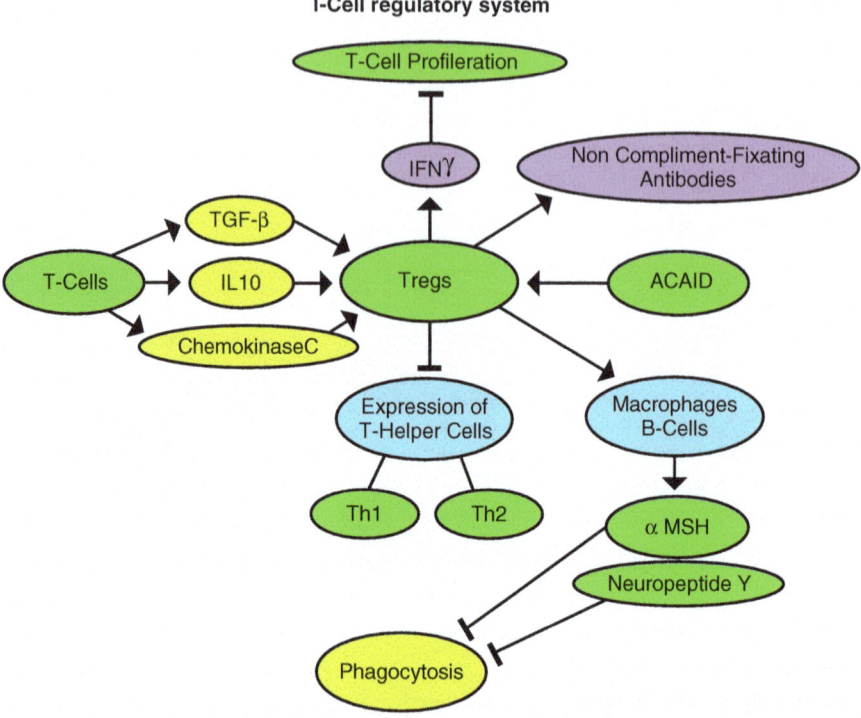

Fig. 6.2 Schematic figure of various pathways of the T-cell regulatory system as part of the immune privilege system of the anterior chamber. Cellular and immunological responses, influences, and interactions, as shown

Regulation of macrophage activity is also an important part of suppression of phagocytosis. The production of neuropeptides alpha MSH and Neuropeptide Y expressed by retinal pigment epithelium induces anti-inflammatory cytokine which suppress phagosomes production, maturation and activation. These neuropeptides also suppress antigen stimulated CD4 T cells to proliferate [1] (Fig. 6.2).

Iris Wound Healing

Wound healing is a very basic and systemic process in order to protect and restore the organism from external or internal assault. These includes trauma, surgery, acute and chronic illnesses.

Most research articles are based on external organs like skin or internal organs such as stomach ulcers. Little or no attention has been paid on healing process of the iris.

Iris assault can happen due to traumatic or iatrogenic injury during eye surgery or by laser surgery for individuals with the narrow angle of the eye to protect them against and to cure acute angle closure glaucoma.

Catastrophic iris damage due to laser ablation for color changing of the iris at other institutions have been observed by the author.

Human iris has unique characteristic that is unlike other tissues in the body, it does not heal after surgical excision such as in peripheral iridectomy or by perforation with laser as in laser peripheral iridotomy.

In order to understand the wound healing process in the iris, we have to again compare it to the skin since the wound healing process in the skin has been well defined and explained.

Since there are different stages of wound healing, we compare each stage between skin and iris and at the end summarize the differences in a table.

The classic wound healing in the skin is the result of interplay of cells, growth factors and cytokines which results in closure of the wound.

The stages and phases of the wound healing is a continuous process which each step is depend on the completion of the previous step.

Interruption or lack of these steps will interfere with the proper wound healing or the lack of wound healing as we see in the iris tissue.

Here we go through each stage of classic skin wound healing process to step by step compare and explain why there is such a drastic difference in iris process of wound healing.

We start each paragraph by the skin wound healing process then we discuss its relevance to the iris (Fig. 6.3) [8].

Stage One: The Vascular Response and Coagulation

Immediately after injury to the skin multiple events happens and this stage is completed within few hours:

- Traumatized vascular and lymphatic vessels flushing the wound to remove microorganisms and antigens. This initial step does not occur in the iris due to the special cuffing of the iris vessels that prevent bleeding after injury or cutting and also the iris does not contain lymphatic vessels.
- Clothing cascade in the skin will initiate: The extrinsic system from the injured skin and intrinsic system aggregation of thrombocytes by exposure to collagen. This also does not happen in iris due to lack of bleeding and cloth formation in the Iris tissue after assault.
- Initial vasoconstriction of injured blood vessels for 5–10 minutes triggered by platelets to Control blood loss. This event can happen in the iris.
- The blood cloth filling up the wound gap in the skin containing cytokines and growth factors. This step does not happen in the Iris due to lack of blood clot formation.
- In certain pathological conditions such as rubeosis or hemangioma bleeding can occur in the iris.

Wound healing process in skin vs. IRIS

	Skin	IRIS
Stage I	Vascular Response Blood Clotting	Lack of Bleeding No Blood Clotting
Stage II	Cellular Response Inflammatory Response	Minimal Cellular Response Minimal or No Inflammation
Stage III	Proliferation & Repair Reepithelialization Vascular Restoration Granulation Tissue Formation	No Proliferation & Repair No Epithelial Cells No Vascular Response No Granulation Tissue Formation
Stage IV	Remodeling Scar Formation	No Remodeling No Scar Formation

Fig. 6.3 Summary of wound healing process comparison between Skin and Iris. Each stage of the healing process is categorized and the red X indicates the lack of function

- The blood clot in the skin contains fibrin, fibronectin, vitronectin and thrombospondins.
- This step does not happen in most situation in the Iris due to lack of blood clot formation.
- Initial formation of provisional matrix as scaffolding structure for migration of leukocytes, keratinocytes, fibroblasts and endothelial cells and reservoir of growth factors. This step does not happen in the Iris due to lack of previous step and lack of keratinocytes in the iris.
- Local perfusion failure and lack of oxygen in the skin will increase glycolysis, PH changes and hypoxia induced factors. This step does not happen in the Iris due to lack of previous step.
- Vasodilation follows vasoconstriction with invasion of thrombocytes. This step can happen in the Iris but irrelevant to the outcome.
- Platelets influence leukocyte infiltration and release of chemotactic factors.

Platelets and leukocytes release cytokines and initiate many steps to continue the process of healing such as:

- Activate inflammatory process such as IL-1alpha, IL-1beta, and TNF-alpha.
- Stimulation of collagen synthesis FGF-2, IGF-1, TGF-beta.
- Activation and transformation of fibroblasts to myofibroblasts by TGF-beta.
- Initiation of angiogenesis by FGF-2, VEGF-A, HIF-1alfa, and TGF-beta.
- Initiation of reepithelization bt EGF, FGF-2, IGF-1 and TGF-alpha.

These steps do not happen in the Iris due to lack of previous steps in the iris.

Stage Two: The Cellular Response and Inflammation

This stage is affected in the iris due to lack of stage one and due to the specific immune privilege of the iris and anterior chamber of the eye that interferes with activation of inflammatory cells and lack of inflammatory response cytokines. Earlier in this chapters we have discussed the process of immune privilege in detail.

In the skin this stage of wound healing has early and late phases which is irrelevant to the iris.

Early phase: Neutrophil recruitment (day 1–3 after injury).

Phagocytosis and production of proteases that kills local bacteria and degrade necrotic tissue.

Production of antimicrobial substances such as:

- Cationic peptides
- Iecosanoids

Production of proteases:

- Elastase
- Cathepsin G
- Proteinase 3
- Urokinase-type plasminogen activator

Production of chemo-attractants for other cells that are involved in inflammatory phase.

Release of TNF-alpha, IL-1beta and IL-6 which stimulate VEGF and IL-8 for repair response.

Changing the phenotype and cytokine profile expression of Macrophages.

Late phase: Appearance and transformation of monocytes (around or after day 3).

Macrophages enter the injury zone to perform:

- Phagocytosis of the pathogens and cell debris.
- Secretion of growth factors such as TGF-beta, TGF-alpha, basic FGF, PDGF and VEGF

- Production of chemokines and cytokines crucial for cell and tissue movement and restoration.
- Activation of resident skin cells for synthesis of extracellular matrix (ECM).
- Activation of the next phase of the healing process.

Stage Three: The Proliferative and Repair Phase

This phase in the skin composed of re-epithelization and resurfacing (day 3–10), Neovascularization and angiogenesis and granulation formation. This stage also does not happen in the iris due to lack of epithelium in the surface, lack of angiogenesis in normal physiological conditions. And lack of granulation formation in the iris due to the lack of previous stages as we mentioned earlier.

The three main events in this stage in the skin are:

- Covering the wound surface
- Restoration of vascular tissue
- Formation of granulation tissue

The process starts with migration of the local fibroblasts along the fibrin network. Re-epithelialization from the wound edges.

Neovascularization and angiogenesis activation by capillary sprouting.

Synthesis of collagen and fibronectin serves as closing the tissue gap.

Synthesis of collagen increase throughout the wound.

Eventually the proliferation of fibroblast decline adjusting the balance between the synthesis and degradation of the ECM.

The steps in the formation of the new vessel formation (Neovascularization) in the skin are:

- The binding of the growth factor to their receptors on the endothelial cells of the existing blood vessels.
- Activation of intracellular signaling cascade.
- Secretion of proteolytic enzymes by activated capillary endothelial cells which dissolves the basal lamina.
- Proliferation and migration of the endothelial cells into the wound (Sprouting)
- Release of matrix metalloproteinases at the front of proliferation, lysing the surrounding tissue for advancement.
- The new sprouts form small tubular canal that interconnect to others, forming a vessel loop.
- Eventually inner vascular ring shrinks, but interconnection between radially arranged vessels will differentiate into mature arteries and venules.

Granulation Tissue Formation is the last step in proliferation phase. Granulation tissue is composed of:

- Fibroblasts
- Granulocytes
- Macrophages

- Capillaries
- Loose collagen bundles.

Granulation tissue is highly vascularized due to the fact that the process of angiogenesis is continues.

Granulation tissue is also packed with fibroblasts to produce collagen and ECM substances such as:

- Fibronectin
- Glycosaminoglycans
- Proteoglycans
- Hyaluronic Acid

At the end of this phase the fibroblasts will differentiate to myofibroblasts and the process of apoptosis will terminate.

It is interesting and should be addressed that the lack of collagen VII in Iris also contribute to its lack of healing process [2].

Stage IV: Remodeling

Remodeling of the skin starts from day 21 to one year after injury. Again, there is no stage four or remodeling of the iris due to lack of all previous steps.

The process of events in the skin are as follows:

- Apoptosis of the granulation tissue
- ECM changes due to replacement of collagen III the product of proliferative phase by collagen type I.
- Myofibroblasts attach to the collagen fibers to cause wound contraction.
- Angiogenesis decreases causes decline in blood flow to the healing area.
- Wound metabolic activity slows down and finally stops

It is not surprising that the healing process does not happen in Iris after this comparative review [7].

The above explanation is based on normal physiologic conditions of the iris.

There are many pathologic conditions that can cause bleeding, Inflammation and scar formation in the iris and healing or closure of iridotomies induces surgically or by laser.

Abnormal bleeding can occur due to iris neovascularization due to ischemia, diabetes and inflammation [4].

Other conditions include trauma, juvenile xantogranuloma, iris hemangioma, iris malignant tumors and metastasis.

Iris Inflammation or iritis and uveitis can start all the inflammatory processes as we discussed earlier and can activate iris healing process. Inflammation can occur due to trauma as in traumatic iritis, Bacterial and viral infections including herpes simplex and herpes zoster and neoplasms, autoimmune conditions Etc.

Granulation tissue does not occur in the iris due to the factors discussed above, however iris tissue can heal by opposing the edges of the wound by suturing it, without scar formation.

Iris scarring also can happen after iris ablation by laser in attempt to change the color of the eye, due to inflammation induced by excessive laser energy.

Bibliography

1. Benque IJ, Xia P, Shannon R, Ng TF, Taylor AW. The neuropeptides of ocular immune privilege, α-MSH and NPY, suppress phagosome maturation in macrophages. Immuno Horizons. 2018;2(10):314–23. https://doi.org/10.4049/immunohorizons.1800049.
2. Guerra L, Odorisio T, Zambruno G, Castiglia D. Stromal microenvironment in type VII collagen-deficient skin: the ground for squamous cell carcinoma development. Matrix Biol. 2017;63:1–10. https://doi.org/10.1016/j.matbio.2017.01.002.
3. Mérida S, Palacios E, Navea A, Bosch-Morell F. Macrophages and uveitis in experimental animal models. Mediators Inflammation. 2015;2015 https://doi.org/10.1155/2015/671417.
4. Moazed K, Albert D, Smith TR. Rubeosis iridis in "pseudogliomas". Surv Ophthalmol. 1980;25(2):85–90. https://doi.org/10.1016/0039-6257(80)90151-4.
5. Naylor A, Hopkins A, Hudson N, Campbell M. Tight junctions of the outer blood retina barrier. International Journal of Molecular Sciences. 2020;21(1):211.
6. Niederkorn JY. The eye sees eye to eye with the immune system: the 2019 Proctor Lecture. Invest Ophthalmol Visual Sci. 2019;60(13):4489–95. https://doi.org/10.1167/iovs.19-28632.
7. Shu DY, Lovicu FJ. Myofibroblast transdifferentiation: the dark force in ocular wound healing and fibrosis. Prog Retinal Eye Res. 2017;60:44–65. https://doi.org/10.1016/j.preteyeres.2017.08.001.
8. Smith PC, Martínez C, Martínez J, McCulloch CA. Role of fibroblast populations in periodontal wound healing and tissue remodeling. Front Physiol. 2019;10 https://doi.org/10.3389/fphys.2019.00270.
9. Sugita S, Ng TF, Lucas PJ, Gress RE, Streilein JW. B7+ iris pigment epithelium induce CD8+ T regulatory cells; both suppress CTLA-4+ T cells. J Immunol. 2006;176(1):118–27. https://doi.org/10.4049/jimmunol.176.1.118.
10. Zhou R, Caspi RR. Ocular immune privilege. F1000 Biol Rep. 2010;2 https://doi.org/10.3410/B2-3.

Chapter 7
Iris Versus Skin

Abstract As was mentioned in previous chapters, the unique structure and characteristics of iris can be better understood by comparing it to the skin. This chapter is to consolidate the information on these differences and present it in a table in order to simplify the concepts.

This table will provide a quick reference to these complex variations at a glance.

These changes are categorized according to the subjects that have been described in the previous 6 chapters. Consideration of these differences are very crucial for the researchers and the pharmaceutical companies for pigment cell research and drug delivery modalities.

In previous chapters, we covered the major differences between the skin and iris, from embryology to anatomy, from histology to electron microscopy and from immunology to wound healing process.

For details on each of these fields of science we recommend the review of each related chapters individually.

Discussion

There are many similarities between skin and Iris, yet these organs have major differences that will be discussed here.

The main similarities are:

- Their embryonic origin, which are both from embryonic surface ectoderm and mesoderm.
- Iris and skin both contain melanocytes that originates from neural crest that migrate to their final destination in these organs.
- They both contain epithelium (Skin epithelium and Iris pigment epithelium).
- They both contain mesodermal connective tissue with blood vessels, nerve supply (Dermal tissue and Iris stroma).

K. T. Moazed, *The Iris*, https://doi.org/10.1007/978-3-030-45756-3_7

- Genetic common genes of oculocutaneous albinism (OCA) which mutations can cause error in melanin synthesis and lack of pigmentation [3].

Major differences between the iris and the skin are their location and function in the body.

- Skin is an external organ located on the surface of the body and its main function is as a protective barrier from external environmental hazards.
- Iris is an internal organ with its major function is to control the amount of light entering the eye.

There are also major differences on the physiology and function of pigment cells (Melanocytes) in these organs that is summarized in the table on Iris vs Skin Melanocytes Differences (Fig. 7.1a, b).

Highlights of each category of differences are described as follows:

Embryology

- The migration of melanocytes from neural crest has different pattern. Iris stromal Melanocytes migrate from Neural Crest via Mesoderm in contrast with Iris Pigment epithelium and the skin Melanocytes migrate from Neural Crest via Surface ectoderm [7].
- Iris has no basement Membrane separating the Fibroblasts from Melanocytes. As we discussed in the embryology chapter, the iris basement membrane is located in both sides of iris pigment epithelium on the posterior surface.
- Skin has basement Membrane that separates Fibroblasts from Melanocytes. In skin the melanocytes are resting in the epithelial basal layer and are separated from dermis and the fibroblasts by basement membrane.

As we mentioned in earlier chapters basement membrane (BM) has a very important effect on melanocytes. Production of laminin and fibronectin by basement membrane harness the melanocytes and control their proliferation and migration.

- In the skin there is a direct contact of melanocytes to the BM which harness them by expression of Laminin and Fibronectin.
- Iris melanocytes are being controlled by adjacent fibroblasts that produce the Laminin and fibronectin like BM. (Detailed discussion in chapter on iris embryology)

Anatomy

- Iris has no epithelium on the anterior surface to cover the melanocytes. Instead there is a thin non continuous and fenestrated meshwork of fibroblasts on the surface of the iris with direct contact to the melanocytes.

- Anatomical position of iris structures from front to the back are: Anterior border, stroma basement membrane, dilator muscle, iris pigment epithelium, Basement membrane.
- Skin has epithelium (Keratinocytes) on the anterior surface. These keratinocytes surround and cover Melanocytes. The skin keratinocytes are in direct contact with melanocytes.
- Anatomical position of skin structures from outward to inward are: Stratum corneum, stratum spinosum, Basal layer & melanocytes, dermis matrix and fibroblasts. (Detailed discussion in chapter on iris anatomy)

IRIS vs. Skin

a

	IRIS	**Skin**
Embryology	• Origin is Neural Crest • Migration via Mesoderm • No Basement Membrane (BM) between Fibroblasts & Melanocytes • Melanocytes are harnessed by Fibroblasts	• Origin is Neural Crest • Migration via Surface Ectoderm • BM between Fibroblasts & Melanocytes • Melanocytes harnessed by BM
Anatomy	• Structure from anterior to posterior: Fibroblasts, Melanocytes, Stroma, BM, Iris Pigment Epithilium (IPE) & BM	• Structure from anterior to posterior: Keratinocytes, Melanocytes, BM & Fibroblasts
Histology	• Melanocytes in direct contact with Stroma connective tissue • Melanocytes surrounded by blood vessels & capillaries • Melanin in Melanocytes & Macrophages	• Melanocytes are separated from connective tissue by BM • Melanocytes not surrounded by blood vessels & capillaries • Melanin in Melanocytes & Keratinocytes
Electron Microscopy	• Melanocytes are round with minimum Dendrite • Melanin production minimal • Melanosome Stages I, II & III (*Blue) • Melanosomes away from nucleus (*) • Melanosomes transferred to Macrophages & Fibroblasts	• Melanocytes are oval with many Dendrite • Melanin production maximum • Melanosome Stages IV • Melanosomes around the nucleus • Melanosomes transferred to Keratinosites
Molecular Biology	• Melanocytes not responsive to UV • Not Influenced by alpha-MSH & ACTH • Non-Functioning MC1R • COX-2 procuction is Endogenous • Only EP Recdptors but no FP Receptors • Melanocyte Receptors: EP, SCF, IL Histomine & Neurotransmitters • Paracrine mainly responding to adjacent Fibroblasts	• Melanocytes highly responsive to UV • Highly influenced by alpha-MSH & ACTH • Highly active MC1R • COX-2 production is Exogenous • Both EP & FP Receptos • Melonocyte Receptors: MC1R, Wnt, Frizzled, ET1, SCF VEGF & HGF • Paracrine Mainly responding to adjacent Keratinocytes

Fig. 7.1 (**a**) Table comparing the healing process after injury to the skin versus iris. The normal four stages of the wound healing process in the skin do not occur in the iris, as is summarized here. (**b**) Table comparing the iris and skin according to specific fields of science

IRIS vs. Skin

b

	IRIS	Skin
Neural Network	• Direct Synapsis of nerve endings with Melanocytes • Neural netork has major impact on function of Melanocytes	• Mostly indirect Synapsis of nerve endings with Melanocytes • Neural netork has minimal impact on function of Melanocytes
Role of Pigment on Emerging Tissue Color	• Epithelium does not correlate to iris color • Color variation not limited to Melanin	• Epithelium directly correlates to skin color • Color variation limited to Melanin
Melanocyte Access Barriers (Drug Delivery)	• Cornea Epithelium, Bowman's Layer, Corneal Srtroma, Descemet's Membrane, Corneal Endithelium & Aqueous Humour • Conjunctiva Epithilium, Tenon's Capsule, Sclera, Anterior Chamber & Aqueous Humour	• Stratum Corneum • Stratum Spinosum
Wound Healing	• No bleeding after insult • No blood clot • No surface epithelium • Lack of collagen VII • Immune compromised environment • No inflammatory response • No granulation tissue • No scar formation	• Bleeding after insult • Blood clot • Surface epithelium involvement • Presence of collagen VII • Non-immune compromised environment • Inflammatory response • Granulation tissue formation • Scar formation

Fig. 7.1 (continued)

Histology

- Iris Melanocytes on the stroma are surrounded and are in direct contact with mesodermal loose connective tissue and macrophages.
- Skin Melanocytes are isolated and separated from dermal connective tissue by the basement membrane.
- Iris Melanocytes have abundant blood vessels and capillaries around them.
- In contrast, epidermal Melanocytes have no blood vessels or capillaries around them since there are no blood vessels in the epidermal tissue in normal physiologic conditions.
- The location of the Iris pigment melanin is in many different parts of the iris. Large number of melanocytes containing pigment are located on the anterior surface of the iris depending of the color of the iris.

Some pigment (melanin) also located deep in stromal Melanocytes again depends on the color of the eye. There are also macrophages containing melanin in the iris stroma.

The posterior pigment epithelium of the iris is packed with melanosomes containing melanin that is independent of the iris color.

Iris Melanocytes scattered in the anterior surface and the iris stroma in different numbers according to the color of the iris.

- In the Skin the pigment melanin is located in the melanocytes and keratinocytes.

   Skin Melanocytes are only located on the basal layer in the average ratio of 1–8 basal cells. (Detailed discussion in chapter on iris histology)

Electron Microscopy

The shape of melanocytes also different in skin versus iris.

- Iris Melanocytes are round and have minimal dendrite formation.
- Skin Melanocytes are oval shape and have many dendritic projections.
- Iris Melanin production minimal (stable) due to the fact that they don't donate pigment to surrounding cells in contrast to skin melanocytes that are constantly producing melanin and are very active.
- In Blue eyes melanosomes are located at the peripheral cytoplasm away from nucleus and contain stages I–III.
- Iris melanin does not transfer from melanocytes to surrounding cells and iris melanocyte have minimal denticity, however the melanosomes can be transferred and discarded by phagocytosis by macrophages and fibroblasts
- Skin melanin is constantly delivered and transfer to keratinocytes via the dendritic projections of the skin melanocytes. As the keratinocytes mature from the basal layer in normal polarization process and constantly being regenerated the pigment transfer will continue permanently. (Detailed discussion in chapter on iris molecular biology)

Molecular Biology

- Iris Melanocytes are not influenced by Hormonal signals (alpha-MSH and ACTH)
- In contrast to skin Melanocytes that are mostly influenced by hormonal signals (ACTH, alpha Melanocortin, Melatonin)
- Iris Melanin production does not get activated by UV exposure and iris color does not change by sun exposure.
- Skin Melanin production is very sensitive to UV exposure and skin color changes in sun exposure as sun tanning.

- Melanocortin1Receptor (MC1R) which is the main cell membrane receptor and the most important participant in melanogenesis in skin.
- Iris melanocytes does not have function (MC1R).
- Iris COX-2 production is endogenous.
- Skin COX-2 production is exogenous [6].
- Iris melanocytes do not express the FR receptors but express EP receptors
- Skin melanocytes express both FP and EP receptors.
- Iris Melanocytes have Minimal Tyrosinase activity due to lack of productivity.
- Skin Melanocytes have very active Tyrosinase level due to their constant melanin production.
- Iris melanocyte surface receptors are: EP, SCF, IL, Histamine, Neurotransmitters.
- Skin melanocyte main surface receptors are: MC1R, Wnt, SCF, Frizzled, ET1, VEGF, HGF [1].
- Iris Melanocytes Paracrine receptors are responding mainly to adjacent Fibroblasts [5].
- Skin Melanocytes Paracrine receptors are mainly responding to adjacent Keratinocytes with different receptors. (Detailed discussion in chapter on iris molecular biology)

Neural Network

- Iris melanocytes have direct Neural synaptic connection to melanocytes.
- Skin melanocyte nerve connection directly and indirectly to melanocytes [2].
- Newly identified skin-neural axis for detecting light by intrinsic UV transduction pathway have been recently described. Melanocytes regulate synapsis transmission via opsin -based photoreceptors [4].

Iris melanogenesis is mostly influenced by Sympathetic system as the lack of sympathetic innervation causes depigmentation of the iris as in Horner's syndrome whereas skin Melanogenesis has minimal influence by Sympathetic system.

Role of Pigment on Emerging Tissue Color

- Iris pigment epithelium at the posterior surface of the iris does not contribute to the color of the iris.
- Skin epithelium pigments directly correlate to the color of the skin.
- Iris variation in color is not limited to the Melanin pigment (Multiple factors are involved).
- Skin color variation directly related to amount of Melanin in keratinocytes and melanocytes.

Wound Healing

The most significant property of iris regarding the lack of wound healing and scar formation in physiological conditions can be explained by:

- Lack of bleeding after surgical incision due to special elastic bands around the iris blood vessels.
- Lack of clot formation necessary for scaffolding platform for healing process.
- Lack of surface epithelium to fill up the wound gap.
- Lack of collagen VII necessary for healing process.
- Immune compromised environment of anterior chamber privilege.
- Lack of inflammatory reaction necessary for wound healing.
- Lack of granulation tissue formation due to absence of previous stages of the wound healing process.
- Lack of scar formation and retraction due to lack of previous stages. (Detailed discussion in chapter on iris wound healing)

Drug Delivery and Barriers

The differences between iris and skin also exist in their potential for drug delivery approaches to the melanocytes and their melanosomes.

These includes delivery of chemicals, drugs, small molecules, peptides, hormones, nanoparticles etc. These deliveries to the melanosomes can be for many different reasons such as therapeutic or cosmetic.

Iris melanosome access barriers are:

- Via cornea, which is trough cornea epithelium, Bowman's layer, corneal stroma, Descemet's membrane and corneal endothelium.
- Via conjunctiva through conjunctiva epithelium, Tenon's capsule and sclera, into the anterior chamber and aqueous humor.

Skin melanosome access barriers are through different layers of epithelium:

- Stratum corneum
- Stratum spinosum

For the above mentioned reasons, Iris Melanocyte access require transport system to deliver

The desired agents to the melanocytes.

Skin access is much simpler and is usually by direct contact vectors such as lotions, creams and ointments.

Bibliography

1. Aoki H, Yamada Y, Hara A, Kunisada T. Two distinct types of mouse melanocyte: differential signaling requirement for the maintenance of non-cutaneous and dermal versus epidermal melanocytes. Development. 2009;136(15):2511–21. Available at: https://dev.biologists.org/content/develop/136/15/2511.full.pdf.
2. Chateau Y, Misery L. Connections between nerve endings and epidermal cells: are they synapses? Exp Dermatol. 2004;13(1):2–4. https://doi.org/10.1111/j.0906-6705.2004.00158.x.
3. Federico JR. Albinism. 2019. Available at: https://www.ncbi.nlm.nih.gov/books/NBK519018/.
4. Law BM. Photobiology of epidermal melanocytes. 2019. Available at: http://nrs.harvard.edu/urn-3:HUL.InstRepos:40620134.
5. Sharif NA, Crider JY. Intracellular signaling in human iridial fibroblasts and iridial melanocytes in response to prostaglandins, endothelin, isoproterenol, and other pharmacological agents. Curr Eye Res. 2011;36(4):310–20. https://doi.org/10.3109/02713683.2010.542869.
6. Wentzel P, Bergh K, Wallin Ö, Niemelä P, Stjernschantz J. Transcription of prostanoid receptor genes and cyclooxygenase enzyme genes in cultivated human iridial melanocytes from eyes of different colours. Pigm Cell Res. 2003;16(1):43–9. https://doi.org/10.1034/j.1600-0749.2003.00001.x.
7. Yamane T, Hayashi SI, Mizoguchi M, Yamazaki H, Kunisada T. Derivation of melanocytes from embryonic stem cells in culture. Dev Dyn. 1999;216(4–5):450–8. https://doi.org/10.1002/(SICI)1097-0177(199912)216:4/5<450::AID-DVDY13>3.0.CO;2-0.

Chapter 8
Iris Genetics

Abstract The genetics and inheritance of the iris regarding its morphology and color is very complex since it is involved in many different genes and their interactions. Recently discovery of SNP (single nucleotide polymorphism) in intron 86 of the gene HERC2 has been discovered. C allele at "rs12913832" leads to decreased expression of OCA2 in blue eyes. Multiple factors are involved in eye color variations and will be discussed in brief, the detailed data and information is way above the scope of this book. The summarized and simplified version is being discussed in this chapter and references are provided for more comprehensive insight to this fast evolving field of science.

Discussion

As the genetic field of science is in a fast evolving with new sequencing technologies and ongoing discoveries that make more information being available as time goes by.

There is a very good review of genetics of human color and patterns published by Strum & Larsson which is highly recommended [8].

At the time of the first human migrations out of Africa 60,000 years ago, our ancestral population had characteristic Dark skin, hair, and eye color to adapt to the high UV radiation around the equator.

As the first settlements moved north away from the equator adaptive mutations happened in the genes carrying pigmentary regulations. There were advantages in the lighter pigments Pheomelanin (Orange/yellow) rather than Eumelanin (Dark Brown) and less pigmentation that helped better absorption of vitamin D which was crucial to their health.

Blue-eyed people share a common ancestor, presumably 6000–10,000 years ago.

A "switch" or a simple change from adenine to guanine mutation at HERC2 happened. This mutation directly affects OCA2 gene, which regulates the pigmentation of eyes, hair and skin, as first described by Professor Hans Eiberg, University of Copenhagen.

Mutation took place north of the Black Sea, among the proto-Indo-Europeans who subsequently spread into Western Europe and later into Iran and India. Ironically, neither the first person to have the mutation, nor his or her children, would have had blue eyes themselves.

Human skin, hair and eye color is a polymorphic phenotype with strong genetic control.

The mutation also produces blond hair and fair skin, which is a survival advantage by increased production of vitamin D, and increases the sexual selections preference as reported.

Discovery of the location of the Blue eye gene (2008–2009) in humans indicates that blue eye color is associated with, and likely caused by, a single nucleotide polymorphism (rs12913832) in an intron 86 of the gene HERC2, which likely regulates expression of the neighboring pigmentation gene OCA2 [3].

There is overwhelming evidence that OCA2 gene region is regulating pigmentation in humans.

- OCA2 is the human homolog of the mouse pink-eyed dilution gene (p).
- Mutation in OCA2 gene leads to oculocutaneous albinism [4].
- OCA2 is divided into 24 exons covering more than 345 kbp of DNA.
- Many polymorphisms and non-synonymous amino acid substitutes in OCA2 gene can occur in different populations.
- HERC2 protein does not directly control the pigmentation pathway, but by indirect controlling the expression of OCA2 [1].
- Both MiTF and HLTF enhancer sequence elements in the region of HERC2 Interon 86 control the expression of OCA2 gene products [2].
- **rs12913832-C** is the blue eye SNP (single nucleotide polymorphism) that has been well identified. C allele at "rs12913832" leads to decreased expression of OCA2 in blue eyes [10].
- SNPs in rs12913832 at the region 406 bp is associated with and affects binding sites for transcription factors HLTF, LEF1 and MITF that are critical for gene regulation in melanocytes.
- Interferon Regulatory Factor 4 (IRF4) cooperate with MITF to activate expression of Tyrosinase the essential enzyme for melanin synthesis. A SNP within an Interon of this gene affects the melanin synthesis [5].
- There are more many mutations and gene variation that is responsible to the variety of human skin, hair and eye color [6].
- Other gene variants in pigment synthesis (melanogenesis) genes have been described such as in tyrosinase (TYR) and Melanocortin1 receptor (MC1R).
- Markers in the OCA2 locus are strongly associated with the eye color.
- 97.3% of light-colored eye people and 92.9% of Dark-colored eye people could be correctly classified through HERC2 (rs12913832)/OCA2 (rs1800407) [7].
- MC1R gene variations: MC1R is a transmembrane G-Protein coupled receptor with high incidence of variation that activates by a-MSH and ACTH to start the signal transduction to produce eumelanin. It has the most influence on the hair color.

- OCA2/HERC2: This complex is associated with blue vs brown eye phenotype presentation. Polymorphism in Intron 86 of HERC2 (rs12913832) influence OCA2 expression by functioning as an enhancer element. The T allele at this locus is associated with increased OCA2 expression with resultant brown eyes. The C allele causes the reduction of OCA2 expression and is associated with blue eyes [6].

     Chromosome: 15
     OCA2 gene: Location 15q12-q13.1
     HREC2 location; Location: 15q13.1
     [9] (Fig. 8.1)

OCA2 controls the synthesis of tyrosinase and Tyrosinase-related protein also maintains the PH of melanosomes.

Genetic variation in combination with resultant pigmentary and anatomical variations attribute to the variety of color differences in human eyes. Due to the vast variety of structural differences in eye color, hypothetically one can expect that there should be many other genes that are involved in inheritance of the iris color. The combination of the genes involved in iris development which affect its structure and morphology and its color for example pigment migration and settlement in the different parts of the iris anterior surface and or iris stroma.

Considering that the color of iris underline the skin has many other factors attributes to it, which perhaps some of these factors can be associated with their own specific genes.

- The amount of Melanin in the melanocytes of the anterior surface of the Iris.
- The type of melanin and its ration between pheomelanin and Eumelanin.
- The number of fibroblasts in the front surface of the iris.
- The amount of collagen on the anterior surface of the iris.
- The number of melanocytes and macrophages in the Iris stroma.
- The location and distance of melanosomes from the nucleus in melanocytes.
- Number and size melanosomes in melanocytes.
- The stages of melanosomes in melanocytes.
- The amount of iris pigment epithelium is the same in all eyes with different colors. yet its existence is essential for reflected light from the iris, as we see a pink reflection from the iris of patients with ocular albinism.
- Tindal effect = scattering in colloidal particles
- Rayleigh Effect = scattering by particles
- Anatomical variations include the thickness of the stroma and its contents.
- Amount of collagen accumulation of the iris stroma.
- Blue shift spectrum absorption of reflected light through the soft tissue, Melanin and air interface
- The participation of collagen content of the cornea as shown by removing the cornea reveals that the color variation is not as appreciable.

For details on each of these subjects we recommend reviewing the related chapters of this book.

Fig. 8.1 Schematic diagram of chromosome 15 with the location of *OCA2* and *HERC2* highlighted in red

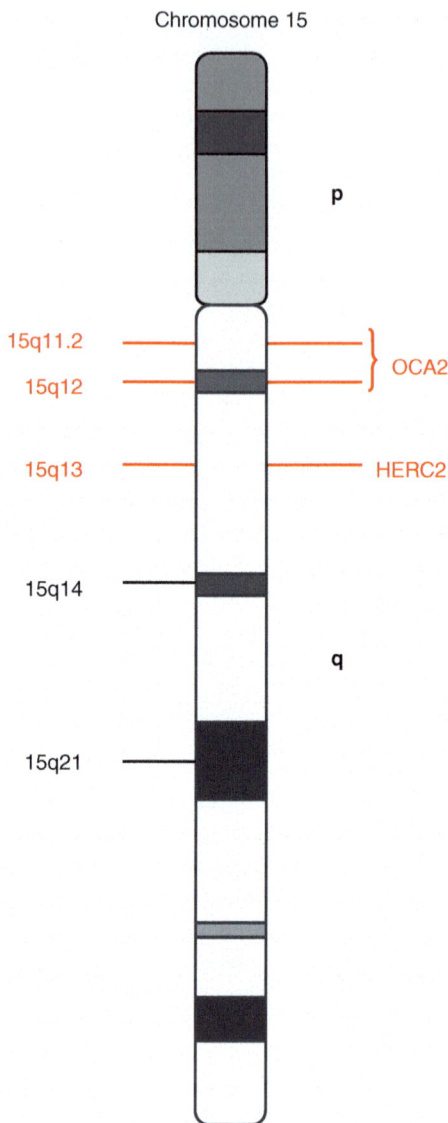

Bibliography

1. Edwards M, Cha D, Krithika S, Johnson M, Cook G, Parra EJ. Iris pigmentation as a quantitative trait: variation in populations of European, East Asian and South Asian ancestry and association with candidate gene polymorphisms. Pigm Cell Melanoma Res. 2016;29(2):141–62. https://doi.org/10.1111/pcmr.12435.
2. Eiberg H, Troelsen J, Nielsen M, Mikkelsen A, Mengel-From J, Kjaer KW, Hansen L. Blue eye color in humans may be caused by a perfectly associated founder mutation in a regu-

latory element located within the HERC2 gene inhibiting OCA2 expression. Hum Genet. 2008;123(2):177–87. https://doi.org/10.1007/s00439-007-0460-x.

3. Hohl DM, Bezus B, Ratowiecki J, Catanesi CI. Genetic and phenotypic variability of iris color in Buenos Aires population. Genet Mol Biol. 2018;41(1):50–8. https://doi.org/10.1590/1678-4685-gmb-2017-0175.

4. Lin Y, Chen X, Yang Y, Che F, Zhang S, Yuan L, Wu Y. Mutational analysis of TYR, OCA2, and SLC45A2 genes in chinese families with oculocutaneous albinism. Mol Genet Genomic Med. 2019;7(7):e00687. https://doi.org/10.1002/mgg3.687.

5. Praetorius C, Grill C, Stacey SN, Metcalf AM, Gorkin DU, Robinson KC, Van Otterloo E, Kim RS, Bergsteinsdottir K, Ogmundsdottir MH, Magnusdottir E. A polymorphism in IRF4 affects human pigmentation through a tyrosinase-dependent MITF/TFAP2A pathway. Cell. 2013;155(5):1022–33. https://doi.org/10.1016/j.cell.2013.10.022.

6. Quillen EE, Norton HL, Parra EJ, Lona-Durazo F, Ang KC, Illiescu FM, Pearson LN, Shriver MD, Lasisi T, Gokcumen O, Starr I. Shades of complexity: New perspectives on the evolution and genetic architecture of human skin. Am J Phys Anthropol. 2019;168:4–26. https://doi.org/10.1002/ajpa.23737.

7. Shapturenko MN, Vakula SI, Kandratsiuk AV, Gudievskaya IG, Shinkevich MV, Luhauniou AU, Borovko SR, Marchenko LN, Kilchevsky AV. HERC2 (rs12913832) and OCA2 (rs1800407) genes polymorphisms in relation to iris color variation in Belarusian population. Forensic Sci Int Genet. 2019; https://doi.org/10.1016/j.fsigss.2019.09.127.

8. Sturm RA, Larsson M. Genetics of human iris colour and patterns. Pigm Cell Melanoma Res. 2009;22(5):544–62. https://doi.org/10.1111/j.1755-148X.2009.00606.x.

9. Wang H, Wan Y, Yang Y, Li H, Mao L, Gao S, Xu J, Wang J. Novel compound heterozygous mutations in OCA2 gene associated with non-syndromic oculocutaneous albinism in a Chinese Han patient: a case report. BMC Med Genet. 2019;20(1):130. Available at: https://bmcmedgenet.biomedcentral.com/articles/10.1186/s12881-019-0850-7.

10. Zaorska K, Zawierucha P, Nowicki M. Prediction of skin color, tanning and freckling from DNA in Polish population: linear regression, random forest and neural network approaches. Hum Genet. 2019;138(6):635–47. Available at: https://link.springer.com/article/10.1007/s00439-019-02012-w.

Chapter 9
Iris Photobiology and Scanning Modules

Abstract In order to evaluate the preferred modules to scan and document the iris structure, it is necessary to discuss the photobiology of the anterior chamber of the eye where the iris is located.

The emerging light has to pass through the 5 layers of the cornea, enter the anterior chamber, pass through the aqueous Humor, reach the iris surface, and then enter the iris stroma.

The absorption, scattering, and reflection of light have a crucial effect on iris's emitted light and as the result its color. The amount of light absorption, scattering and light reflection is discussed in this chapter. Photobiology of melanin also plays a crucial role on the light absorption as well as scavenging of the reactive oxygen species (ROS).

The scanning modules for evaluating the microstructure of iris are discussed with an emphasis on optical coherence tomography (OCT) with the specific requirement of elaborating the unique iris tissue properties.

Iris Photobiology

Accessibility of the Iris to Light Radiation

The iris is covered by 5 layers of cornea: Epithelium, Bowman's membrane, stroma, Descemet's membrane and endothelium, and floats in the aqueous humor in the anterior chamber of the eye. Most visible light (400–750 nm) can pass through the cornea and the aqueous humor and reaches the anterior surface of the iris. Virtually all UV radiation below 295 nm (UV-C and part of UV-B) is blocked by the cornea and does not reach the iris (Fig. 9.1) [3, 8].

The transmission of UV radiation at 290–400 nm (UV-A and UV-B) through the cornea and the aqueous humor can be expressed by two different parameters: the direct transmittance and the total transmittance.

© Springer Nature Switzerland AG 2020
K. T. Moazed, *The Iris*, https://doi.org/10.1007/978-3-030-45756-3_9

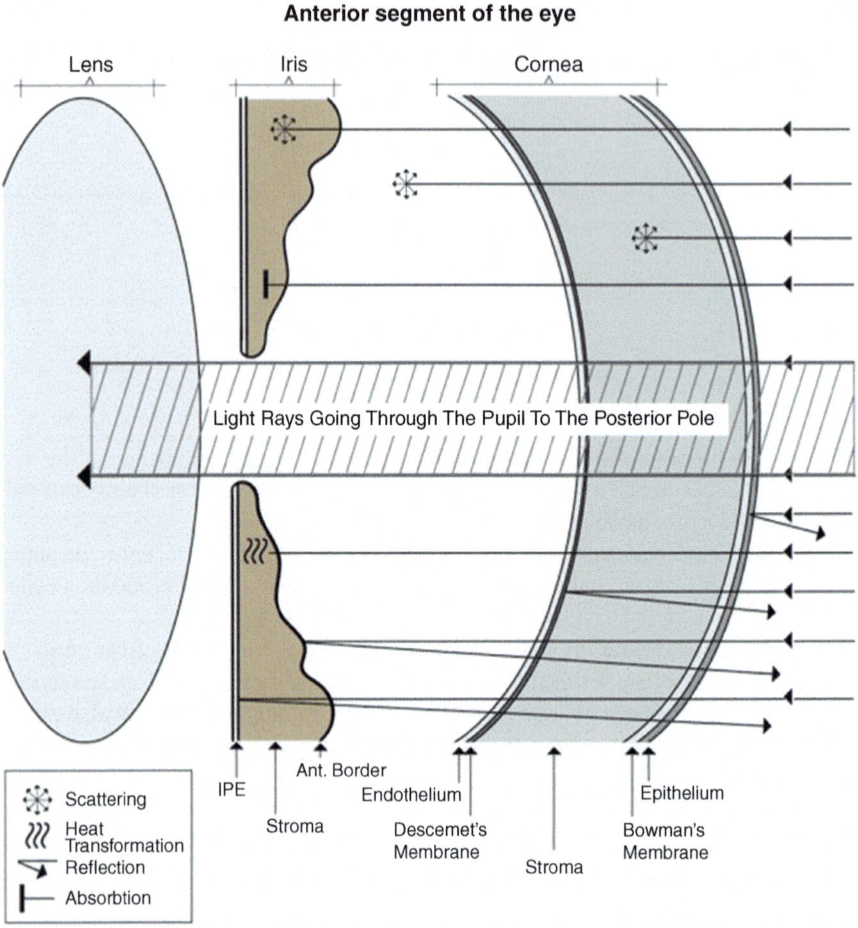

Anterior segment of the eye

Fig. 9.1 Light rays entering the anterior segment of the eye. The central light rays pass through the anterior chamber then passes through the pupil and to the posterior pole. Some rays are reflected by different surfaces, and other rays are scattered, absorbed, and transformed into heat

When light passes through the ocular medium, different interactions may occur:

- Direct transmission through the medium
     Light passes through the medium without interacting with it.
- Absorption by the medium
- The light is absorbed by the medium and turned into heat.
- Reflection by the medium
- The light is reflected by the medium, note that this includes internal reflections where the light is reflected more than once.
- Scattering by the medium
     The light is absorbed and immediately reemitted by the medium in all directions.

The total transmittance of radiation combines both the direct transmission, and indirect transmission through the scattered radiation.

UV Light Transmission

The direct and total transmittance of UV radiation that pass through the cornea and aqueous humor are:

- 32–42% at 350–400 nm (UV-A)
- 20–50% at 320–350 nm (UV-B)

Age affects the UV transmission through the cornea and aqueous humor. The percentages of light transmitted according to age and the wavelength are shown below.

Age	320 nm	350 nm	400 nm
8	20%	80%	98%
24	19%	50%	60%
80	17%	32%	40

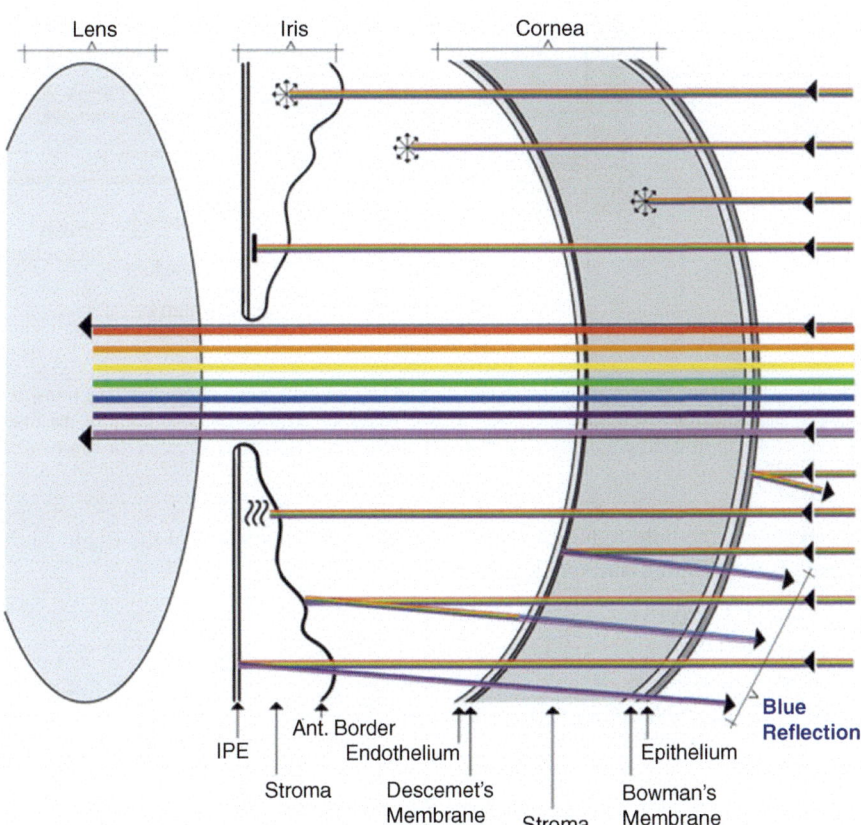

Anterior segment of the blue eye

Fig. 9.2 The full spectrum light enters the eye and undergoes scattering, absorption, heat transformation, and reflection. Reflected spectrum of light would be affected by absorption of the red portion of the spectrum by the collagen components of the iris and cornea, and only the blue wavelength would be reflected out

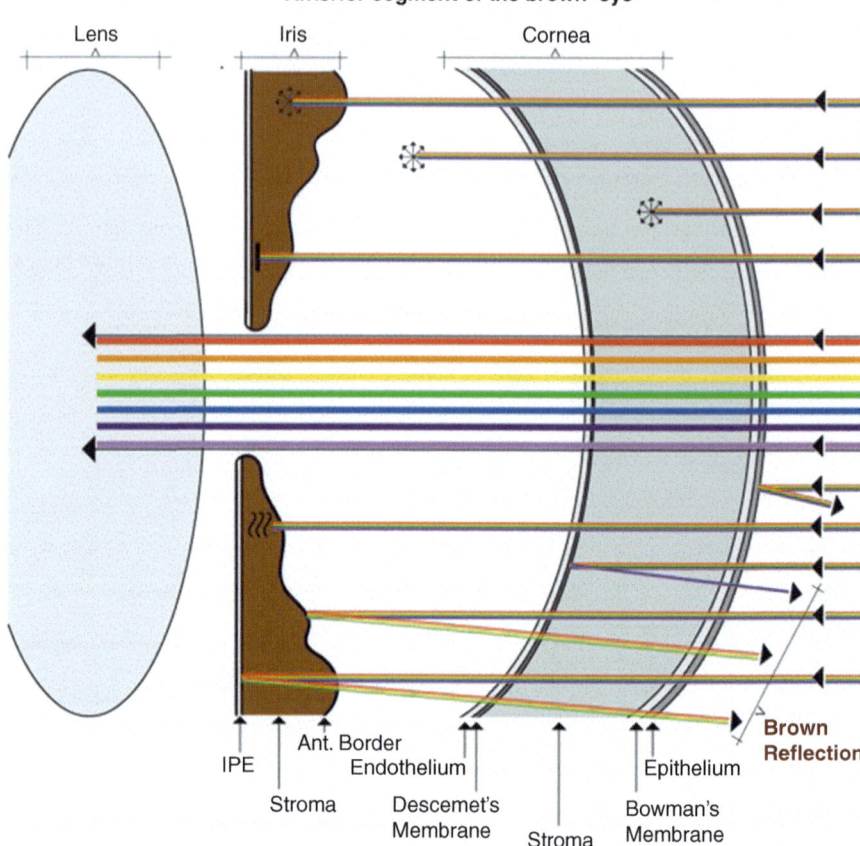

Fig. 9.3 The full spectrum light enters the eye and undergoes scattering, absorption, heat transformation, and reflection. Reflected spectrum of light would be affected by absorption of the blue portion of the spectiuon by melanocytes of the iris stroma, and only the red/green (brown) wavelength would be reflected out

Therefore, the light radiation that reaches the anterior surface of the iris in adult human being is approximately less than:

- 5% of all UV-C
- 5–20% of UV-B
- 20–60% of UV-A
- 60–90% of visible light [3] (Figs. 9.2 and 9.3)

Transmission of Light Radiation Through the Iris

The iris is a specific tissue containing various pigments, mainly melanin, hemoglobin, collagen, and intercellular matrix. Therefore, the iris can absorb and scatter a larger proportion of visible light and UV radiation entering its surface, and functions as a light screen [8].

Most biological soft tissues have relatively low light absorption property in the visible and near infrared (NIR) spectral regions, especially between 600 nm and 1300 nm. This spectral range is known as a "tissue optical window" or "therapeutic window".

Outside of this region, light is greatly absorbed by tissue pigments (such as hemoglobin and melanin) in the visible spectral region, and by tissue water content in the long wavelength NIR spectral region [28].

Fibronectin, a plasma protein immunologically identical with a major surface protein of normal fibroblasts and basement membrane (BM) bind to collagen and gelatin [5]. This combination absorbs the longer wavelength (red) part of the spectrum which results in the reflected light containing more of the shorter wavelength (blue) of the spectrum. For example, the deep located nevus in the dermis will look blue (blue nevus) or the reflection of the blood vessels on human body look blue whereas the blood has a red color. Similarly, the iris reflected light in blue eye population looks blue whereas there is no blue color or dye in the eye (Figs. 9.2 and 9.3).

The absorption spectrum of collagen powder is measured between 610 and 1040 nm by time-resolved transmittance spectroscopy [27].

Photobiology of Melanin

Melanin has a protective effect on the cells and tissues that contain it, or are near it, which consists of the photo-screening effect and the biophysical/biochemical effect [18].

- The effect of uveal melanin is related to its location. In the anterior segment (the iris), which is exposed to sunlight and UV radiation, the photo-screening effect dominates. Melanin absorbs near-infrared, visible light, and UV radiation, with absorption increasing at the shorter wavelengths.
- In the iris, the pigment epithelium and the melanocytes absorb and block visible light and UV radiation, thus, they possess photoprotective and light screen effects.

There are two chemical forms of melanin, eumelanin and pheomelanin. Several studies have compared the reactivity of eumelanin and pheomelanin.

- Both types of melanin act as a free radical scavenger and inhibit UV-induced lipid peroxidation. However, when pheomelanin is complexed with Fe (III), it stimulates UV-induced lipid peroxidation, whereas eumelanin does not [13].
- The antioxidant property of melanin is related to the type of melanin: the greater the ratio of eumelanin to pheomelanin, the better the antioxidant capacity of the melanin [4].
- The higher the melanin and eumelanin content of cultured melanocytes the better the rate survival after UVB irradiation [16].
- UV irradiation of pheomelanin may also generate reactive oxygen species whereas eumelanin tends stabilize and eradicate it [26].

• Pheomelanosmes are more prooxidant than eumelanosomes and this difference is attributed to the pigment content of the melanosome, whether containing eumelanin or pheomelanin.

Skin Melanin, Hemoglobin, and Light Scattering Properties can be Quantitatively Assessed In Vivo Using Diffuse Reflectance Spectroscopy [30].

Iris Optical Coherence Tomography (IOCT) and Scanning Modules

For scanning the iris, similar to scanning of the retina/macula, there is a need for specific and different modules, equipment and software programing. Recently, the technologies for imaging of retinal pigment epithelium (RPE) melanin have been reviewed [15]. The standard view of iris with anterior segment OCT (AS-OCT) can be observed in (Fig. 9.4).

Comparison of brown & blue Iris oct

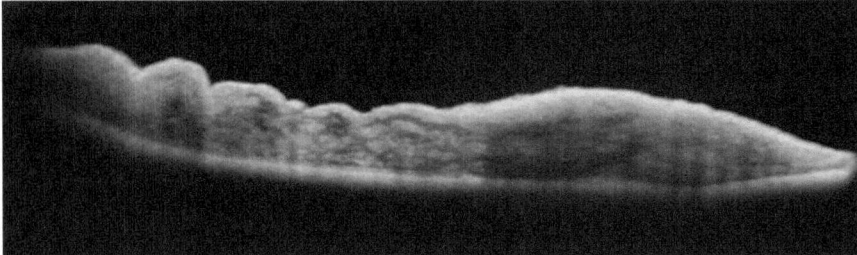

OCT of Brown Iris

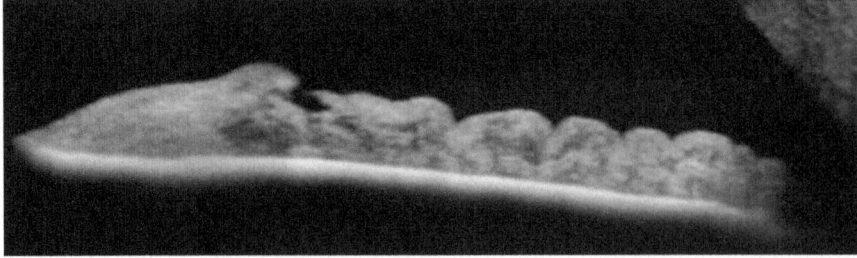

OCT of Blue Iris

Fig. 9.4 OCT of both brown and blue irides. The pigment on the anterior border of the brown iris is noticeable in OCT. The absence of pigment is easily recognized on the blue iris anterior border

There are many different ways of scanning the ocular tissues.

- Line scan: gives the option of getting multiple parallel lines with the length of 12 mm to cover the iris. The axis of the lines can rotate 360 degree and the distance varied as needed.
- Radial Scan: consists of multiple equally spaced line scan that pass through the central common axis, with its center in the center of the pupil.
- Iris thickness map: The same as radial but with a fixed diameter.
- Fast iris thickness map: A quick protocol that takes a short time to acquire limited scans for volume analysis.
- Raster lines: Multiple parallel lines placed over a rectangular region that can be adjusted to cover the area of pathology.
- Stromal scan: This protocol is composed of spoke pattern configuration with equally spaced scan lines. The color coding represents the different iris thicknesses. The elimination of posterior double layers of Iris Pigment Epithelium (IPE) by demarcation line between the posterior surface of the stroma and IPE can be used, and its elimination.
- 360 Iris topography by continuous axial scanner in a rotating manner.
- Surface topography of the iris as in corneal topography by combination modes and reconstruction software.

For the very dark Irides and in evaluation of iris pigment epithelium, the thickness' measurements can be very important specially in conditions such as pigment dispersion syndrome.

The iris pigment epithelium thickness also can be measured as will be discussed with different types of OCT based on multiple scans of one same point obtaining an image in which will suppress the noise generated by individual images. Also using longer wavelength will produce a greater penetration without losing detection sensitivity.

A Biophysically-Based Spectral Model of Light Interaction with Human Skin have been reported and discussed [12].

A Predictive Light Transport Model for the Human Iris to simulate the light scattering and absorption occurring within the Iris tissue has been designed and reported [14]. We found the conclusions and the comments that was posted in this study very beneficial. Spacially we found the following quotation very relevant:

"The ocular tissues, especially those forming the human iris, pose the most challenging modeling problems which are often associated with data scarcity". The proposed and discussed model was algorithmically simulating the light scattering and absorption processes occurring within the iris and computes the spectral radiometric responses. the spectral results provided by the model are evaluated through comparisons with actual measured iridial data, and its integration into frameworks is illustrated through the generation of images depicting iridial chromatic variations [14].

Glaucoma and Oct with Topography of the Iris, as a Unit for Laser Intervention

There are many types and subtypes of glaucoma. The main category is the Open angle glaucoma and angle closure glaucoma. OCT can be very essential to evaluate different types at each category.

• In classic chronic open angle glaucoma, the treatment usually starts with topical application of medications (eyedrops), the use of laser in addition may be needed to be included to control the intra ocular pressure. The evaluation of the angle structure of the eye that is in part the base of the iris, can be a very valuable source for therapeutic planning for future treatment. The standard laser treatments for this condition includes ALT and SLT.
• Pigmentary glaucoma is a condition that is associated with iris atrophy and thinning. The iris moves back and forth and releases the pigment which clogs the meshwork that drains the Aqueous Humor from the eye. The increase in the intraocular pressure causes damage to the optic nerve and eventually blindness. Combination of medical treatment and surgery/laser intervention (Iridotomy) is very beneficial to make a small hole in the iris to make a new connection between the anterior and the posterior chamber of the eye.
• The standard treatment of acute angle Closure Glaucoma is laser iridotomy which prevent the capture of the aqueous humor in the posterior chamber and prevent an acute increase in intra ocular pressure referred to as "acute narrow wangle glaucoma" which can cause blindness.

The laser iridotomy is a preferred mode of treatment for this condition and is performed by using Argon laser or YAG laser to which would make a full thickness hole as a safety valve on the iris.

The laser iridotomy is also indicated for the patients with narrow iridocorneal angle as a preventative procedure to protect them against the angle closure glaucoma attack.

The standard evaluation of the angle is a part of standard examination of the eye by the eye specialists and is called Gonioscopy. This is done by placing a contact mirrors with an angle to provide view of the angular structures (Gonio-lens).

Recently there has been an increasing role for OCT in management of glaucoma.

For example, in open angle glaucoma the OCT of the optic disc reveals the changes in the thickness of the nerve fiber layer (NFL) of the retina as the consequence of glaucoma and the topography of the optic disc documents the cup to disc ratio as it increases by progression of the glaucoma.

As in narrow angle glaucoma, the anterior segment OCT (AS-OCT) reveals the angular degree of the eye which is the angle between the iris root and the cornea periphery [23].

There is need for OCT hardware and software program to give 3-dimensional topography of the iris with thickness assessment in order to locate the best possible spot for laser iridotomy.

The existing 3d models do not reflect the histology of the iris, and there is no high-resolution topography of the iris available at present.

Indications for the need for specific iris OCT:

- Studying histologic iris structure in glaucoma patients.
- Identify and diagnose abnormalities and diseases of the iris.
- Monitoring the benign and malignant tumors of the iris such as Iris nevus, diffuse iris nevus, amelanotic iris nevus, iris melanocytosis, metastatic or malignant transformation of melanocytes (Malignant melanoma).
- Monitoring the course of treatment on acute and chronic inflammatory conditions such as pigment dispersion syndrome, essential iris atrophy, or iritis. This includes viral induced iritis. Many viruses can affect the iris such as Herpes Simplex and Herpes Zoster (HSV-HZV) others include Cytomegalovirus (CMV), and Rubella.
- Post-operative evaluation of surgical or laser surgical cases such as patency of the aqueous shunt after glaucoma surgery.
- Locating the optimal location and power setting for laser surgery on Iris. This includes therapeutic laser surgeries as in glaucoma laser surgeries or cosmetic laser surgeries for iris color change.
- Detecting iris neovascularization Rubeosis Iridis (RI) in diabetic patients, or after central retinal vein occlusion or post radiation treatment.
- Identifying the population, melanin density and anatomical location of melanocytes in iris tissue by ultrahigh resolution high speed OCT can locate exact plane of stroma for destruction of melanin by femto laser that does not produce heat with complete within few microns' accuracy.
- Participation in automated and robotic surgeries in the iris for the above discussed conditions.
- Performing remote-operated operations and laser surgeries in the remote places on earth or in the space, moon or planets or space stations.
- Combining with virtual reality equipment for intra operative interactions in the future.
- Due to the fact that melanin pigment storing zinc it can be used as contrast in iris.
- There is an existing patent that describes the use of zinc in OCT [31].

As for now, one of the most effective use of laser surgery in ophthalmology is for the treatment of glaucoma.

Glaucoma is one of the leading causes of blindness in the world. It is estimated that there is over 60 million people are affected worldwide and the numbers are increasing [22].

Primary Angle Closure Glaucoma (PACG) is the second most common type of glaucoma.

The main mechanism of (PACG) is the blockage of aqueous flow from the posterior chamber to the anterior chamber of the eye by the iris which is called pupillary block. This would cause the iris to move forward and close the iridocorneal angle which is responsible for the drainage of the aqueous humor outside the globe.

As the result the pressure inside the eye increases to the point that would cause permanent damage to the optic nerve that will cause blindness.

The treatment of this condition before the laser era was to take these patients to the operating room and perform a surgical incision at the limbus of the eye to enter the anterior chamber. Then with special iris forceps the peripheral iris is pinched and pulled out of the eye and is cut with a small scissors and the surgical wound is then closed with a suture. This was called peripheral iridectomy and still is used during the glaucoma filtering surgery of the eye.

By introduction of the laser the procedure can be done much faster without the need to opening the eye due to penetration of the laser energy through the clear cornea.

However, there are problems with laser iridotomy which can be minimized by creating a special type of interactive process to identify and localize the feasible area for laser treatment.

There are many factors involved in laser iridotomy procedure:

– Corneal transparency can be affected by corneal edema or aging opacities (Arcus Senilis).
– Iris thickness, location of the crypts and folds and furrows, ridges, rings, iris corona, freckles, and a zigzag shaped collarette.
– Iris color, pigment absorbs the laser energy and can affect the outcome. The darker the color of the eye the more laser energy is needed.
– Ethnic background: There is a large racial difference in the color and the thickness of the iris and the incidence of the PACG is much higher in Indian and Asian eyes [6].

Location Identification for Laser Surgery

The iridotomy specially if it is large can affect the vision and causes major discomfort for the patient (Dysphotopsia). There are many references on the best location for the peripheral iridotomy. The most practical is to use a small hole around 0.2–0.3 mm in size and locate it between 11 and 1 O'clock to be covered by the upper eyelid to prevent extra image on the retina through the newly induced hole. There have been disagreements about the location of the iridotomy on the iris but recent studies have confirmed that the visual symptoms will disappear after 6 months regardless of the location [25].

The procedure can be very difficult and not successful if the iris is thick or the iridotomy is at the wrong area. The complications will increase if the patient is at high risk of bleeding or can induce iatrogenic iritis due to excess laser energy to the eye that result painful red eye.

There is a definit need for an OCT equipment that is capable of performing both iris topography and 3D volume calculation.

A detailed iris surface topography to identify all the structural specifications of the iris, as mentioned above, can be extremely helpful. The installed software can identify and mark the structural variations. The 3D scanner can measure the thickness of the iris and match it to the topographic scan and mark the thinnest area for laser intervention. The information can then be processed by the software due to priority of the favorable sites for treatment. The best location can then be calculated by the primary locations at the periphery of the iris and then towards secondary locations closer to the center. The pupillary area will be on the red zone which is not considered practical due to residual visual disturbances (Dysphotopsia).

The software can also calculate the amount of laser energy that is needed to penetrate the iris at each location according to the database archives that matches that area.

In the future the robotic laser equipment can be programmed to automatically scan the eye make a diagnosis and treat the eye by performing the necessary laser procedure at the best possible location without any intervention.

Specific Types of OCT by Focusing on Histology and Molecular Biology of the Iris

The standard OCT imaging is able to produce micron scale images in the depth of 1–2 mm. This is very convenient for study of iris since the thickness of the iris is varying in different parts averaging from about 400 to 600 microns [9].

The OCT specifications and criteria is on a constant change due to fast improvement in technology and science.

Due to the fact that several variations of OCT have been developed recently, none has the specifics that is needed for the evaluation of iris and they do not address the organ/tissue specifics that is needed.

The Perfect OCT for evaluating the iris should have the ability to perform different tasks in a same unit which is a possible software/hardware engineering challenge. The Following are very essential in evaluating the iris.

The ideal OCT equipment for the iris (I-OCT) should be able to:

1. Documentation of the color of the iris.
2. Surface topography of the entire iris.
3. 3D configuration and mapping of the iris.
4. Identification and thickness measurement of the iris anterior border, Iris stroma, iris muscles and the posterior iris pigment epithelium.
5. Thickness identification of all areas of the iris from center to the periphery or reverse.
6. Identification and location and measurement of the Ruff, Collarette, Furrows, crypts of fuchs, Iris freckles and Wolfflin nodules.

- To Perform Spectroscopic OCT to locate the location and the amount of pigmentation in the stroma of the iris [7].
- To identify inflammatory cells/necrotic cells and their location in the iris.

7. Histological identification:

   (a) Identification and thickness measurement of collagen layer on the anterior surface of the iris.
   (b) Identification and thickness measurement of the melanocytes and the cell population (number) of the melanocytes in the iris anterior border and in the stroma.
   (c) Identification of the borders and location and the thickness measurement of the sphincter and dilator muscles.
   (d) Identification of the borders and of the thickness measurement of the posterior double layers of iris pigment epithelium.
   (e) Performing Spectroscopic OCT to locate the exact location and the amount of pigmentation in the stroma of the iris.
   (f) To identify inflammatory cells/necrotic cells and their location in the iris

8. Molecular identification of:

Melanin: Melanin accumulation in malignant and non-malignant conditions such as iris nevus or Melanoma can be evaluated and the progression of them can be documented.

Zinc: Metallothioneins (MTs) are zinc-ion-binding proteins that have antioxidant properties. They decrease by aging and inflammatory conditions which releases the Zn that is toxic to the tissue.

Copper: (Kayser-Fleischer ring) CU accumulation in the Iris periphery in the Descemet membrane (1–2 mm thick) as a green-brown ring as a characteristic for Wilson disease which associates with neurological symptoms in 98% of the patients.

The proposed OCT also should be able to perform Doppler OCT to locate the vascular structure of the iris as was described by swept source OCT [21].

Molecular biology and melanin content of the iris can be evaluated by Pump-Probe OCT (PPOCT) [10].

Melanin molecule is a polymer and does not have a single molecular structure. There are different groups of melanin such as Eumelanin which is the most abundant and is dark brown in color, the Pheomelanin which is yellow orange and neuromelanin located in neural tissue. Each group has different species with different physical properties and biochemical functions. The PPOCT sensitive to melanin can be used to diagnose or monitor pigmentary changes in the iris such as pigmentary glaucoma, iris melanoma, pigment dispersion syndrome, Essential iris atrophy etc [11].

The use of designed two-color Fourier domain OCT system has been described for measurement of melanin in porcine iris.

Polarization sensitive OCT is also yet another way to evaluate the melanin content of the Iris. Bernhard B. et al. has reported PSOCT as a functional extension of OCT due to polarization properties of melanin on his article [2].

In 2015, OCT angiography of iris melanoma was described by Skalet et al. with collaboration with MIT and Carl Zeiss Meditec company using anterior segment OCT system operating at 1050 nm wavelength at 100 KHz axial repetition rate [24].

Considering unique properties of OCT makes it a valuable tool for ophthalmology.

- OCT is a near-microscopic instant imaging source
- It can be used in live subjects
- There is no need for preparation of the patients
- There is no need for anesthetics
- There is no need for histology specimen (Processing, cutting and staining)
- Its performance is without using ionizing radiation
- It is noninvasive and no contact with the patient is necessary

Background

The concept of OCT started to develop in eighties. The first one dimensional image reported in 1991. Two dimensional images were developed in 1993, followed by 3 dimensional images and by 1994 the anterior segment OCT was introduced and since then, many different types and versions have been emerged and the technology continues to be improved.

The main source of interest at first was retina. This was followed by OCT of the optic nerve which has become a standard module to evaluate glaucoma progression and then the cornea OCT followed by the anterior segment which was added to the menu with the emphasize on the angle structure to measure the degree of the angle structure.

A good review of the history and development of OCT was described by Schuman (Schuman, 2008). Many more advancement in technology have been made since then and yet more to be developed.

The introduction of cataract surgery using Femto laser and anterior segment OCT facilitate the initial stages of the operation is becoming popular in recent years.

In summary the common use of OCT in ophthalmology at present are:

- Anterior segment OCT for evaluation of:

- Diseases of the cornea.
- Evaluation of the angle of the eye.
- Femto laser-assisted cataract surgery.
- Iris doppler angiography for neovascularization and neoplasm.

- Posterior segment OCT for evaluation of:

  - Retina in diabetic patients
  - Macula in macular diseases such as macular edema or degeneration.
  - Optic nerve for glaucoma patients.
  - Retinal angiography for neovascularization for example as in diabetic retinopathy

  Slit lamp adapted OCT (SL-OCT) is basically mounting the OCT on the examining slit lamp.

The basic concept of the OCT can be summarized in a figure which would be easy to understand (Fig. 9.5). However, here are many different variations of the original OCT which each have their own restrictions and benefits:

- Time Domain OCT (TD-OCT) using moving mirror which results in slow image formation.
- Spectral Domain OCT (SD-OCT) no moving mirror high resolution and fast.
- Polarization sensitive OCT (PS-OCT) useful for topography and pigmented tissue.
- Swept source OCT (SS-OCT) using longer wavelength for better tissue penetration and can be used in pigmented tissue.
- Fourier Domain OCT (FD-OCT) Distributing different optical frequencies into the detector stripe.
- Enhanced depth image OCT (EDI-OCT) which is useful for evaluation of choroid.

At present recent OCT equipment are capable of:

- Scan speed of 100,000 scan/second
- Resolution of 2–3 micrometer
- Scan depth of 2–2.9 micrometer
- Tunable laser as light source which can provide wavelengths from 840 nm to up to 1065 nm.

There are many companies working on newer and better imaging devices with little interest in iris histology. The main companies that have been working on the anterior segment OCT are:

- Heidelberg from Germany (Spectralis)
- Carl Zeiss Meditec Inc. form USA/Germany (Cirrus HD)
- Optovue from USA (RTVue)
- Tomey from Germany with 3 D images of anterior chamber (Casia)
- Topcon from Tokyo, Japan

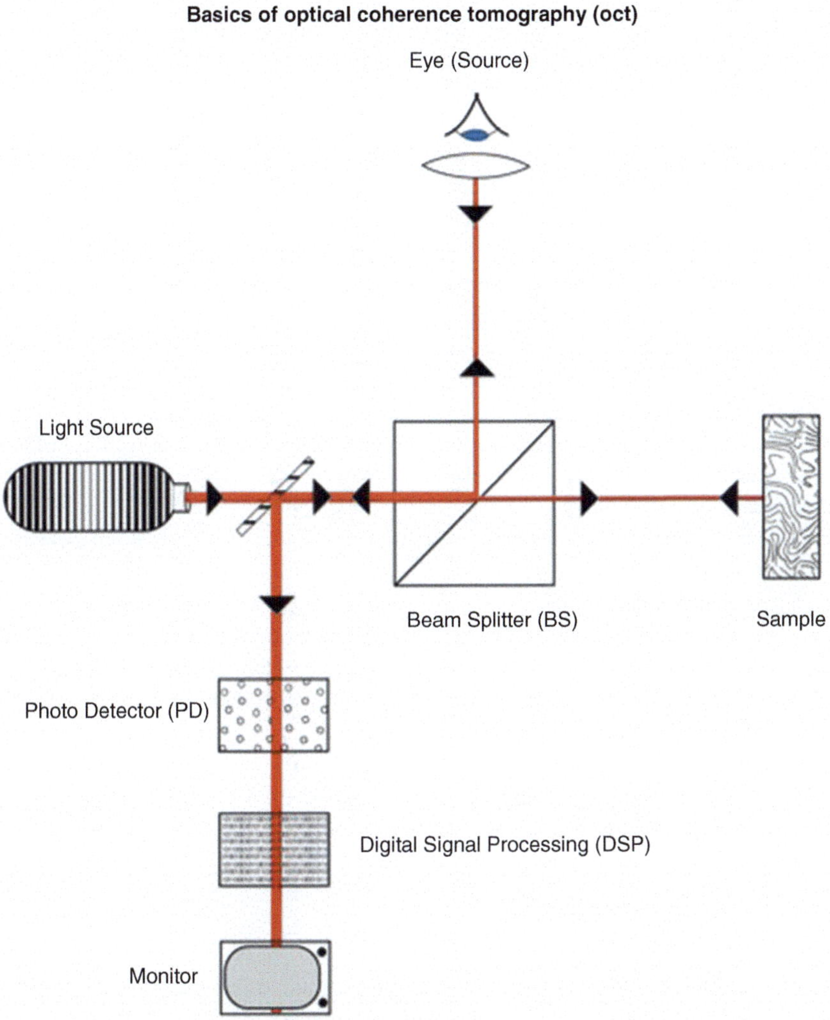

Basics of optical coherence tomography (oct)

Eye (Source)

Light Source

Beam Splitter (BS)   Sample

Photo Detector (PD)

Digital Signal Processing (DSP)

Monitor

Fig. 9.5 The basics of OCT are presented in this diagram. The emitted light source is divided by the beam splitter and enters both the sample and the source. The reflected light, detected by the photo dector, is then transported through the digital signal processor, the results of which become visible images on the monitor

These devices are not designed and are not programmed to evaluate the iris histology. As the result the iris images are crude and nonspecific.

Also, there are unique iris tissue specifications that are not like any other part of the eye. The closest comparable tissue is the choroid yet there exist many differences.

Specifications of iris tissue related to OCT:

1. Movement

    Unlike the other parts of the eye (not referring to the globe movement), the iris is constantly moving. This can overcome by

    • Using pilocarpine eye drops 20 minutes before to immobilize and constrict the pupil
    • Using the fast OCT system.
    • Using standard tracking software

2. Variability

    The iris unlike retina, optic nerve and cornea Iris have a very large structural variations in different individuals.

3. Irregular surface

    The surface of the iris is very irregular and is missing in certain parts make it difficult to target. These irregularities are due to the folds and craters such as Crypts of Fuchs, collarette, and on the back surface of the iris the radial Folds of Schwalbe, etc.

4. Size and shape

    The iris shape and size are dependent on the status of the iris in dilation state or miotic state.

5. Pigmentation and freckles

    The most variable part is the amount of pigment on the anterior surface of the iris and the stroma. The range from no pigment in blue eyes to the darkly pigmented stroma in brown eyes which requires the different range of setting to be available in the same OCT equipment.

6. Vascularity

Iris is a highly vascularized organ and would require the availability of the Doppler imaging technique to be added to the device.

As was mentioned earlier there are many similarities between the iris and choroid which needs to be addressed:

• Embryology and origin [29].
• Like in the Iris, Choroid blood vessels are originated from mesoderm. Pigment cells and pericytes are originated from Neural crest.
• Vascularization: Both organs are highly vascularized.
• Pigmentation: Choroid is highly pigmented whereas iris stromal pigmentation varies according to its color (except for iris pigment epithelium that has constant amount of pigmentation in all)
• Anatomical Location: Iris is located in the anterior part of the eye in front of the lens. Choroid is located at the most posterior part of the eye behind the retina and retinal pigment epithelium (RPE).
• Visibility: Iris is visible directly through the clear cornea, but choroid is covered with clear retina and darkly pigmented RPE.

• Accessibility: Iris front surface has no membrane or epithelium and is exposed to aqueous humor. Choroid has cornea, lens, retina, Iris pigment epithelium and the 5 layered Bruch's membrane in front of it.

It is important to address the fact that highly pigmented iris in dark brown iris is very similar to the choroid with its high vascularity and pigment. The concept of functional OCT parameters that has been experimented on choroid should be functional also for iris.

In publication of Jan. 2016, speckle-noise free 1050 nm swept source optical coherence tomography has been used for measuring small choroidal melanocytic tumors [17].

Swept Source OCT (SS-OCT) is standard in most ophthalmic systems with specifications that are higher scanning speed with higher sensitivity. It has no moving mirrors and has minimal signal drop-off with depth.

Also, using Frequency domain low-coherence interferometer with SS-OCT increases the performance to a very high scanning speed up to 20 kHz and higher and maintain the sensitivity. The fact that it may lose sensitivity with increase depth may not be a major downfall since the surface and the stroma of the iris are very thin approximately around

Average 100–300 micrometer.

The standard eye tracking software and locating the focus spot at the correct location will also improve the image quality.

Due to recent interest and many studies in progress regarding the iris pigmentation there is a desperate need for an OCT capable of distinguishing detail anatomy and histology of the iris and locate the amount and location of pigment melanin on the stroma and the anterior surface of the iris.

The posterior 2 layers of iris pigment epithelium which is constant can be identified by software and can be separated from the rest of the iris. The main interest should be emphasized on the surface and stroma.

For measuring choroidal thickness, the original OCT probe light of 800 nm is not feasible due to high back scattering of retinal pigment epithelium (RPE). In recent studies the use of longer higher probe light wavelength up to 1060 nm has been used with much better results using with high spectral Source OCT (SS-OCT) [17].

Iris Neovascularization "Rubeosis Irides" (RI)

RI is a very aggressive and devastating phenomena that leads to blindness in diabetic patients or in other conditions that associates with ischemia (lack of oxygen) to the eye and/or chronic inflammation that originally reported by the current author [19].

As newly generated blood vessels grows at the angle of the eye where the drainage of the aqueous occurs, the angle gets zipped by contraction of the new fibrovascular tissue. This will cause the obstruction of the outflow of the aqueous from the eye. As the result the aqueous that has been secreted by the nonpigmented layer of the ciliary epithelium at ciliary processes cannot exit the globe and as the result the intraocular pressure will rises and build up intra-ocular pressure which causes the damage to the optic nerve and resulting in blindness.

The combination of pan-retinal photocoagulation by laser is to be combined with the use of intravitreal injection of Anti VEGF (Vascular Endothelial Growth Factor).

The first anti VEGF developed by the use of recombinant humanized monoclonal antibody blocks the formation of new blood vessels by inhibiting its growth factor. The growth of new blood vessels is the main reason for complications in the ocular tissue as it retracts and breaks that cause anatomical changes like angle closure and by causing hemorrhage with its devastating consequences.

The use of anti VEGF drugs such as Bevacizumab (Avastin) was originally approved for treatment of colon cancer by FDA in 2004 later on its benefit in ophthalmology was recognized for treatment of neovascularization conditions in the eye such as wet type macular degeneration and Rubeosis. Later on, another drug Ranibizumab (Lucentis) was introduced in the market and now there are many newer generations of Ant-VEGF that arrived or in the process of research and development at present [1].

Eylea (Aflibercept) is another anti-VEGF treatment that is available to control neovascularization process in the eye.

There is an urgency and the need for early detection and treat iris neovascularization by specific iris focused OCT with capability of Doppler angiography which can protect the eye against blindness.

New Parameters for Iris Specific OCT (ISP-OCT)

There is no standard and specific parameter software to evaluate the iris of the eye. The current OCT models lack the ability to precisely define the structure anatomy and histology of the iris for research and development and to address the anomalies and the diseases of iris including glaucoma. At present anterior segment OCT (ASOCT) is being used to evaluate the iris (Fig. 9.4) [20].

The latest version of anterior chamber OCT by Carl Zeiss/Meditec (Visante) has given clear images of the anterior segment of the eye. The anterior chamber can evaluate and measure pre and post operatively after image acquisition, using the analysis mode of the system's software.

Also, the anterior chamber diameters and depth and angle structures can be measured.

One of the major limitations of AC OCT is the inability to image through the heavily pigmented Iris Pigment epithelium (IPE) and also very highly pigmented Irides of dark colored eyes. As a result, the volume of the entire iris cannot be accurately measured.

Another important factor is that there is no standard analytical software for the iris, which makes it difficult to compare the different studies on Iris volume and structure.

Due to the fact that there are no specific parameters for iris evaluation and anatomy, there is a major need for new set of software for anatomical compartmentalization of different parts of the iris.

Iris compartments have different anatomical properties and thicknesses. This will allow to establish physical and physiological boundaries that are important to evaluate different normal variation and pathological conditions to be analyzed by OCT.

We also set a standard for future research and development studies to be compatible with each other.

Demarcations

From Periphery to the center the software should be able to use concentric circles based on the anatomy of the iris.

From periphery to the center the delineation circles should be:

- Cornea-scleral line (Limbus)
- The thinnest peripheral cornea that is part of the angle structure.
- The peripheral iris
- The collarette
- The ciliary Zone

Bibliography

1. Amadio M, Govoni S, Pascale A. Targeting VEGF in eye neovascularization: what's new? A comprehensive review on current therapies and oligonucleotide-based interventions under development. Pharmacol Res. 2016;103:253–69. https://doi.org/10.1016/j.phrs.2015.11.027.
2. Baumann B, Baumann SO, Konegger T, Pircher M, Götzinger E, Schlanitz F, Schütze C, Sattmann H, Litschauer M, Schmidt-Erfurth U, Hitzenberger CK. Polarization sensitive optical coherence tomography of melanin provides intrinsic contrast based on depolarization. Biomed Opt Express. 2012;3(7):1670–83. https://doi.org/10.1364/BOE.3.001670.
3. Boettner EA, Wolter JR. Transmission of the ocular media. Invest Ophthalmol Visual Sci. 1962;1(6):776–83. Available at: https://iovs.arvojournals.org/article.aspx?articleid=2122713.
4. Chedekel MR, Agin PP, Sayre RM. Photochemistry of pheomelanin: action spectrum for superoxide production. Photochem Photobiol. 1980;31(6):553–5. https://doi.org/10.1111/j.1751-1097.1980.tb03745.x.
5. Engvall E, Ruoslahti E. Binding of soluble form of fibroblast surface protein, fibronectin, to collagen. Int J Cancer. 1977;20(1):1–5. https://doi.org/10.1002/ijc.2910200102.
6. George R, Paul PG, Baskaran M, Ramesh SV, Raju P, Arvind H, McCarty C, Vijaya L. Ocular biometry in occludable angles and angle closure glaucoma: a population based survey. Br J Ophthalmol. 2003;87(4):399–402. https://doi.org/10.1136/bjo.87.4.399.

7. Harper DJ, Konegger T, Augustin M, Schützenberger K, Eugui P, Lichtenegger A, Merkle CW, Hitzenberger CK, Glösmann M, Baumann B. Hyperspectral optical coherence tomography for in vivo visualization of melanin in the retinal pigment epithelium. J. Biophotonics. 2019;12(12).

8. Hu DN, Simon JD, Sarna T. Role of ocular melanin in ophthalmic physiology and pathology. Photochem Photobiol. 2008;84(3):639–44. https://doi.org/10.1111/j.1751-1097.2008.00316.x.

9. Invernizzi A, Giardini P, Cigada M, Viola F, Staurenghi G. Three-dimensional morphometric analysis of the iris by swept-source anterior segment optical coherence tomography in a Caucasian population. Invest Ophthalmol Visual Sci. 2015;56(8):4796–801. https://doi.org/10.1167/iovs.15-16483.

10. Jacob D, Shelton RL, Applegate BE. Fourier domain pump-probe optical coherence tomography imaging of Melanin. Opt Express. 2010;18(12):12399–410. https://doi.org/10.1364/OE.18.012399.

11. Kim J, Brown W, Maher JR, Levinson H, Wax A. Functional optical coherence tomography: principles and progress. Phys Med Biol. 2015;60(10):R211. Available at: https://iopscience.iop.org/article/10.1088/0031-9155/60/10/R211/pdf.

12. Krishnaswamy A, Baranoski GV. A biophysically-based spectral model of light interaction with human skin. In Computer graphics forum 2004 Sep (Vol. 23, No. 3, pp. 331-340). Oxford, UK and Boston, USA: Blackwell Publishing, Inc. 10.1111/j.1467-8659.2004.00764.x.

13. Krol ES, Liebler DC. Photoprotective actions of natural and synthetic melanins. Chem Res Toxicol. 1998;11(12):1434–40. https://doi.org/10.1021/tx980114c.

14. WY Lam M, VG Baranoski G. A predictive light transport model for the human iris. In Computer graphics forum 2006 Sep (Vol. 25, No. 3, pp. 359-368). Oxford, UK and Boston, USA: Blackwell Publishing, Inc. https://doi.org/10.1111/j.1467-8659.2006.00955.x.

15. Lapierre-Landry M, Carroll J, Skala MC. Imaging retinal melanin: a review of current technologies. J Biol Eng. 2018;12(1):29. https://doi.org/10.1186/s13036-018-0124-5.

16. De Leeuw SM, Smit NP, Van Veldhoven M, Pennings EM, Pavel S, Simons JW, Schothorst AA. Melanin content of cultured human melanocytes and UV-induced cytotoxicity. J Photochem Photobiol. 2001;61(3):106–13. https://doi.org/10.1016/S1011-1344(01)00168-3.

17. Maloca P, Gyger C, Hasler PW. A pilot study to compartmentalize small melanocytic choroidal tumors and choroidal vessels with speckle-noise free 1050 nm swept source optical coherence tomography (OCT choroidal "tumoropsy"). Graefe's Arch Clin Exp Ophthalmol. 2016;254(6):1211–9. https://doi.org/10.1007/s00417-016-3270-9.

18. d'Ischia M, Wakamatsu K, Cicoira F, Di Mauro E, Garcia-Borron JC, Commo S, Galván I, Ghanem G, Kenzo K, Meredith P, Pezzella A. Melanins and melanogenesis: from pigment cells to human health and technological applications. Pigm Cell Melanoma Res. 2015;28(5):520–44. https://doi.org/10.1111/pcmr.12393.

19. Moazed K, Albert D, Smith TR. Rubeosis iridis in "pseudogliomas". Surv Ophthalmol. 1980;25(2):85–90. https://doi.org/10.1016/0039-6257(80)90151-4.

20. Peterson JR, Blieden LS, Chuang AZ, Baker LA, Rigi M, Feldman RM, Bell NP. Establishing age-adjusted reference ranges for iris-related parameters in open angle eyes with anterior segment optical coherence tomography. PLoS One. 2016;11(1) https://doi.org/10.1371/journal.pone.0147760.

21. Pijewska E, Sylwestrzak M, Gorczynska I, Tamborski S, Pawlak MA, Szkulmowski M. Blood flow rate estimation in optic disc capillaries and vessels using Doppler optical coherence tomography with 3D fast phase unwrapping. Biomed Opt Express. 2020;11(3):1336.

22. Quigley HA, Broman AT. The number of people with glaucoma worldwide in 2010 and 2020. Br J Ophthalmol. 2006;90(3):262–7. https://doi.org/10.1136/bjo.2005.081224.

23. Radhakrishnan S, Goldsmith J, Huang D, Westphal V, Dueker DK, Rollins AM, Izatt JA, Smith SD. Comparison of optical coherence tomography and ultrasound biomicroscopy for detection of narrow anterior chamber angles. Arch Ophthalmol. 2005;123(8):1053–9. https://doi.org/10.1001/archopht.123.8.1053.

24. Skalet A, Li Y, Lu CD, Jia Y, Lee B, Hornegger J, Fujimoto JG, Huang D. A pilot study of OCT angiography of iris melanomas. Invest Ophthalmol Visual Sci. 2015;56(7):3365. Available at: http://iovs.arvojournals.org/article.aspx?articleid=2333225.
25. Srinivasan K, Zebardast N, Krishnamurthy P, Kader MA, Raman GV, Rajendrababu S, Venkatesh R, Ramulu PY. Comparison of new visual disturbances after superior versus nasal/temporal laser peripheral iridotomy. Ophthalmology. 2018;125(3):345–51.
26. Kowalczuk C, Priestner M, Baller C, Pearson A, Cridland N, Saunders R, Wakamatsu K, Ito S. Effect of increased intracellular melanin concentration on survival of human melanoma cells exposed to different wavelengths of UV radiation. Int J Radiat Biol. 2001;77(8):883–9. https://doi.org/10.1080/09553000110062521.
27. Taroni P, Comelli D, Pifferi A, Torricelli A, Cubeddu R. Absorption of collagen: effects on the estimate of breast composition and related diagnostic implications. J Biomed Opt. 2007;12(1):014021. https://doi.org/10.1117/1.2699170.
28. Tsai CL, Chen JC, Wang WJ. Near-infrared absorption property of biological soft tissue constituents. J Med Biol Eng. 2001;21(1):7–14. Available at: http://www.jmbe.org.tw/files/13/public/13-930-1-PB.pdf.
29. Zhao S, Overbeek PA. Regulation of choroid development by the retinal pigment epithelium. Mol Vis. 2001;7:277–82. Available at: http://www.molvis.org/molvis/v7/a39.
30. Zonios G, Bykowski J, Kollias N. Skin melanin, hemoglobin, and light scattering properties can be quantitatively assessed in vivo using diffuse reflectance spectroscopy. J Invest Dermatol. 2001;117(6):1452–7. https://doi.org/10.1046/j.0022-202x.2001.01577.x.
31. https://patents.google.com/patent/US7075658B2/en.

Chapter 10
Eye Color Change

Abstract In recent years there have been many modalities to change and enhance the color of the eye. Many studies have been reported on anthropological and evolutionary significance of the eye color. There is a significant market in cosmetic industry for eye color change as exist with skin whitening, Hair color products and nail polishes. At present, the eye color change options have become available by introduction of colored contact lenses, laser intervention and surgical implants, also other small molecules and topical applications are in the process of investigation by research and commercial institutions. Here, each option has been discussed and their benefits and disadvantages were reviewed. The benefits and side effects as are summarized in relevant tables.

The theoretical comparison of the colored contact lens, the iris implant and hypothetical eye drops have been shown in the figure below (Figs. 10.1 and 10.2):

The eye color has many direct and indirect effect in our social interactions and the desire of being able to change the color of the eye in the same way as changing the hair color is very appealing to general public.

The anthropological studies on eye color describes the spreading pattern of the eye color mutation in humans [2, 5].

A very good literature review on forensic aspect of the eye color is published recently [7].

Another good review of genetic patterns can be found in Strum article [12].

The universal desire for attractiveness and the perception of "beauty" by the brain has been an important day to day task which was referred to in recent article [13].

The effect of eye color on evolutionary mate selection and sexual preferences have been reported in the literature and sociobiological studies such as the attraction of blue-eyed men for blue-eyed women [9].

© Springer Nature Switzerland AG 2020

207

K. T. Moazed, *The Iris*, https://doi.org/10.1007/978-3-030-45756-3_10

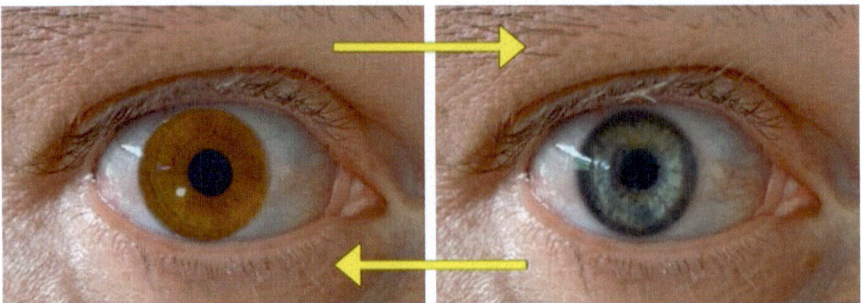

Fig. 10.1 Typical presentation of brown and blue irides

Benefits	Contact Lens	Surgical Implant	Hypothetical Drops
Non-invasive	+	−	+
Easily reversible	+	−	+
Patient can be dialated	+	−	+
Natural looking	−	−	+
Relatively inexpensive	+	−	+
Gradual color change	−	−	+
Night vision unaffected	−	−	+
Immediate results	+	+	−

Fig. 10.2 Comparison of different approaches to eye color change. The benefits and disadvantages of the above three different approaches to eye color change have been summarized here

Also, many studies suggest that the Father's eye color in women can influence their choice of selecting partners [1].

Other studies have evaluated the consistency of mate choice by hair and eye color [10].

The psychological aspect of the eye color have been studied and reported frequently, for instance the trustworthy-Looking face has been associated more with the brown eye rather than the blue eye people [8].

The statistics on desire to change the color of the eye have been discussed in the addendum at the end of this book.

The blue eye gene mutation has happened by a single nucleotide polymorphism (SNP) mutation by a switch of a single change from adenine to guanine in (rs12913832) in an intron 86 of the gene Herc2 which regulates the expression of the neighboring pigment gene OCA2 on chromosome 15 long arm (q) [11].

The mutation also produces blond hair and fair skin, which is a survival advantage by increased production of vitamin D in the skin in the geographic locations with lower amount of UV exposure [6].

The histological variation of different color irides have been discussed in detail in previous chapters in this book.

Recently, there have been many different approaches to achieve the goal of changing the eye color, yet none have been resulting in a perfect outcome.

The most desirable theoretical way would be to create an eye drop that gradually change the eye color while it is being used and then, the possibility of the eye color to return to its original color by stopping the use of the eye drops. Of course, the safety and side effects have to be studied trough the standard processes and the final approval by the FDA.

Color Contact Lenses

Color contact lenses has been around for many years and has been improved dramatically by better quality as the advancing technology. However, the color change is not very satisfactory and does not look natural specially in people with the dark color irides. There are also many limitations on using color contact lenses, for instance, many cannot tolerate contact lenses due to pre-existing conditions such as allergy, dry eyes, uveitis, etc.

Laser Ablation Color Procedure

Laser color change is still under investigation by research organizations and pharmaceutical companies. There are many safety issues and non-reliable results due to anatomical and histological differences in the structure of iris that has been discussed in previous chapters. The outcome of these procedures has not been completely evaluated. One of the problems with this method is that it is a permanent procedure and the result and the final outcome is not guaranteed and it cannot be reversed. There are theoretical concerns as it may cause pigment dispersion syndrome, iris scarring, iritis and glaucoma which can occur as complications after laser iris ablation. Also, in very dark brown irides the location of the pigment is not limited to the surface of the iris, but trough the entire stroma. The ablation of the entire iris will cause major complications such as glaucoma, scarring and deformity of the iris. This also will associate with blurry vision due to lack of iris motility due to the scarring. Also, the resultant color of the eye will not be satisfactory after laser ablation of the iris as it is not possible to remove entire pigment cells from the stroma without damaging the iris structure.

Surgical Iris Implant Insertion

Surgical Iris implants have been developed originally for aniridia (lack of iris) or colobomas (lack of sector of iris and for treatment of severe traumatic iris injury). Recently it has been used as a cosmetic procedure for color changing of the eye. There have been many complications associated with iris implants which have ended up with removal of the implant due to severe consequences, such as implant induced Iritis or glaucoma. This procedure is not safe at present and yet to be investigated, studied and improved in the future.

Chemical and Small Molecule Iris Color Intervention

Chemicals and small molecules have been under investigation for the past few years. There have been no final results that can be marketed and the results are not yet available. There is a need for research in this field but there have been great relutance by major pharmaceutical companies and investors to sponsor these projects due to many factors for example:

These projects are very time consuming since it may take many years form "theory to the market".

Studies are very expensive, the cost of running laboratories, staff, scientists, technicians, animal trials, human trials, and final FDA approval.

The very high Expense of the eye color drops projects, the long process of research from theory to market, and the Possibility of illegal copying of the final products for a cheap internet sale have influenced investors to be reluctant to support these studies. However, the revenue for such a desirable entity would be huge and would be similar to the hair color companies and other compatible cosmetic companies.

The evolutionary advantage has made the blue eyes to spread around the world and multiply in numbers. It was explained as being exotic and unusual which make it desirable. There is a survey at the end of this book in the addendum that randomly asked 3000 people in US about the preference in the color of the eye. The results have been shown in different graphs.

The factors involved in the desire of changing the eye color are many including:

- Today society of change, with desire to try new possibilities.
- Ability to be able to intervene the racial borders.
- Sexual preferences as confirmed in the survey, most people preferred light color eyes Green/Blue for their partners.

Controversial social aspect of eye color:

- The role of white sclera and large pupil "Bella Donna"
- Role of colonialization and European supremacy.
- Racial profiling in US
- Art history and the European paintings with angels with blue eyes.
- Advertising icons until recently.

Conclusion

A safe way to change the color of the eye is a very desirable and financially beneficial for the companies to invest in. It can be as popular as hair color that is being used today in every Country and by diverse human skin melanin contents from dark skin to very fair. It can blur the racial differences and bring equality and ability to change as desired by individuals.

Bibliography

1. Bressan P. Fathers' eye colour sways daughters' choice of both long- and short-term partners. 2018. Retrieved from Scientific Reports: https://www.nature.com/articles/s41598-018-23784-7.
2. Edwards M. Analysis of iris surface features in populations of diverse ancestry. 2015. Retrieved from Royal Society Open Science: https://doi.org/10.1098/rsos.150424.
3. Frost P. Sexual selection and human geographic variation. 2008. Retrieved from Journal of Social, Evolutionary, and Cultural Psychology https://doi.org/10.1037/h0099346.
4. Frost P. Sexual selection and human geographic variation. 2008. Retrieved from Journal of Social, Evolutionary, and Cultural Psychology,: https://psycnet.apa.org/fulltext/2010-01935-003.html.
5. Frost P. The puzzle of European hair, eye, and skin color. 2014. Retrieved from Scientific Research: http://www.scirp.org/journal/aa, https://doi.org/10.4236/aa.2014.42011.

6. Jablonski NG. Evolution of human skin color and vitamin D. 2018. Retrieved from vitamin D (Forth Edition): https://doi.org/10.1016/B978-0-12-809965-0.00003-3.
7. Karsara MA. True colors: a literature review on the spatial distribution of eye and hair pigmentation. 2019. Retrieved from FSI: Genetics: https://doi.org/10.1016/j.fsigen.2019.01.001.
8. Kleisner K. Trustworthy-looking face meets brown eyes. 2013. Retrieved from PLOS: https://doi.org/10.1371/journal.pone.0053285.
9. Laeng B. Why do blue-eyed men prefer women with the same eye color?. 2007. Retrieved from Behavioral Ecology and Sociobiology: https://link.springer.com/article/10.1007/s00265-006-0266-1.
10. Stebovar Z. Consistency of mate choice in eye and hair colour: testing possible mechanisms. 2019. Retrieved from Evolution and Human Behavior: https://doi.org/10.1016/j.evolhumbehav.2018.08.003.
11. Strum RA. A single SNP in an evolutionary conserved region within Intron 86 of the HERC2 gene determines human blue-brown eye color author links open overlay panel. 2008. Retrieved from AJHG: https://doi.org/10.1016/j.ajhg.2007.11.005.
12. Sturm RA. Genetics of human iris colour and patterns. 2009. Retrieved from Pigment Cell & Melanoma: https://doi.org/10.1111/j.1755-148X.2009.00606.x.
13. Yarosh DB. Perception and deception: human beauty and the brain. 2019. Retrieved from Behav Sci: https://doi.org/10.3390/bs9040034.

Addendum: Eye Color Survey

Eye Color Preference Survey

Material & Method

We used three survey questionnaires to conduct three separate surveys: May 21, 2017/June 5, 2017/June 19, 2017.

There were 1049 responses on the first survey, followed by 1136 responses for the second survey and finally 1033 responses for the last survey.

The age of participants is categorized by 4 groups:

- Below 18 years
- 18–35 years
- 35–55 years
- Above 55 years

The gender was categorized by 3 groups:

- Male
- Female
- Other

US regions used for the study:

- New England
- Middle Atlantic
- East North Central
- West North Central
- South Atlantic
- East South Central
- West South Central
- Mountain
- Pacific

© Springer Nature Switzerland AG 2020

K. T. Moazed, *The Iris*, https://doi.org/10.1007/978-3-030-45756-3

Survey Device Type:

- IOS phone/tablet
- Android phone/tablet
- Other phone/tablet
- Windows desktop/laptop
- Mac OS desktop/laptop
- Other

Results

The survey results images are self-explanatory and in the format of pie charts and graphs.

Survey study number one – May 21, 2017

Q1 Are you satisfied with your current eye color?

Answered: 1,049   Skipped: 0

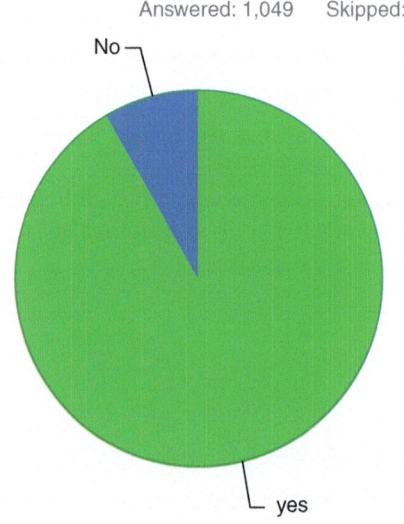

ANSWER CHOICES	RESPONSES	
Yes	91.90%	964
No	8.10%	85
TOTAL		1,049

Q2 Would you like to change your eye color?

Answered: 83   Skipped: 966

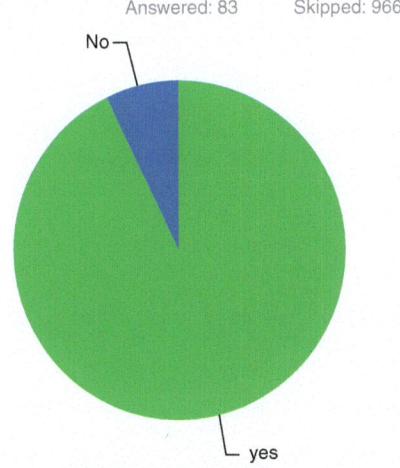

ANSWER CHOICES	RESPONSES	
Yes	92.77%	77
No	7.23%	6
TOTAL		83

Q3 What color eye would you prefer to have?

Answered: 76   Skipped: 973

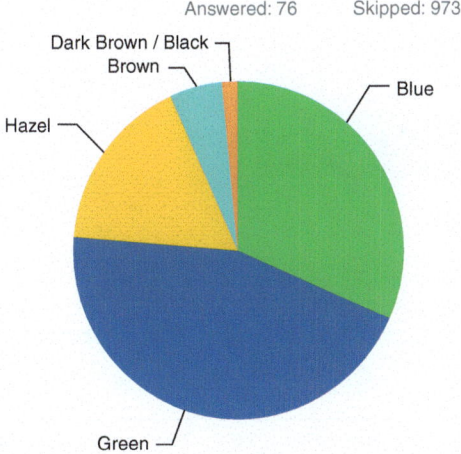

ANSWER CHOICES	RESPONSES	
Blue	31.58%	24
Green	44.74%	34
Hazel	17.11%	13
Brown	5.26%	4
Dark Brown / Black	1.32%	1
TOTAL		76

Q4 Do you prefer temporary or permanent eye color change?

Answered: 76   Skipped: 973

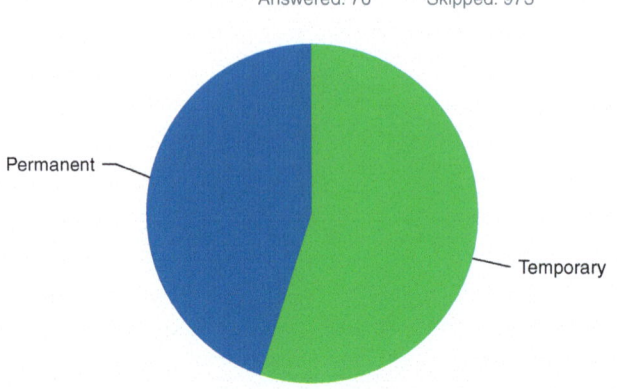

ANSWER CHOICES	RESPONSES	
Temporary	55.26%	42
Permanent	44.74%	34
TOTAL		76

Q5 What types of treatment would you be willing to undergo?

Answered: 76   Skipped: 973

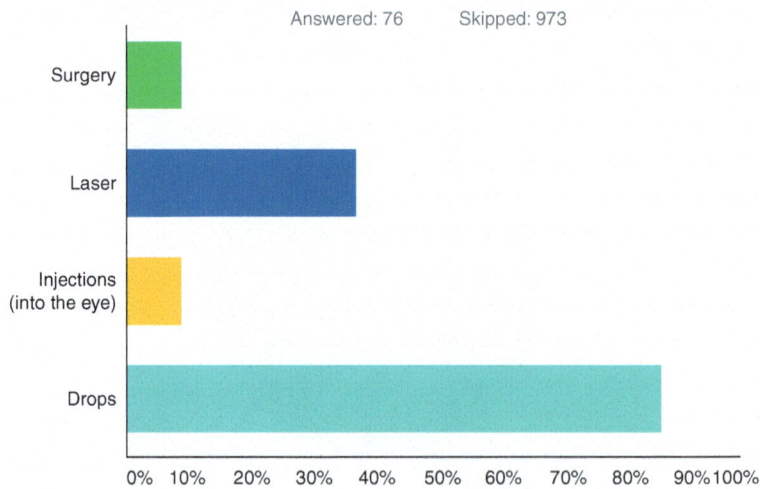

ANSWER CHOICES	RESPONSES	
Surgery	9.21%	7
Laser	36.84%	28
Injections (into the eye)	9.21%	7
Drops	85.53%	65
Total Respondents: 76		

Q6 What is the maximum you would be willing to pay?

Answered: 76   Skipped: 973

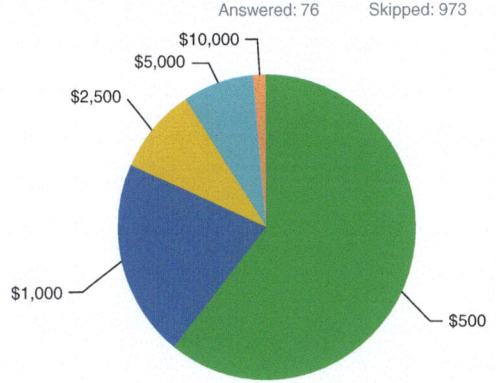

ANSWER CHOICES	RESPONSES	
$500	60.53%	46
$1,000	21.05%	16
$2,500	9.21%	7
$5,000	7.89%	6
$10,000	1.32%	1
More than $10,000	0.00%	0
TOTAL		76

Q7 Which of the following is closest to your natural hair color?

Answered: 1,006   Skipped: 43

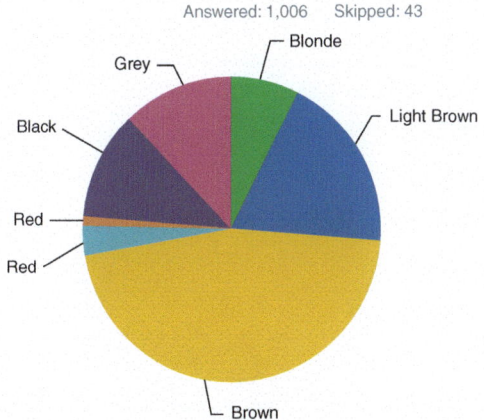

ANSWER CHOICES	RESPONSES	
Blonde	7.36%	74
Light Brown	18.89%	190
Brown	46.02%	463
Red	3.18%	32
Red	0.89%	9
Black	11.73%	118
Grey	11.93%	120
TOTAL		1,006

Q8 If you dye your hair, what color is it currently?

Answered: 1,006   Skipped: 43

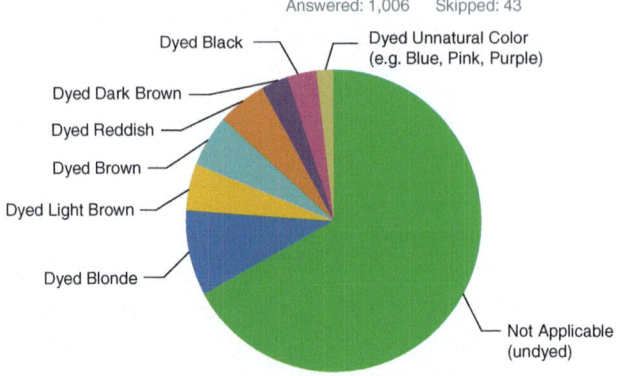

ANSWER CHOICES	RESPONSES	
Not Applicable (undyed)	66.90%	673
Dyed Blonde	9.24%	93
Dyed Light Brown	5.07%	51
Dyed Brown	5.37%	54
Dyed Reddish	5.57%	56
Dyed Dark Brown	2.88%	29
Dyed Black	3.28%	33
Dyed Unnatural Color (e.g. Blue, Pink, Purple)	1.69%	17
TOTAL		1,006

Q9 What is your skin color?

Answered: 1,006   Skipped: 43

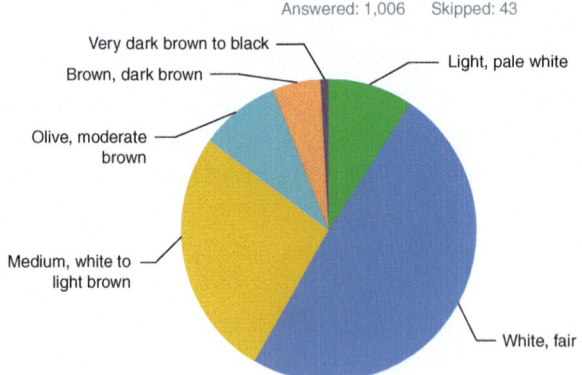

ANSWER CHOICES	RESPONSES	
Light, pale white	9.05%	91
White, fair	49.20%	495
Medium, white to light brown	27.14%	273
Olive, moderate brown	8.55%	86
Brown, dark brown	5.27%	53
Very dark brown to black	0.80%	8
TOTAL		1,006

Q10 What color eyes do you prefer for your spouse or partner?

Answered: 1,006   Skipped: 43

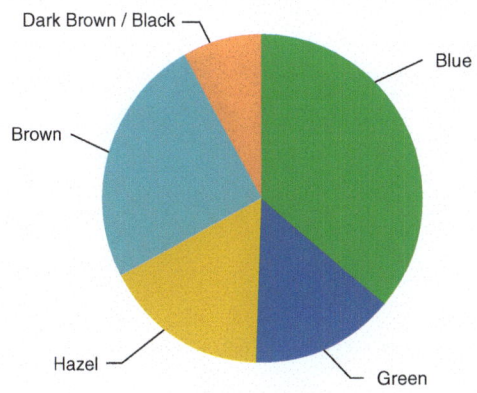

ANSWER CHOICES	RESPONSES	
Blue	36.18%	364
Green	14.41%	145
Hazel	16.80%	169
Brown	24.55%	247
Dark Brown / Black	8.05%	81
TOTAL		1,006

Q11 If you are currently being treated for glaucoma, are you concerned about darkening of your iris?

Answered: 1,006   Skipped: 43

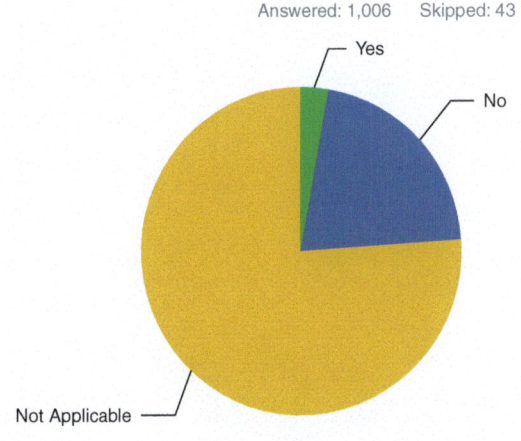

ANSWER CHOICES	RESPONSES	
Yes	2.78%	28
No	21.27%	214
Not Applicable	75.94%	764
TOTAL		1,006

Q12 What is your age?

Answered: 1,001   Skipped: 48

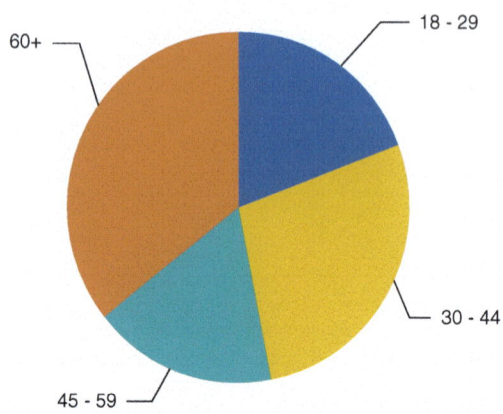

ANSWER CHOICES	RESPONSES	
Under 18	0.00%	0
18 - 29	19.28%	193
30 - 44	27.67%	277
45 - 59	17.38%	174
60+	35.66%	357
TOTAL		1,001

Q13 What is your gender?

Answered: 1,001   Skipped: 48

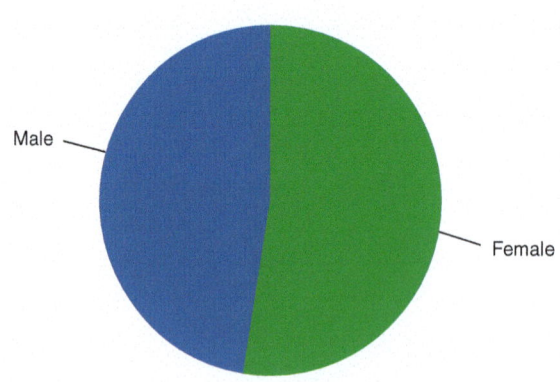

ANSWER CHOICES	RESPONSES	
Female	52.75%	528
Male	47.25%	473
TOTAL		1,001

Q14 How much total combined money did all members of your HOUSEHOLD earn last year?

Answered: 1,000   Skipped: 49

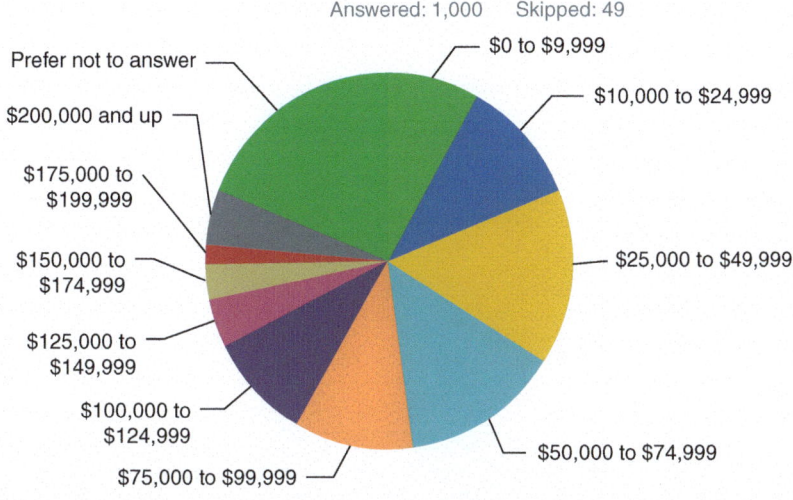

ANSWER CHOICES	RESPONSES	
$0 to $9,999	8.30%	83
$10,000 to $24,999	10.60%	106
$25,000 to $49,999	15.20%	152
$50,000 to $74,999	13.80%	138
$75,000 to $99,999	10.50%	105
$100,000 to $124,999	9.20%	92
$125,000 to $149,999	4.10%	41
$150,000 to $174,999	3.10%	31
$175,000 to $199,999	1.70%	17
$200,000 and up	4.70%	47
Prefer not to answer	18.80%	188
TOTAL		1,000

Q15 US Region

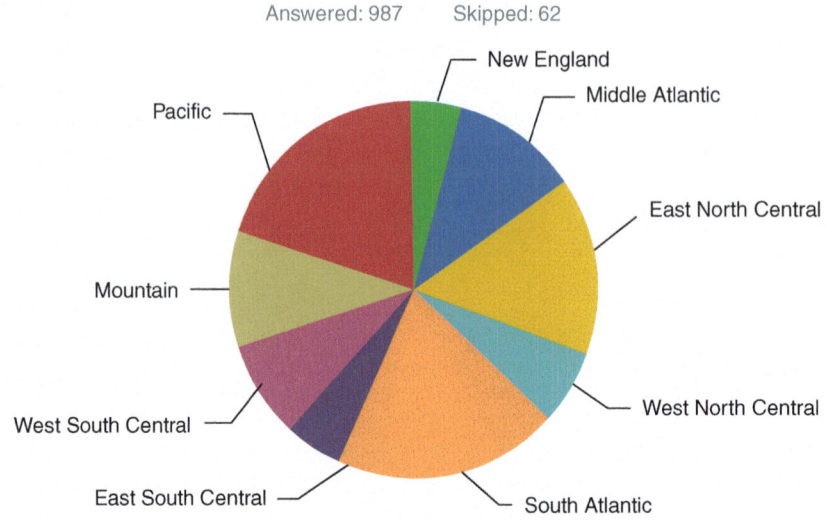

ANSWER CHOICES	RESPONSES	
New England	4.26%	42
Middle Atlantic	11.14%	110
East North Central	15.40%	152
West North Central	6.18%	61
South Atlantic	19.96%	197
East South Central	4.96%	49
West South Central	8.21%	81
Mountain	9.93%	98
Pacific	19.96%	197
TOTAL		987

Q16 Device Types

Answered: 1,001   Skipped: 48

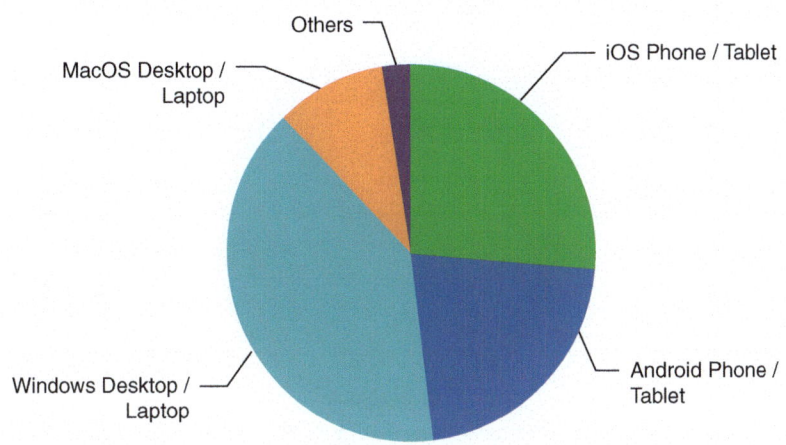

ANSWER CHOICES	RESPONSES	
iOS Phone / Tablet	26.57%	266
Android Phone / Tablet	21.68%	217
Other Phone / Tablet	0.00%	0
Windows Desktop / Laptop	39.66%	397
MacOS Desktop / Laptop	9.59%	96
Other	2.50%	25
TOTAL		1,001

Survey study number two – June 5, 2017

Q1 Are you satisfied with your current eye color?

Answered: 1,136   Skipped: 0

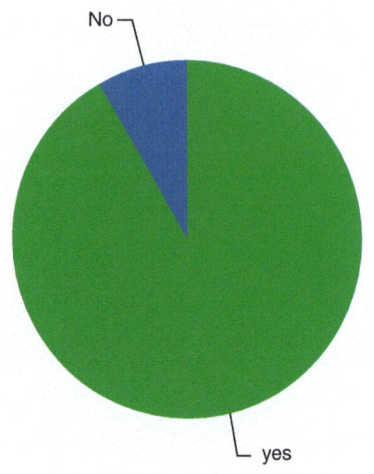

ANSWER CHOICES	RESPONSES	
Yes	90.93%	1,033
No	9.07%	103
TOTAL		1,136

Q2 Would you like to change your eye color?

Answered: 1,134   Skipped: 2

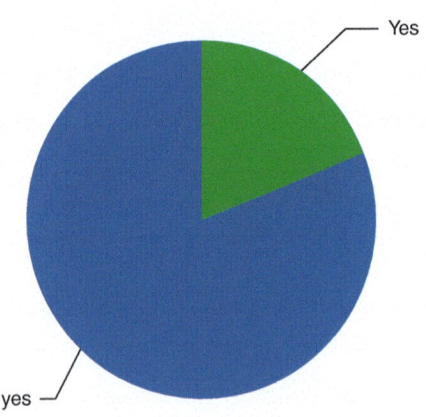

ANSWER CHOICES	RESPONSES	
Yes	19.05%	216
No	80.95%	918
TOTAL		1,134

Q3 If you were to change the color of your eye, what color would you prefer?

Answered: 1,055   Skipped: 81

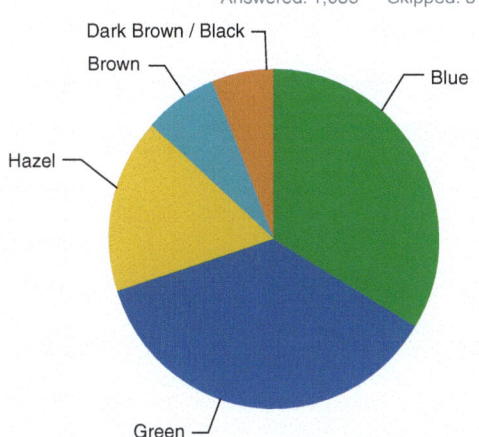

ANSWER CHOICES	RESPONSES	
Blue	33.84%	357
Green	36.40%	384
Hazel	16.59%	175
Brown	7.20%	76
Dark Brown / Black	5.97%	63
TOTAL		1,055

Q4 If you were to change the color of your eyes, would you prefer it to be temporary or permanent?

Answered: 1,055   Skipped: 81

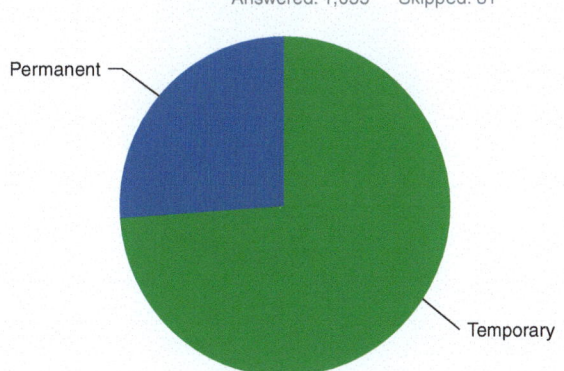

ANSWER CHOICES	RESPONSES	
Temporary	73.93%	780
Permanent	26.07%	275
TOTAL		1,055

Q5 If you were to change the color of your eyes, what types of treatment
would you be willing to undergo?

Answered: 1,055   Skipped: 81

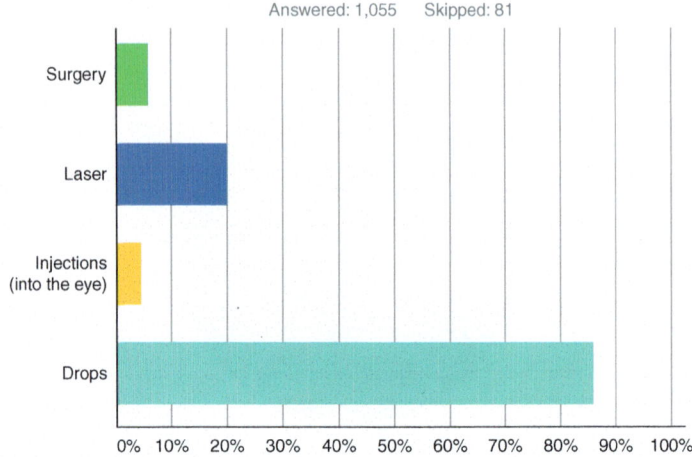

ANSWER CHOICES	RESPONSES	
Surgery	6.73%	71
Laser	19.72%	208
Injections (into the eye)	5.12%	54
Drops	83.70%	883
Total Respondents: 1,055		

Q6 What is the maximum you would be willing to pay?

Answered: 1,055   Skipped: 81

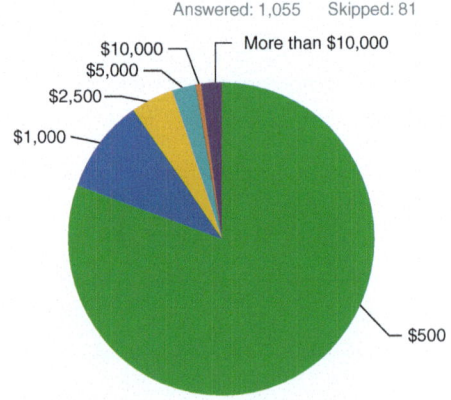

ANSWER CHOICES	RESPONSES	
$500	80.57%	850
$1,000	9.76%	103
$2,500	4.55%	48
$5,000	2.37%	25
$10,000	0.76%	8
More than $10,000	1.99%	21
TOTAL		1,055

Q7 Which of the following is closest to your natural hair color?

Answered: 1,033   Skipped: 103

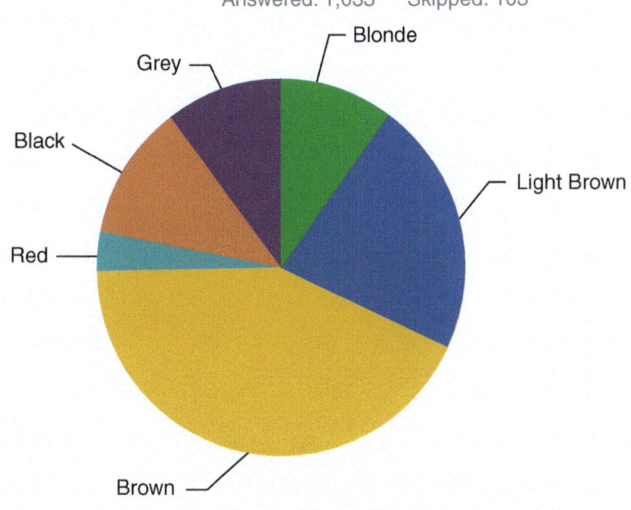

ANSWER CHOICES	RESPONSES	
Blonde	10.07%	104
Light Brown	22.07%	228
Brown	42.79%	442
Red	3.29%	34
Black	11.62%	120
Grey	10.16%	105
TOTAL		1,033

Q8 If you dye your hair, what color is it currently?

Answered: 1,033   Skipped: 103

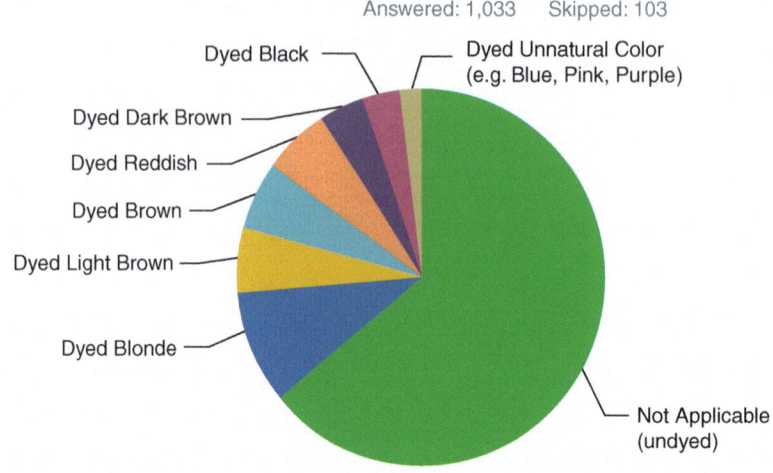

ANSWER CHOICES	RESPONSES	
Not Applicable (undyed)	64.09%	662
Dyed Blonde	9.58%	99
Dyed Light Brown	5.71%	59
Dyed Brown	5.71%	59
Dyed Reddish	6.00%	62
Dyed Dark Brown	3.87%	40
Dyed Black	3.10%	32
Dyed Unnatural Color (e.g. Blue, Pink, Purple)	1.94%	20
TOTAL		1,033

Q9 What is your skin color?

Answered: 1,033   Skipped: 103

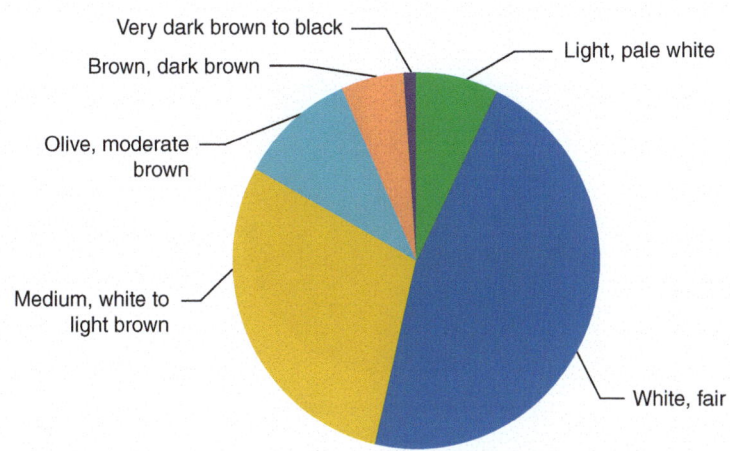

ANSWER CHOICES	RESPONSES	
Light, pale white	7.45%	77
White, fair	46.18%	477
Medium, white to light brown	29.53%	305
Olive, moderate brown	10.45%	108
Brown, dark brown	5.42%	56
Very dark brown to black	0.97%	10
TOTAL		1,033

Q10 What color eyes do you prefer for your spouse or partner?

Answered: 1,033   Skipped: 103

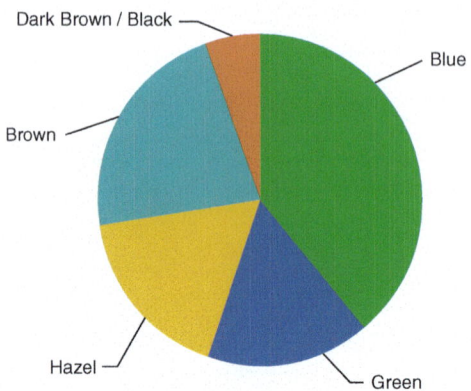

ANSWER CHOICES	RESPONSES	
Blue	39.01%	403
Green	16.36%	169
Hazel	17.13%	177
Brown	21.97%	227
Dark Brown / Black	5.52%	57
TOTAL		1,033

Q11 If you are currently being treated for glaucoma, are you concerned about darkening of your iris?

Answered: 1,033   Skipped: 103

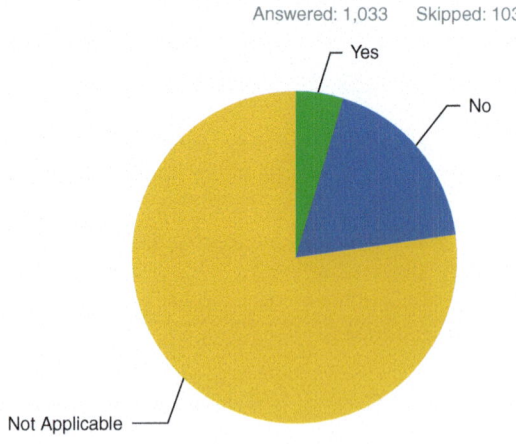

ANSWER CHOICES	RESPONSES	
Yes	4.94%	51
No	18.01%	186
Not Applicable	77.06%	796
TOTAL		1,033

Q12 What is your age?

Answered: 1,023   Skipped: 113

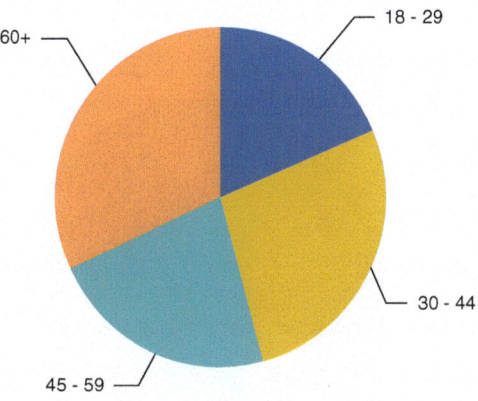

ANSWER CHOICES	RESPONSES	
Under 18	0.00%	0
18 - 29	18.87%	193
30 - 44	26.98%	276
45 - 59	22.39%	229
60+	31.77%	325
TOTAL		1,023

Q13 What is your gender?

Answered: 1,023   Skipped: 113

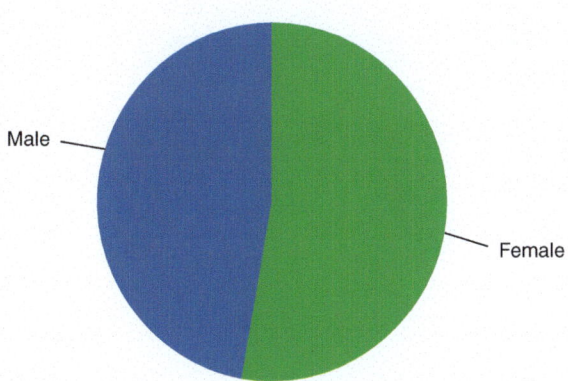

ANSWER CHOICES	RESPONSES	
Female	52.98%	542
Male	47.02%	481
TOTAL		1,023

Q14 How much total combined money did all members of your HOUSEHOLD earn last year?

Answered: 1,023   Skipped: 113

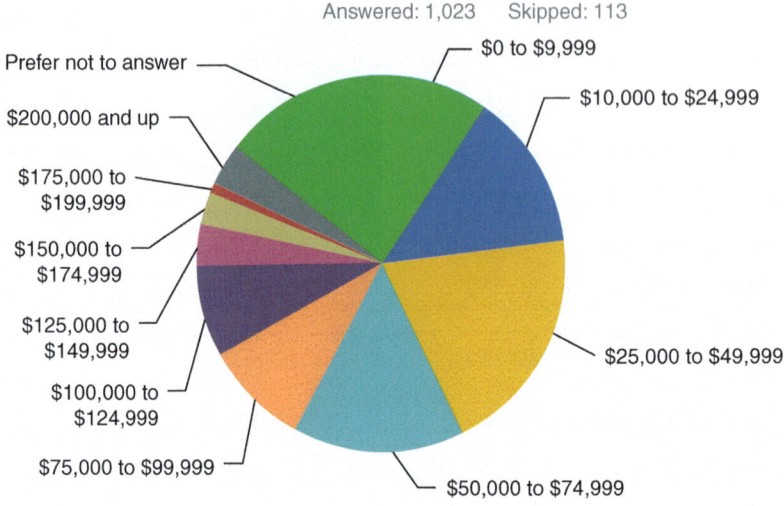

ANSWER CHOICES	RESPONSES	
$0 to $9,999	9.68%	99
$10,000 to $24,999	13.39%	137
$25,000 to $49,999	19.94%	204
$50,000 to $74,999	15.05%	154
$75,000 to $99,999	8.90%	91
$100,000 to $124,999	8.02%	82
$125,000 to $149,999	3.62%	37
$150,000 to $174,999	2.54%	26
$175,000 to $199,999	1.08%	11
$200,000 and up	3.62%	37
Prefer not to answer	14.17%	145
TOTAL		1,023

Q15 US Region

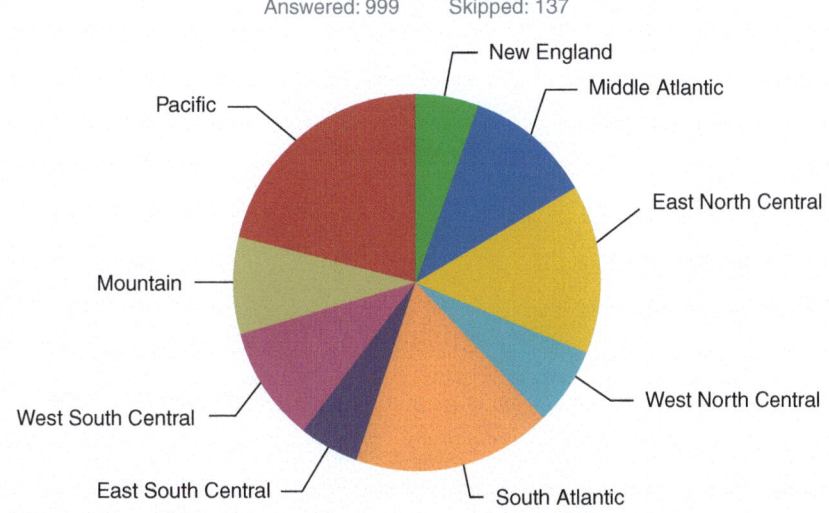

Answered: 999   Skipped: 137

ANSWER CHOICES	RESPONSES	
New England	5.61%	56
Middle Atlantic	11.31%	113
East North Central	14.41%	144
West North Central	6.51%	65
South Atlantic	17.72%	177
East South Central	5.11%	51
West South Central	10.11%	101
Mountain	8.21%	82
Pacific	21.02%	210
TOTAL		999

Q16 Device Types

Answered: 1,023   Skipped: 113

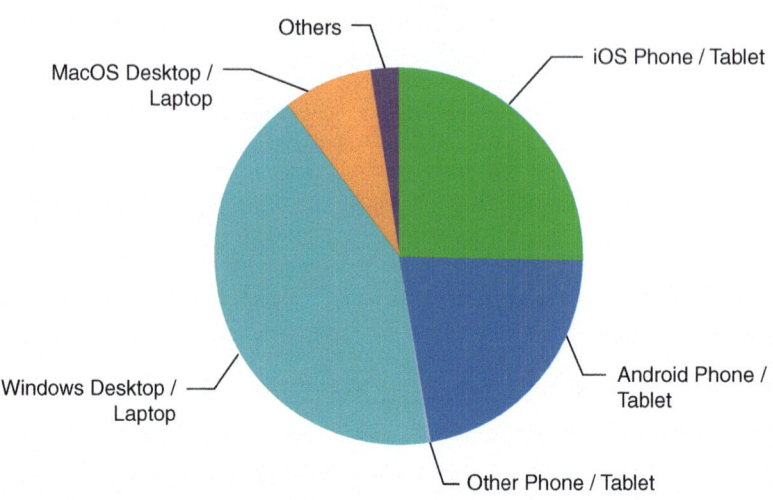

ANSWER CHOICES	RESPONSES	
iOS Phone / Tablet	25.51%	261
Android Phone / Tablet	21.99%	225
Other Phone / Tablet	0.10%	1
Windows Desktop / Laptop	42.23%	432
MacOS Desktop / Laptop	7.92%	81
Other	2.25%	23
TOTAL		1,023

Survey study number three – June 19, 2017

Q1 Would you like to have the ability to change your eye color?

Answered: 1,034   Skipped: 0

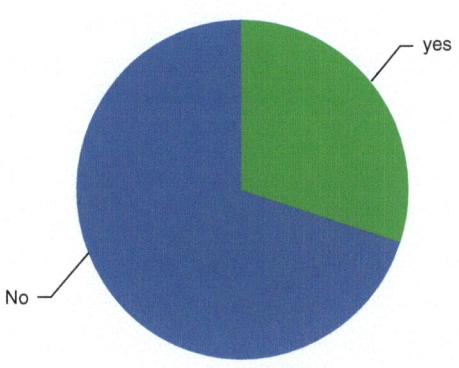

ANSWER CHOICES	RESPONSES	
Yes	30.17%	312
No	69.83%	722
TOTAL		1,034

Q2 If you were to change the color of your eye, what color would you prefer?

Answered: 1,034   Skipped: 0

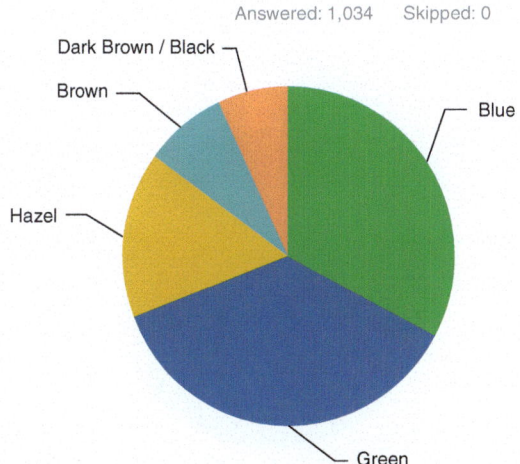

ANSWER CHOICES	RESPONSES	
Blue	32.88%	340
Green	36.36%	376
Hazel	15.96%	165
Brown	8.12%	84
Dark Brown / Black	6.67%	69
TOTAL		1,034

Q3 What is your natural eye color?

Answered: 1,034   Skipped: 0

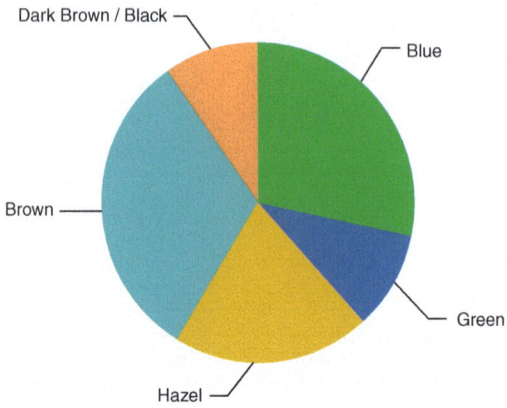

ANSWER CHOICES	RESPONSES	
Blue	28.43%	294
Green	10.06%	104
Hazel	20.31%	210
Brown	31.53%	326
Dark Brown / Black	9.67%	100
TOTAL		1,034

Q4 If you could choose, which eye color would you wish you were born with?

Answered: 1,034   Skipped: 0

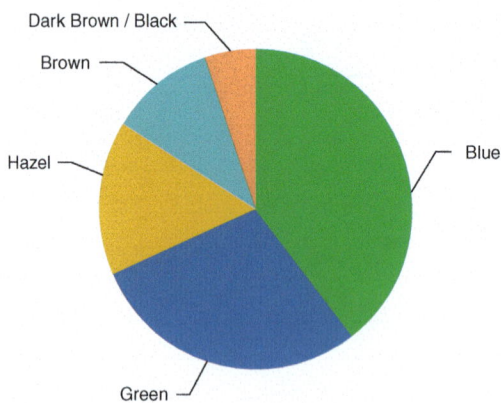

ANSWER CHOICES	RESPONSES	
Blue	39.46%	408
Green	28.92%	299
Hazel	15.67%	162
Brown	10.74%	111
Dark Brown / Black	5.22%	54
TOTAL		1,034

Q5 If you were to change the color of your eyes, would you prefer it to be temporary or permanent?

Answered: 1,034   Skipped: 0

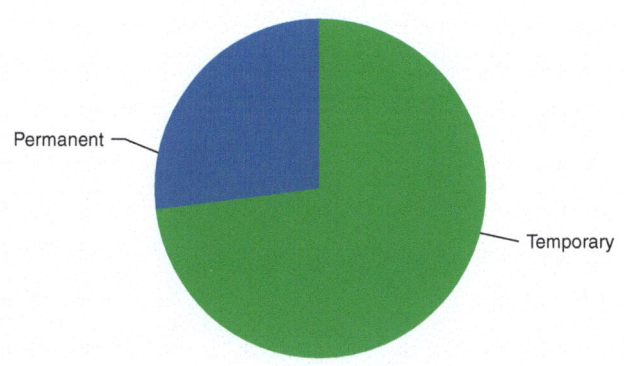

ANSWER CHOICES	RESPONSES	
Temporary	73.11%	756
Permanent	26.89%	278
TOTAL		1,034

Q6 If you were to change the color of your eyes, what types of treatment would you be willing to undergo?

Answered: 1,034   Skipped: 0

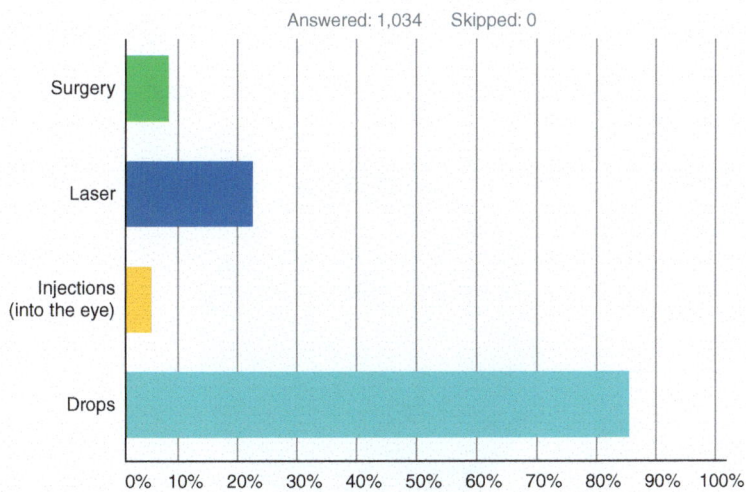

ANSWER CHOICES	RESPONSES	
Surgery	5.71%	59
Laser	21.08%	218
Injections (into the eye)	4.74%	49
Drops	83.46%	863
Total Respondents: 1,034		

Q7 What is the maximum you would be willing to pay?

Answered: 1,034   Skipped: 0

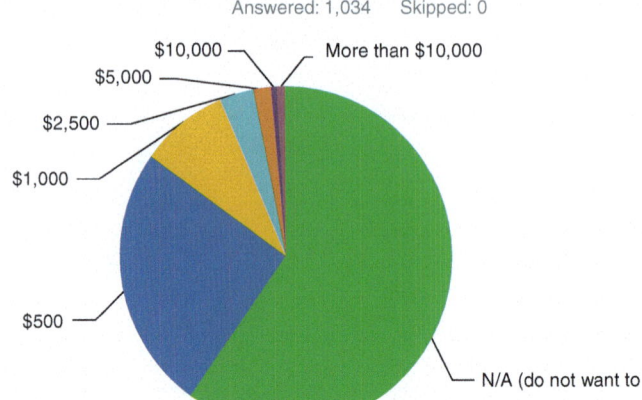

ANSWER CHOICES	RESPONSES	
N/A (do not want to change eye color)	59.77%	618
$500	25.34%	262
$1,000	8.61%	89
$2,500	3.29%	34
$5,000	1.64%	17
$10,000	0.68%	7
More than $10,000	0.68%	7
TOTAL		1,034

Q8 Have you ever tried color contact lenses?

Answered: 1,034   Skipped: 0

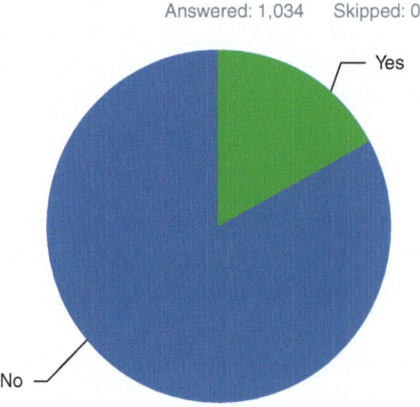

ANSWER CHOICES	RESPONSES	
Yes	17.02%	176
No	82.98%	858
TOTAL		1,034

Q9 Which of the following is closest to your natural hair color?

Answered: 1,034   Skipped: 0

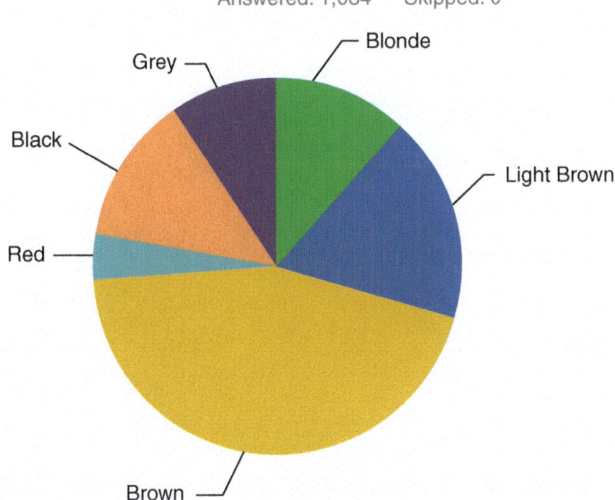

ANSWER CHOICES	RESPONSES	
Blonde	11.80%	122
Light Brown	17.89%	185
Brown	44.39%	459
Red	3.97%	41
Black	12.67%	131
Grey	9.28%	96
TOTAL		1,034

Q10 If you dye your hair, what color is it currently?

Answered: 1,034   Skipped: 0

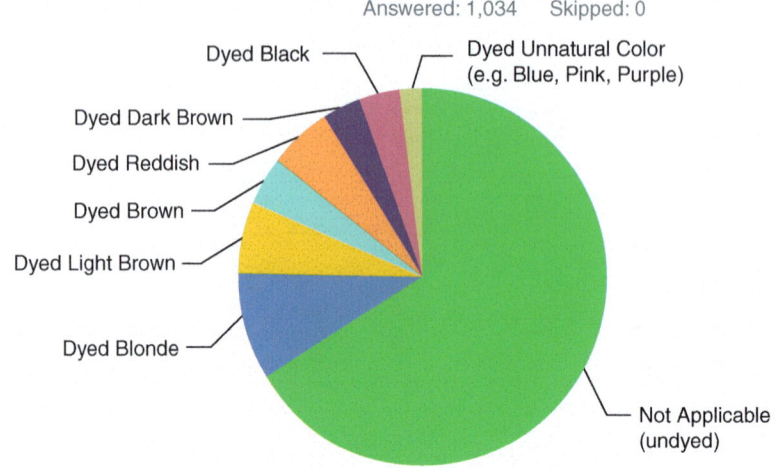

ANSWER CHOICES	RESPONSES	
Not Applicable (undyed)	66.34%	686
Dyed Blonde	8.99%	93
Dyed Light Brown	6.09%	63
Dyed Brown	4.35%	45
Dyed Reddish	5.51%	57
Dyed Dark Brown	3.19%	33
Dyed Black	3.58%	37
Dyed Unnatural Color (e.g. Blue, Pink, Purple)	1.93%	20
TOTAL		1,034

Q11 What is your skin color?

Answered: 1,034   Skipped: 0

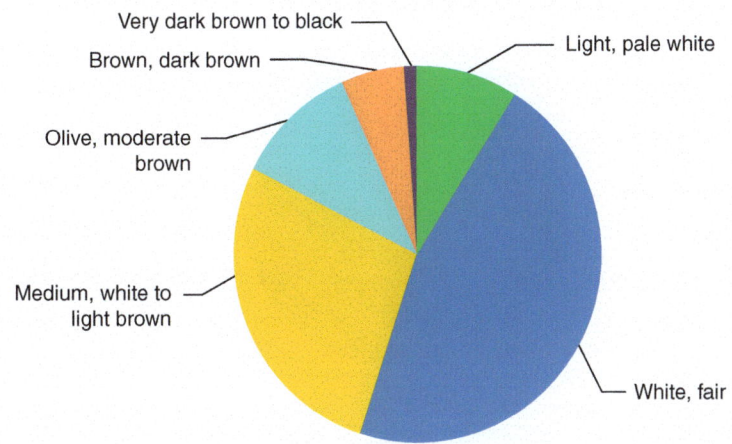

ANSWER CHOICES	RESPONSES	
Light, pale white	9.09%	94
White, fair	45.94%	475
Medium, white to light brown	27.76%	287
Olive, moderate brown	10.64%	110
Brown, dark brown	5.71%	59
Very dark brown to black	0.87%	9
TOTAL		1,034

Q12 In your personal opinion, which eye color is more attractive to you?

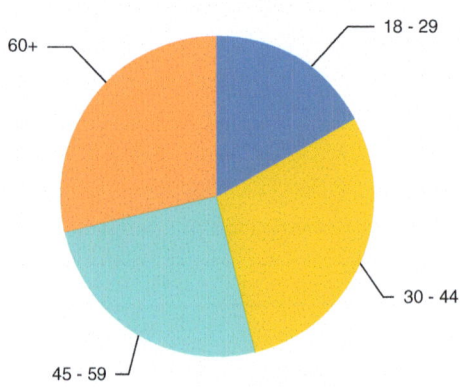

ANSWER CHOICES	RESPONSES	
Blue	45.65%	472
Green	26.40%	273
Hazel	13.64%	141
Brown	10.06%	104
Dark Brown / Black	4.26%	44
TOTAL		1,034

Q13 What is your age?

ANSWER CHOICES	RESPONSES	
Under 18	0.00%	0
18 - 29	17.04%	175
30 - 44	29.11%	299
45 - 59	25.32%	260
60+	28.53%	293
TOTAL		1,027

Q14 What is your gender?

Answered: 1,027   Skipped: 7

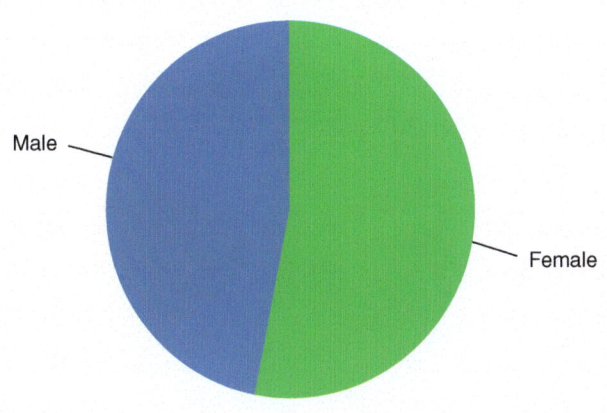

Male

Female

ANSWER CHOICES	RESPONSES	
Female	53.07%	545
Male	46.93%	482
TOTAL		1,027

Q15 How much total combined money did all members of your HOUSEHOLD earn last year?

Answered: 1,027   Skipped: 7

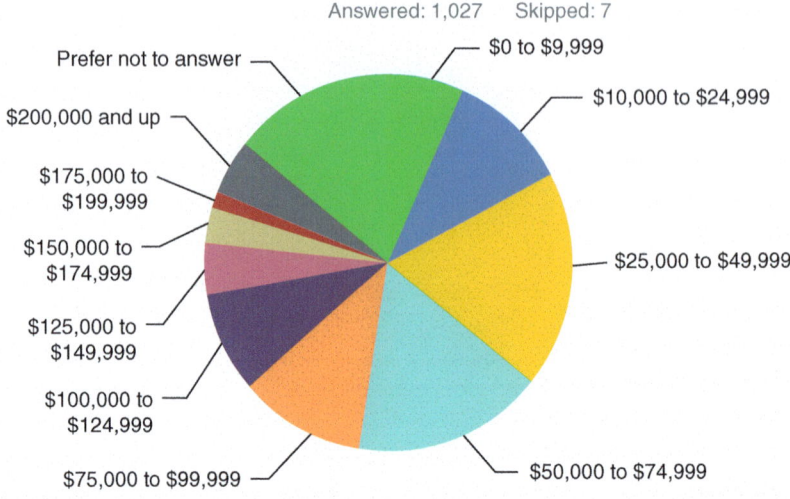

ANSWER CHOICES	RESPONSES	
$0 to $9,999	6.91%	71
$10,000 to $24,999	10.52%	108
$25,000 to $49,999	18.50%	190
$50,000 to $74,999	16.75%	172
$75,000 to $99,999	11.00%	113
$100,000 to $124,999	8.67%	89
$125,000 to $149,999	4.38%	45
$150,000 to $174,999	3.12%	32
$175,000 to $199,999	1.46%	15
$200,000 and up	4.77%	49
Prefer not to answer	13.92%	143
TOTAL		1,027

Q16 US Region

Answered: 1,009   Skipped: 25

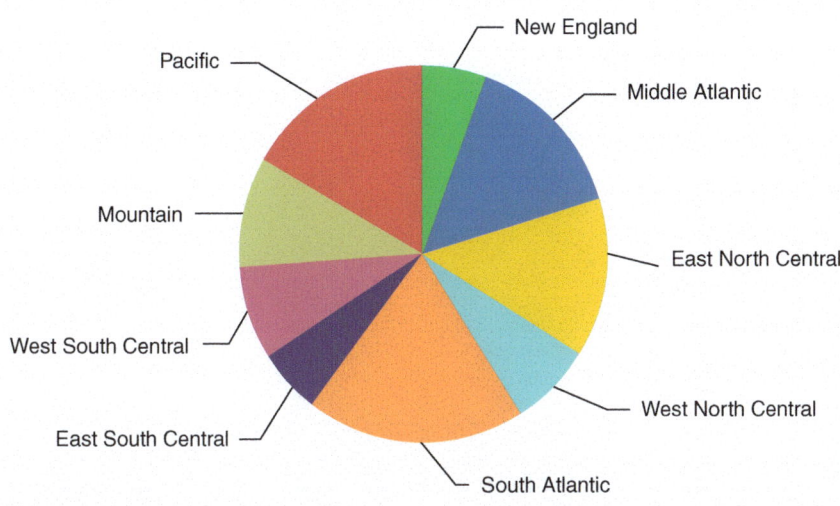

ANSWER CHOICES	RESPONSES	
New England	5.75%	58
Middle Atlantic	14.67%	148
East North Central	13.58%	137
West North Central	7.23%	73
South Atlantic	19.13%	193
East South Central	5.75%	58
West South Central	8.03%	81
Mountain	9.32%	94
Pacific	16.55%	167
TOTAL		1,009

Q17 Device Types

Answered: 1,027   Skipped: 7

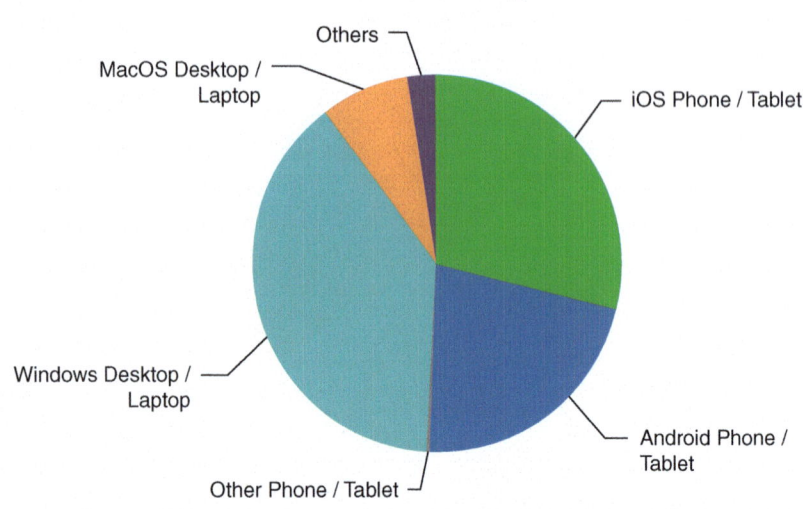

ANSWER CHOICES	RESPONSES	
iOS Phone / Tablet	29.02%	298
Android Phone / Tablet	21.81%	224
Other Phone / Tablet	0.10%	1
Windows Desktop / Laptop	39.05%	401
MacOS Desktop / Laptop	7.79%	80
Other	2.24%	23
TOTAL		1,027

Index

The manufacturer's authorised representative in the EU is Springer
Nature Customer Service Centre GmbH, Europaplatz 3, 69115 Heidelberg,
Germany. If you have any concerns regarding our products, please
contact ProductSafety@springernature.com

Printed and bound by CPI Group (UK) Ltd, Croydon, CR0 4YY

29/04/2026
02099451-0011